Stratton/Wiebelt An Atlas of Removable Partial Denture Design

An Atlas of Removable Partial Denture Design

Russell J. Stratton, D.D.S., M.S.
Professor and Dean
College of Dentistry, University of Oklahoma
Oklahoma City, Oklahoma

Frank J. Wiebelt, D.D.S.
Associate Professor and Chairman
Department of Removable Prosthodontics
College of Dentistry, University of Oklahoma
Oklahoma City, Oklahoma

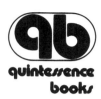

quintessence
books

Quintessence Publishing Co., Inc. 1988
Chicago, London, Berlin, São Paulo, Tokyo, and Hong Kong

Library of Congress Cataloging-in-Publication Data

Stratton, Russell J.
  An atlas of removable partial denture design.

  Bibliography: p.
  Includes index.
  1. Partial dentures, Removable—Atlases.   2. Partial
dentures, Removable—Design—Atlases.   I. Wiebelt,
Frank J.   II. Title. [DNLM: 1. Dental Prosthesis
Design—atlases.   2. Denture, Partial, Removable—
atlases. WU 17 S911a]
RK665.S76   1988   617.6'92   87-7257
ISBN 0-86715-190-0   13-digit ISBN 978-0-86715-190-9

© 1988 by Quintessence Publishing Co, Inc

Quintessence Publishing Co, Inc
4350 Chandler Drive
Hanover Park, IL 60133
www.quintpub.com

Composition: The Clarinda Co., Clarinda, IA
Printing and Binding: Edwards Brothers Inc.

Printed in U.S.A.

Contents

Preface

The current practice of dentistry in the area of removable partial denture design has been described as confusing, illogical, and difficult, if not impossible, to understand. Out of frustration, many dentists elect not to render partial denture service while others delegate excessive responsibility to the laboratory technician. As a result, master casts are often submitted to laboratories with work authorizations which simply say "make partial." Unfortunately, even if the laboratory technician has the educational background needed to develop a logical design, he or she does not have the diagnostic information (e.g., radiographs and periodontal charting) necessary to determine the best design for the particular patient. The resulting prosthesis may be successful or may ultimately damage or destroy the remaining teeth and supporting structures.

It appears that, in spite of excellent research, textbooks, and educational programs, the overall ability of dentists to design removable partial dentures has improved very little over the last several decades. This lack of improvement has been and continues to be a major concern to the dental profession and particularly to educators.

At least three factors contribute to the current predicament. First, the complexity of the task is enormous because minute changes in tooth or tissue contours, periodontal condition, or esthetic requirements may appreciably alter a design.

Second, most dental students receive very little experience in design. Few complete more than four partial dentures prior to graduation. The preparatory periodontal, endodontic, and restorative treatment is often so time-consuming that only limited clinical experience is possible. To compensate, many schools incorporate design exercises on study casts as part of the preclinical teaching program. Seldom does the combined preclinical and clinical design exposure exceed more than 15 to 20 partial dentures. As a result, the graduating dentist is not sufficiently experienced and often feels inadequate or uncomfortable with the design process.

Third, although there are many excellent textbooks currently available, most either deal with generalizations or provide information that must be collected, organized, and correlated in order to develop a specific design for a specific patient. If the individual has the time and motivation, repetition of this process will eventually produce a practitioner who is proficient in design. Frequently, the ladder to experience is too tall and too difficult to climb.

Because neither the complexity of the subject nor the exposure in dental school can be appreciably altered, it appears that the problem must be attacked by improved teaching techniques and reference materials. That is the reason for the development of this book. We hope that with its aid, the student or practitioner can be part way up the ladder when he or she begins the journey to "experience."

The emphasis of this text is on design because it is one of the major weak links in the process of total care. The fact that collection and interpretation of diagnostic data are not discussed in no way decreases their importance. The results of a detailed clinical and radiographic examination *must* dictate the ultimate design of the prosthesis.

It is assumed that all necessary diagnostic information (including study casts) has been collected and is at the dentist's disposal when designing begins. No more than emergency treatment and the initial phase of periodontal therapy should be completed prior to formulation of a tentative partial denture design.

It is also assumed that the practitioner has a dental surveyor. *If the practitioner does not, he or she should not be rendering partial denture service.* The surveyor is just as necessary to removable prosthodontics as reamers and files are to endodontics or burs are to operative dentistry.

Part I of the text discusses surveying, general design principles, and mouth preparation. Although clinical phases of treatment have generally been omitted, the subject of mouth preparation is included because it relates so closely to the principles and function of the design.

Part II is an atlas of designs for various partially edentulous arches. An "ideal" design is given for each situation and possible modifications follow. The goal is to begin with a generally acceptable design and proceed through an organized, step-by-step consideration of the specific components. Modification of the design will depend on diagnostic information collected by the practitioner. The final result should be a design suited to the individual patient. For the beginner, the process will undoubtedly be tedious and slow. However, as he or she gains experience, he or she will be able to produce an acceptable design without prompting on each aspect. The more experienced practitioner may have one or two questionable areas and thus may need to trace references and information related only to those factors.

An effort has been made to consider the most commonly occurring partially edentulous dental arches. Because it is impossible to discuss every situation, some extrapolation from similar designs will be necessary when there are unusual combinations of remaining teeth.

Discussion is limited to conventional partial denture design (i.e., extracoronal clasping) because it is the design concept that is best suited to the majority of patients, general practitioners, and laboratory technicians. The design philosophy recommended is one that combines broad stress distribution, minimal tooth and tissue coverage by the framework, and, whenever possible, retentive elements that release during functional movement of the prosthesis. Although the mesial rest/I-bar/guide plate concept is favored for extension removable partial dentures, other designs are included where applicable.

It is hoped that the material presented will decrease frustration for the practitioner, improve dentist/laboratory communications and understanding, and ultimately help to produce optimal quality partial denture service for the patient.

Acknowledgments

A great many people directly or indirectly contributed to the writing of this textbook. They include those who provided our education years ago and others who more recently assisted in the minute details of preparing the manuscript.

We would like to express our gratitude to our former teachers for the knowledge and inspiration they provided during our specialty training. Dr. Stratton extends his appreciation to the faculty at the Naval Graduate Dental School, especially to Drs. Noel Wilkie, Robert Leupold, Dean Johnson, Ronald Granger, Richard Grisius, and Dorsey Moore. Dr. Wiebelt would like to thank Drs. Frank Kratochvil, Theodore Berg, David Benson, and the remainder of the faculty at UCLA.

Appreciation is also extended to members of the Department of Removable Prosthodontics at the University of Oklahoma for their advice and for their willingness to assume extra duties when preparation of the book created pressures on the routine business of dental education. The wisdom and encouragement of Drs. Dean Johnson and Herbert Shillingburg were particularly important and contributed immensely to the sustained effort required to complete the project.

A very special thank you must be given to our secretary, Tina Parker, for her assistance with typing, copying, proofreading, and a myriad of minor details. Her cheerfulness and enthusiasm never waned, even when our demands were added to her already busy schedule.

And last but not least, the authors would like to express their appreciation to their families for the tolerance and patience they exhibited when the preparation of the manuscript interfered with those things which husbands and fathers are normally expected to do.

PART I
DESIGN CONCEPTS

Introduction

A number of years ago, several longitudinal studies reached the alarming conclusion that removable partial dentures (RPDs) often led to caries, gingival inflammation, increased sulcus depth, and mobility of abutments. Examination of the studies revealed that the prostheses were fabricated without control over design and inserted in spite of unresolved periodontal problems and poor patient home care. In addition, recall programs were often inadequate or nonexistent.

Later studies indicated that quite different results could be expected with thorough diagnosis and treatment planning, systematic design based on sound principles, meticulous periodontal and restorative treatment, optimal home care, and adequate follow-up recall. The incidence of caries was low, and there was no significant deterioration in the periodontal condition. The long-term prognosis was excellent when well-made partial dentures were provided under properly controlled circumstances.

The contrasting results and conclusions of these studies emphasize those factors that are particularly significant in the success of RPD treatment. It is apparent that adequate mouth preparation and follow-up care are essential if the prosthesis is expected to function without actively contributing to the demise of the remaining oral structures. The design of the partial denture must emphasize stress control so that the forces generated during function will lie within the physiologic limits of the supporting structures. In addition, the technical aspects of fabrication must be meticulously carried out so that the prosthesis performs in the planned manner.

A properly designed RPD in combination with well-planned comprehensive treatment will contribute to the preservation of the remaining teeth, bone, and gingiva by maintaining tooth position and occlusion, and restoring or maintaining vertical dimension of occlusion. It will also improve mastication and speech and enhance appearance.

Steps in the treatment of an RPD patient

1. Collection of information
   a. Document clinical findings, including charting of caries and periodontal condition.
   b. Take appropriate panoramic, bite-wing, and periapical radiographs.
   c. Make and mount diagnostic casts.
2. Diagnosis and treatment planning
   a. Evaluate data collected in step 1.
   b. Formulate a sequential treatment plan.
   c. Develop a tentative RPD design.
3. Mouth preparation: phase I
   a. Perform extractions, modification of the existing natural occlusal scheme, and definitive periodontal therapy.
   b. Perform endodontics, operative dentistry, and fixed prosthodontics.
4. Formulation of the final RPD design
   a. Obtain new mounted diagnostic casts if tooth or tissue contours have been significantly altered during phase I of mouth preparation.
   b. Review and modify original diagnostic information as necessary.
   c. Survey new casts and modify the tentative design if necessary.
5. Mouth preparation: phase II
   a. Perform tooth alterations (guide surfaces, rest preparations, and so on) on the diagnostic cast.
   b. Using the designed and modified diagnostic cast as a "road map," perform tooth alterations in the mouth.
   c. Make an alginate impression, pour the impression in quick-set plaster, and recheck the preparations with the aid of a surveyor.
   d. Modify the preparations as necessary, and make a final impression.
6. Fabrication of the RPD
   a. Survey and tripod the master cast.

b. Write an accurate work authorization.
c. Submit the designed diagnostic cast, opposing cast, work authorization, and surveyed and tripoded master cast to the laboratory for framework fabrication.
d. Try-in the framework and modify it as necessary.
e. Make an altered cast impression if indicated.
f. Make occlusal records for mounting casts if the casts cannot be accurately articulated by hand.
g. Arrange or prescribe for arrangement of artificial teeth.
h. Proceed with esthetic try-in if anterior teeth are replaced.
i. Prescribe for processing of the denture base and submit the work authorization to the laboratory.
j. Insert the RPD, make appropriate alterations, review patient instructions, and arrange for adjustment appointments.
7. Recall and maintenance
a. Short-term recall: when possible, see the patient the day following insertion. Anticipate at least one additional appointment for adjustment.
b. Long-term maintenance: the necessity for recall is highly variable depending on the nature of the periodontal and restorative therapy rendered, the type of RPD fabricated, and the patient's level of home care; however, consider specific arrangements an essential component of comprehensive treatment.

Although this text focuses on the design process involved in steps 2c and 4c, step 5, "Mouth preparation: phase II," is also included because it is so intimately linked to the success of the design. The fact that other diagnostic and clinical phases are not discussed in detail does not imply a lack of importance. All phases of treatment must be meticulously performed if the prosthesis is to function optimally without damaging the remaining oral structures.

Development of a framework design

No single design philosophy can be considered "correct" over all others. Variations are possible as long as diagnostic information and good mechanical principles form the basis for the design.

There has been little controversy over the design for tooth-supported RPDs because no functional motion occurs. Rests may be placed on any teeth capable of serving as suitable abutments. Retentive tips may be located in almost any accessible recesses.

Designs for extension RPDs, on the other hand, have generated considerable debate. It is generally agreed, however, that extension RPDs should provide broad stress distribution, minimal tooth and tissue coverage by the framework (except where necessary for support or stabilization), and retentive arms that either release or flex during functional movements of the bases. This text will regard the mesial rest, buccal I-bar, and distal guide plate as the preferred clasp assembly for distal extension RPDs. It is believed that this design will (1) reduce torquing forces on the abutment teeth, (2) result in a more apical resolution of vertical forces applied to the artificial teeth, and (3) increase the radius of rotation of the base, thus distributing functional loads more evenly. Other designs are considered when terminal abutments are mesially inclined or the retentive recesses are not in appropriate locations for I-bars.

The sequence used for the development of a design is, like the design itself, subject to some variation. The experienced dentist will, in fact, make decisions regarding several steps or elements concurrently. His mind will function like a computer, switching between steps as the situation demands. The sequence that follows is recommended as a starting point because it tends to encourage a logical and systematic process:

1. Selection of abutments and surveying
2. Location of rests
3. Location of guide plates
4. Selection of a major connector
5. Placement of minor connectors
6. Selection of retentive, bracing, and reciprocating elements
7. Placement of denture base retentive elements
8. Selection of replacement teeth

Chapter 1

Surveying

Surveying is a diagnostic procedure that analyzes the dimensional relationships of the oral hard and soft tissues. Surveying must be accomplished in association with decisions regarding the selection of abutments and the location of rests. Analyzing the dimensional relationships among anatomic features must be completed prior to removable partial denture (RPD) design or any other definitive treatment. Surveying is an *essential component* of RPD therapy.

The purposes of surveying are to:

1. Determine the most advantageous path of insertion/removal (insertion/dislodgement) for the RPD
2. Locate proximal tooth surfaces that are or can be made parallel to act as guiding surfaces
3. Locate and measure recesses or undercuts for mechanical retention
4. Identify areas of potential hard or soft tissue interferences
5. Determine a path of insertion/dislodgement consistent with esthetic requirements
6. Delineate the height of contour of the abutment teeth and identify areas of undercut that must be avoided, reduced, blocked out, or preserved
7. Help in planning restorative procedures
8. Record the most ideal cast position for future reference
9. Establish a formal plan for the RPD design and the required mouth preparation

The dental surveyor

A dental surveyor (Fig. 1-1) is used to determine the relative parallelism of two or more surfaces of a cast of the dental arch. The surveyor consists of two major components, the surveying stand and the table on which the cast is placed. The surveying stand is composed of a base, a fixed vertical support arm, a horizontal arm, a movable vertical arm, and a chuck at the lower end of the movable vertical arm. Analyzing, measuring, and marking styli (Fig. 1-2) are secured in the chuck. The upper segment of the surveying table (the mounting platform) holds the cast and is attached to the base by a swivel coupling that controls the tilt of the cast.

A surveyor is used to survey the diagnostic cast, to contour wax patterns and crowns, to place or form intracoronal retainers in crowns, and to survey the master cast prior to framework fabrication.

Determining the path of insertion/dislodgement

The path of insertion/dislodgement is dependent upon *(1)* potential guide surfaces, *(2)* undercuts for direct retention, *(3)* hard and soft tissue interferences, and *(4)* esthetic considerations. Although ideal conditions may not be achieved for each of the determinants, the final path of insertion/dislodgement should be optimal for the determinants as a group.

Begin by attaching the diagnostic cast to the surveying table and orienting the mean occlusal plane parallel to the base of the surveyor stand. The final orientation should seldom vary more than 10° from this position. Place the analyzing rod in the chuck at the lower end of the movable vertical arm, and evaluate the positions of the proximal surfaces of

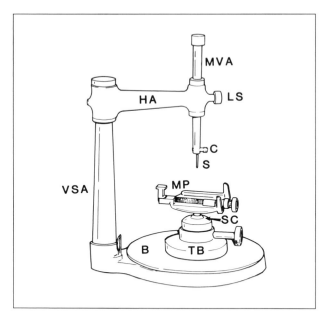

Fig. 1-1 The dental surveyor. Stand base *(B)*; vertical support arm *(VSA)* (fixed); horizontal arm *(HA)*; movable vertical arm *(MVA)*; locking screw *(LS)*; chuck *(C)*; stylus *(S)*; table base *(TB)*; swivel coupling *(SW)*; mounting platform *(MP)*.

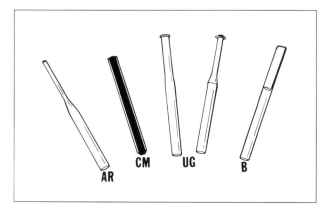

Fig. 1-2 Styli for the dental surveyor. Analyzing rod *(AR)*; carbon marker *(CM)* (in metal sleeve); undercut gauges *(UG)*; blade *(B)* for contouring wax patterns.

the abutments for parallelism (Fig. 1-3). Adjust the anteroposterior tilt of the cast until maximal parallelism is obtained. By aligning the majority of proximal walls, the need for alteration of tooth contours is reduced. (Also see chapter 3 and chapter 9.)

Next, without altering the anteroposterior tilt, vary the side-to-side tilt of the cast until the recesses that are to receive clasp tips are approximately equal (Fig. 1-4). Using the undercut gauges, assess the location and depth of the recesses. Lower the movable vertical arm of the surveyor until the lip of the undercut gauge is beneath the amount of undercut desired (Fig. 1-5a). Place the stem of the gauge against the abutment and gradually raise the gauge until the lip just touches the tooth (Fig. 1-5b). When viewed from the side, a small triangle of light should be evident between the abutment and the gauge. Both the stem and the lip of the gauge must be touching the tooth. The point at which the lip of the gauge touches the abutment represents the deepest position in which the metal of the retainer may contact the tooth. Refine the tilt until the undercuts are correct for the configuration and material of the planned clasp. Reassess the guide plane alignment. Remember, mechanical retainers will only function as planned if the path of insertion/dislodgement is dictated by contact of vertical tooth surfaces with rigid components of the RPD framework.

Continue the surveying process by evaluating hard and soft tissue prominences and corresponding recesses that may interfere with insertion or removal of the rigid portions of the metal framework or acrylic resin denture flanges (Fig. 1-6). Examples include lingual surfaces of lingually tilted premolars and mandibular tori that would interfere with proper positioning of the major connector (Fig. 1-7). Also examine the height of contour of the abutments where circumferential clasps originate (Figs. 1-8a and b). The rigid originating portion of a circumferential clasp cannot be placed in an undercut and must not be so near the occlusal surface that it will interfere with the opposing occlusion. After interferences have been located and analyzed, one of the following corrective procedures must be selected: *(1)* maintain the established orientation of the cast and eliminate the interferences by surgery and/or recontouring of the involved teeth, or *(2)* avoid interferences by altering the tilt

Fig. 1-3 *(left)* Analyzing rod being used to evaluate the proximal surface of a mandibular premolar abutment. The preliminary anteroposterior orientation of the cast should minimize the need for alteration of proximal tooth contours.

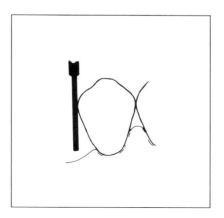
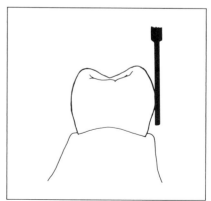

Fig. 1-4 *(right)* Analyzing rod being used to evaluate the buccal undercut of a mandibular premolar. The orientation of the cast is altered until the recesses that are to receive clasp tips are approximately equal.

Fig. 1-5a *(left)* Use of an undercut gauge *(UG)* to determine the location of the desired undercut. The gauge is initially positioned so that its side touches the tooth at the survey line *(SL).*

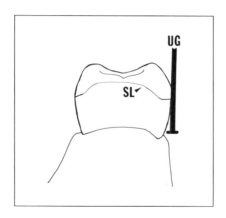
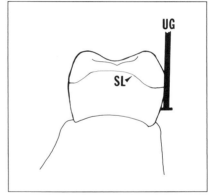

Fig. 1-5b *(right)* The gauge is raised until the stem and the lip *both* touch the tooth. The point of contact of the lip and the tooth represents the deepest position in which the metal of the retainer may contact the tooth.

Fig. 1-6 *(left)* Analyzing rod being used to assess tissue contours. Large buccal prominences contraindicate the use of infrabulge retainers.

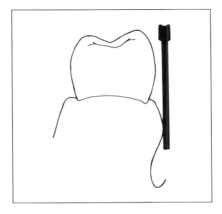
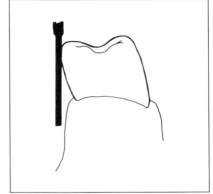

Fig. 1-7 *(right)* Analyzing rod being used to evaluate possible interferences. The lingually tilted mandibular premolar shown would interfere with proper positioning of a lingual bar major connector.

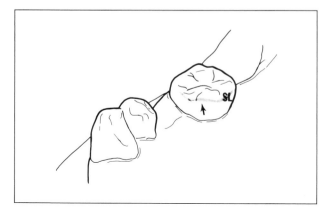

Fig. 1-8a Survey line *(SL)* indicates a height of contour that would interfere with placement of a circumferential retentive arm.

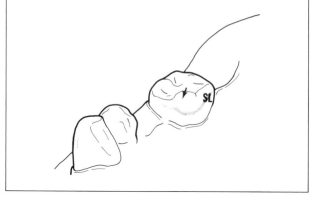

Fig. 1-8b After recontouring, the rigid portion of the arm can be placed above the survey line *(SL)*.

of the cast, thus accepting a compromise from the optimal orientation established for guide surfaces and retention.

Last, consider the esthetic requirements, particularly if anterior replacement teeth are necessary. If there is no tissue undercut, if the anterior teeth can be "butted" against the ridge, or if a short flange can be used, alteration in the path of insertion/dislodgement is usually not required. However, if there is residual ridge loss and the patient exhibits a high lip line, a full flange is necessary and the path of insertion/dislodgement may need to be altered slightly to allow the flange to pass over the tissue prominences. Also, the labial extent of guide planes on anterior teeth must be limited to the linguoproximal surfaces so that metal of the guide plates will not be visible between the natural and artificial teeth.

Placing the survey line

After the orientation is established, the analyzing rod is replaced with a carbon marker and the height of hard and soft tissue contours is marked on the cast. It is *absolutely essential* that survey lines be scribed by the *side* of the carbon marker and not the tip (Fig. 1-9). If the tip touches the cast, erroneous and misleading information will be produced (Figs. 1-10a and b).

The carbon marker is now replaced by the appro-

priate undercut gauge. After the gauge is properly positioned against the abutment, a sharp instrument is used to make a scratch on the stone abutment tooth at the lower edge of the lip of the gauge. The cast is moved away from the gauge and the mark is accented with the tip of a sharpened red pencil. The above procedures are repeated for the remaining abutment teeth, changing undercut gauges as necessary.

Tripoding the cast

Tripoding is a procedure that records the tilt of the cast. It provides a mechanism whereby the practitioner or laboratory technician can reestablish the desired path of insertion/dislodgement.

The carbon marker is placed in the chuck and the vertical arm is lowered until the tip of the marker touches the cast at three widely separated points. The arm is *locked* in position so that no vertical movement is possible. A line 2 to 3 mm long is made at each of three points on the cast, and the lines are circled in red (Fig. 1-11). To avoid confusion, the tripod marks should be placed in areas that will not be involved in the framework design.

A second method of tripoding is accomplished by drawing a vertical line on three sides of the diagnostic cast. The carbon marker or analyzing rod is lowered and placed against the side of the cast. A pencil is then used to draw a vertical line parallel

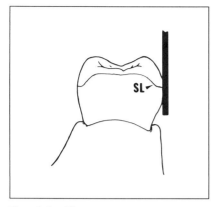

Fig. 1-9 The survey line (SL) must be scribed by the side of the carbon marker.

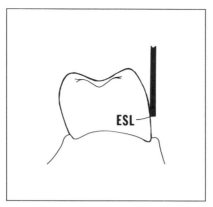

Fig. 1-10a If the tip of the carbon marker is allowed to touch the abutment, an erroneous survey line (ESL) is produced.

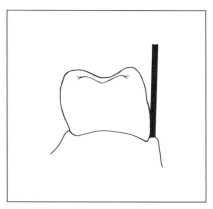

Fig. 1-10b Correct positioning of the marker shows that no undercut exists.

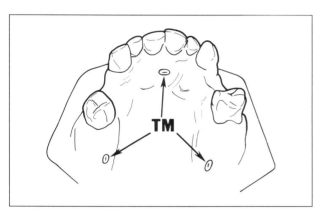

Fig. 1-11 Three tripod marks (TM) should be widely separated and must be made with the vertical arm and the mounting table locked in position.

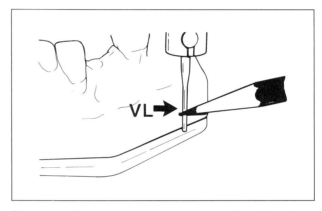

Fig. 1-12 Tripoding may also be accomplished by drawing a vertical line (VL) parallel to the side of the analyzing rod on three sides of the cast. The three lines should be as widely separated as possible.

to the marker or rod (Fig. 1-12). The procedure is repeated on two widely separated areas on other sides of the cast.

Creating a formal plan for the RPD design and mouth preparations

After surveying has been completed, the design of the partial denture framework should be drawn on

the diagnostic cast. Areas of tooth modification should be marked in red.

It is also recommended that recontouring to eliminate interferences and preparation of guide surfaces and rests be performed on the diagnostic cast. If the cast is not removed from the surveying table when these procedures are performed, the reductions may be easily reevaluated on the surveyor. When the recontouring and preparations are completed, the tooth reduction areas are marked in red. The clearly marked and prepared cast will now be a valuable reference for mouth preparation.

Surveying the master cast

The master cast, made following mouth preparation, is surveyed in the same manner described for the diagnostic cast. Because the recontouring and preparations may not have exactly duplicated those planned on the diagnostic cast, it is advisable to follow the same steps described under "Determining the path of insertion/dislodgement." If major discrepancies are noted, it may be necessary to refine the mouth preparations and make a new final impression.

The master cast must be surveyed and tripoded and may have the final design drawn on it. However, it is usually less confusing for the laboratory technician if the design is submitted on the diagnostic cast. The technician can then transfer the design to the master cast in a manner consistent with the procedures of his particular laboratory.

Chapter 2

Rests

A rest is a rigid extension of a partial denture that contacts a remaining tooth (or teeth) to dissipate functional forces.

The functions of rests are to:

1. Prevent movement of the removable partial denture (RPD) framework in a cervical direction
   a. Prevent trauma to the mucosa located around the abutments and beneath the framework (Fig. 2-1)
   b. Maintain the retentive portions of clasps in the prescribed positions (Figs. 2-2a to c)
2. Assist in distribution of occlusal loads over several teeth
3. Force the retentive elements to function in the planned manner, when used as indirect retainers on extension RPDs
4. Restore occlusion on abutments that exhibit tilting or infraocclusion (overlay rest) (Fig. 2-3)
5. Prevent extrusion of unopposed abutments (Fig. 2-4)
6. Direct food away from tooth contacts and embrasure areas
7. Provide lingual bracing on anterior teeth (Fig. 2-5)
8. Determine the correct orientation of the framework to the abutment teeth for altered cast impressions and relining procedures
9. Determine the axis of rotation for extension RPDs (Fig. 2-6)

A rest must be located in a *prepared* occlusal, cingulum, or incisal recess (rest preparation) on the abutment tooth. Ideally, rests should transmit forces along the long axis of the abutment teeth and, therefore, must not be located on inclined surfaces. Rest location, when possible, should

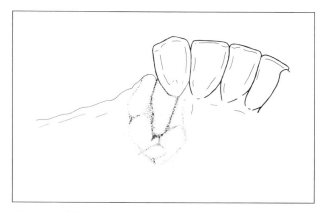

Fig. 2-1 Mandibular left canine showing "stripping" of the lingual gingiva caused by a mandibular RPD without rests (vertical stops).

avoid habitual contact areas. The occlusal surface of the rest should duplicate the natural occlusal morphology of the abutment tooth. It should have sufficient metal thickness to prevent breakage, especially where it joins the minor connector, an area where fracture is common (Fig. 2-7). Tsao (1970) reported that the minimum acceptable thickness is 1.38 mm for stellite alloys and 1.43 mm for cast gold (assuming an occlusal load of 80 kg).

Types of rests

Occlusal rest

An occlusal rest is an extension of the framework that contacts an occlusal surface of a tooth to provide support for an RPD (Fig. 2-8). An occlusal rest

19

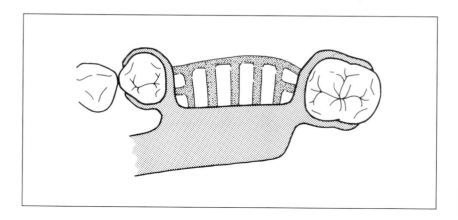

Fig. 2-2a Tooth-supported segment of mandibular RPD without rests present.

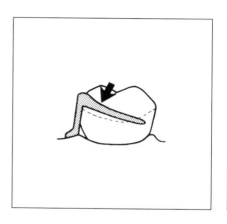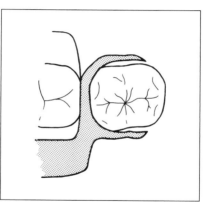

Fig. 2-2b *(left)* Circumferential clasp on molar. Note that the originating portion of the arm *(arrow)* lies above the survey line.

Fig. 2-2c *(right)* Configuration of clasp assembly following wear of the completed RPD. Because no rest was present, vertical forces were transferred to those portions of the arms above the survey line, and the arms spread away from the tooth.

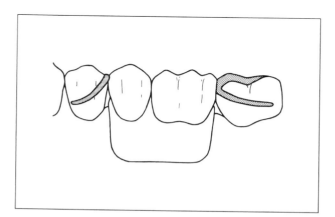

Fig. 2-3 Overlay rest on mandibular left second molar.

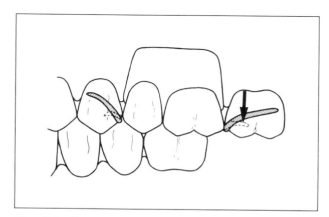

Fig. 2-4 Tooth-supported segment of maxillary RPD. The rest *(arrow)* will prevent extrusion of the unopposed second molar.

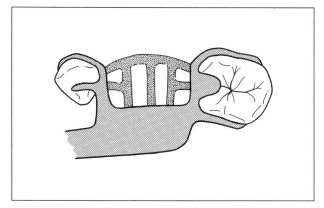

Fig. 2-5 Tooth-supported segment of mandibular RPD. Although the cingulum rest will not provide true reciprocation, it will contribute to horizontal stabilization and will help to counteract stress applied by the retentive arm when the RPD is in place. (*Note:* The retentive arm should be passive when the appliance is fully seated. However, such is not always the case, particularly if the clasps have been adjusted following initial insertion.)

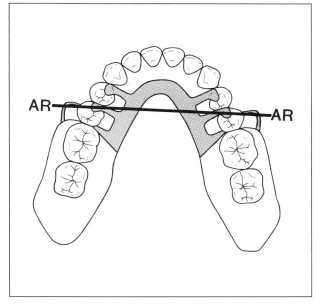

Fig. 2-6 In a distal extension RPD, the axis of rotation *(AR)* passes through the most distal rests when functional forces are directed toward the residual ridge over the bases.

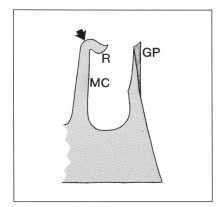

Fig. 2-7 Guide plate *(GP)*, minor connector *(MC)*, and rest *(R)* assembly for a mandibular premolar. The thickness of metal at the junction of the rest and the minor connector *(arrow)* should be at least 1.5 mm.

must form an angle of less than 90° with its minor connector (Fig. 2-9). Vertical forces will then tend to seat the rest in its corresponding recess and minimize the transmission of horizontal stresses to the abutment.

Cingulum (lingual) rest

A cingulum rest is an extension of the framework that contacts the lingual surface of a tooth to provide support for an RPD. Since all lingual surfaces

present inclined planes, it is paramount that lingual rests be located in *prepared* recesses on abutment teeth (Figs. 2-10a and b). Cingulum rests are most commonly used on maxillary and mandibular canines (occasionally on maxillary central and lateral incisors, and rarely on mandibular incisors). The lingual slope on mandibular canines is often so steep that some type of restoration is necessary to ensure a definite vertical stop. Restorations may also be required in maxillary anterior teeth when extreme vertical overlap dictates that the entire

21

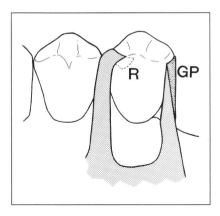 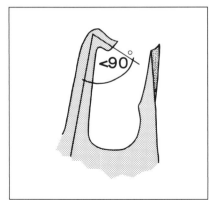

Fig. 2-8 *(left)* Rest *(R)* and guide plate *(GP)* in place on mandibular right second premolar.

Fig. 2-9 *(right)* The common plane of the rest must make an angle of less than 90° with the minor connector.

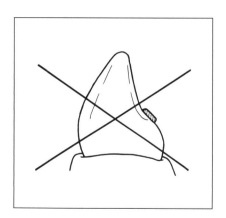 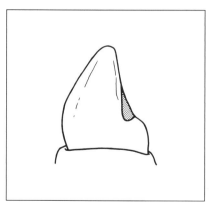

Fig. 2-10a *(left)* Cingulum rest located on an incline without a rest seat.

Fig. 2-10b *(right)* Cingulum rest located in a properly prepared rest seat.

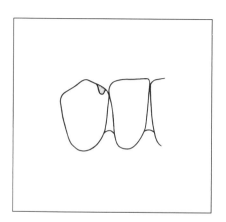 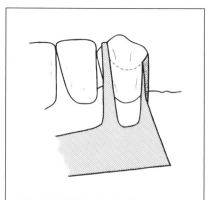

Fig. 2-11a *(left)* Incisal rest on a mandibular canine, facial view.

Fig. 2-11b *(right)* Lingual view. The dotted line on the lingual view represents the superior extent of the metal if plating is to be used.

rest be located within the natural contour of the lingual surface of the tooth. When possible, cingulum rests are preferred over incisal rests because they *(1)* are esthetically superior, *(2)* apply stress at a lower level and thus decrease the effect of horizontal and rotational forces, and *(3)* are less subject to breakage.

Incisal rest

An incisal rest is an extension of the framework that contacts an anterior tooth at the incisal edge to provide support for an RPD (Figs. 2-11a and b). Incisal rests are usually used only on mandibular anterior teeth. Their unesthetic appearance and potential for interference against the incisal edges of the mandibular teeth preclude their use on maxillary anteriors. The mesiodistal location of the rest on the incisal edge is determined by esthetic requirements and the condition of the incisal edge (e.g., avoid placement over large incisoproximal restorations or wear facets).

Rest location

Most decisions related to rest location depend on evaluation of considerable diagnostic data (radiographic findings, periodontal information, occlusion, and so on). Although rest location obviously varies considerably depending on the configuration of the remaining teeth, some generalizations can be made. In *tooth-supported RPDs,* rests are usually located adjacent to the edentulous areas, thus avoiding additional minor connectors and gingival coverage (Fig. 2-12). If diagnostic information indicates that these areas cannot be used, other locations characterized by good access and acceptable occlusal form should be selected. In *extension RPDs,* rest location is intimately related to the design and function of the clasp assemblies employed. However, as a general rule, the primary rests are usually located away from the extension areas (Figs. 2-13a and b). In this way, torquing of the abutment tooth during function can be minimized.

Rest location is intimately related to the type of clasp selection. Refer to chapter 6 for additional information.

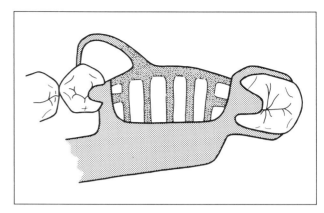

Fig. 2-12 On a tooth-supported segment of an RPD, rests are usually located adjacent to the edentulous area.

Figs. 2-13a and b On extension RPDs, terminal rests *(arrows)* are usually located on occlusal surfaces or incisal edges away from the edentulous area.

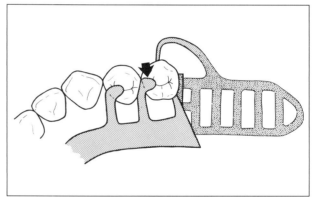

Fig. 2-13a Mandibular distal extension RPD.

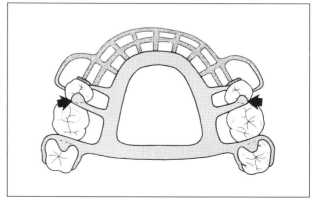

Fig. 2-13b Maxillary anterior extension RPD.

Chapter 3

Guide Surfaces and Guide Plates

Guide surfaces and guide plates (Figs. 3-1a to c) are, respectively, vertical parallel tooth surfaces and corresponding vertical metal struts, which, if properly located and contoured, may act together to determine the path of insertion/dislodgement of a removable partial denture (RPD). Although guide plates are minor connectors, they are considered separately because of their unique form and function.

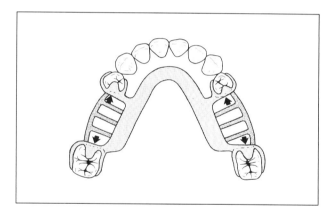

Fig. 3-1a Mandibular Class III RPD framework. Arrows indicate areas of guide surface–guide plate contact.

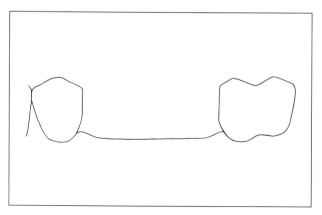

Fig. 3-1b Facial view of proximal guide surface preparations.

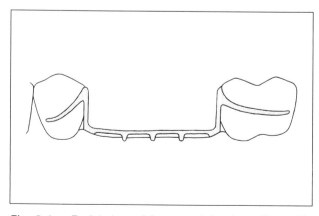

Fig. 3-1c Facial view of framework in place. The guide surface–guide plate relationship determines the path of insertion/dislodgement.

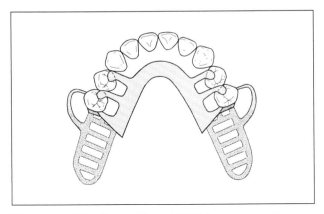

Fig. 3-2a Mandibular Class I RPD framework. The two guide plates present do not determine a definite path of insertion/dislodgement. However, if the tips of the I-bars are placed slightly in front of the greatest mesiodistal curvature of the facial surface of the abutments, there is resistance to dislodgement in all directions.

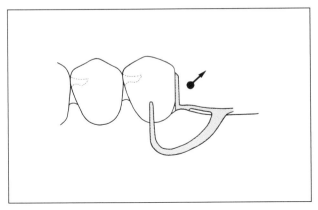

Fig. 3-2b Facial view of clasp assembly in which the I-bar is located exactly at the greatest mesiodistal curvature of the facial surface. Retention will be lacking if the retentive arm can move upward and backward without being forced to flex.

Terminology and concept

The subject of guide surfaces and guide plates has been characterized by ambiguity, uncertainty, misconception, and wide variations in opinion. The term *guide plane* (guiding plane) is a misnomer because, by geometric definition, a plane must be *flat.* Almost all guide planes have at least some buccolingual curvature. Thus, *guide surface* is a more appropriate term.

The *Glossary of Prosthodontic Terms* (1977) defines guiding plane as "two or more vertically parallel surfaces of abutment teeth so oriented as to direct the path of placement and removal of removable partial dentures." However, practically speaking, it is the direction of the path of insertion and dislodgement that is clinically important. In addition, two parallel surfaces frequently *do not* direct a path of insertion/dislodgement (Figs. 3-2a and b). Yet, they are still referred to as *guiding planes.* The corresponding portions of the frameworks are also called *guide plates.*

Guide plate does not appear in the *Glossary of Prosthodontic Terms.* Occasionally in the dental literature and frequently in speech, the term guiding plane is used to describe both the surface of the tooth and the metal plate that contacts the surface. Krol (1973) used the term *proximal plate* and defined it as "a plate of metal in contact with the proximal surface of an abutment tooth usually comprising a part of a clasp assembly." Although proximal plate is certainly acceptable, it represents only one type of guide plate, that which contacts a proximal surface. Several vertical metal plates, rigidly connected, can contact curved surfaces and control, or aid in controlling, the path of insertion/dislodgement. Linguoplating of posterior teeth may serve this function (Figs. 3-3a and b). Additionally, if the curves are converted to parallel surfaces by way of recontouring or restoration, the vertical segments of metal may be shorter occlusogingivally and still assist in ensuring a controlled path. Thus, rigid bracing elements and originating portions of circumferential clasp arms may assist in controlling the path of insertion/dislodgement if their locations are correct relative to prepared parallel surfaces (Fig. 3-3c).

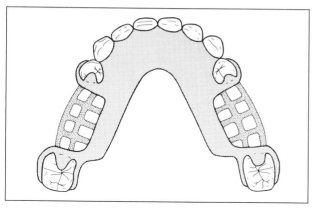

Fig. 3-3a Mandibular Class III RPD framework with a linguoplate major connector.

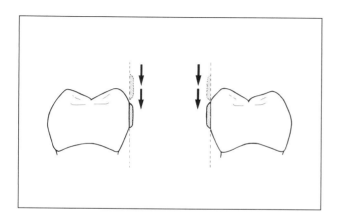

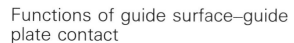

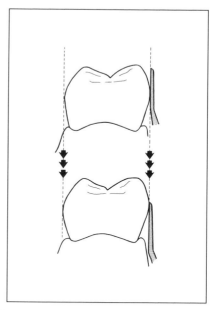

Fig. 3-3b The linguoplate on the premolars may also aid in controlling the path of insertion/dislodgement.

Fig. 3-3c The bracing arms on the molars may also aid in controlling the path of insertion/dislodgement.

Functions of guide surface–guide plate contact

The following functions have been attributed to guide surface–guide plate contact:

1. Provide for one path of insertion/dislodgement
2. Improve retention by creating frictional contact, resisting dislodgement in any direction other than that directed by guide surface–guide plate contact, and ensuring the planned action of retentive, reciprocal, and bracing components
3. Along with other metal components that contact vertical surfaces, aid in stabilizing or bracing the prosthesis against horizontal forces
4. Provide reciprocation
5. Reunite and stabilize the arch and aid in stabilizing individual teeth
6. Reduce the amount of blockout needed in areas of severe undercut, minimizing the amount of space between the denture and the tooth, thus reducing gross food traps
7. Make insertion and removal of the prosthesis easier for the patient
8. Eliminate detrimental strain on abutment teeth and framework components when placing and removing the prosthesis
9. Minimize wedging stresses on the abutment teeth

In addition, guide surface preparations on anterior teeth may be used to restore the normal width between teeth where drifting has reduced the size of the edentulous space; however, the guide plate should not be placed so far labially that the metal will be seen in the finished prosthesis.

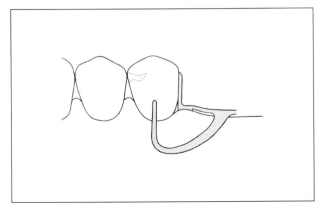

Fig. 3-4a Recommended relationship of guide surfaces, guide plates, and mucosa according to Kratochvil.

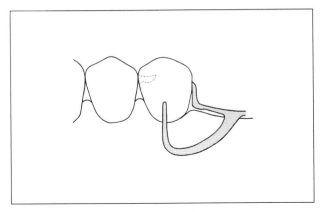

Fig. 3-4b Recommended relationship of guide surfaces, guide plates, and mucosa according to Krol.

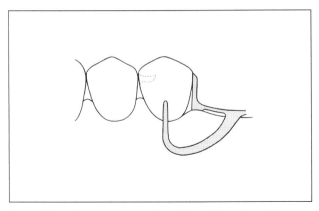

Fig. 3-4c Recommended relationship of guide surfaces, guide plates, and mucosa according to Demer.

Development of the mesial rest–I-bar–guide plate philosophy

Most of the controversy surrounding the guide surface–guide plate relationship concerns extension RPDs. Kratochvil (1963) advocated an extension guide surface preparation to eliminate space between the guide plate and the abutment (Fig. 3-4a). Maximum contact of the guide surface and the guide plate was desired. A 2 to 3 mm metal foot extended from the base of the guide plate onto the mucosa of the residual ridge. Binding of the guide plate against the abutment during function (move-

ment of the extension base toward the tissue when biting force is applied over the base) was prevented by physiologic relief of the metal at the framework try-in stage.

Ten years later, Krol (1973) modified Kratochvil's design and created the term *RPI clasp* (rest–proximal plate–I-bar, Fig. 3-4b). He recommended a much smaller guide surface preparation (2 to 3 mm in height; located in the occlusal third of the proximal surface) and a guide plate that contacted only the bottom 1 mm of the guide surface. Binding or torquing of the abutment was prevented by retaining a small space below the guide surface (into which the guide plate could move during function). The portion of the guide plate in contact with the gingival tissue was relieved.

Demer (1976) proposed another alteration in the design (Fig. 3-4c). He concurred with Krol that a slight undercut should be retained below the guide surface. However, he felt that the more gingival location of the guide plate would create the potential for food entrapment between the occlusal aspects of the abutment and the artificial tooth. He recommended that the guide plate contact the proximal surface of the abutment only at the top of the guide surface. Demer also extended the guide plate lingually far enough so that, in combination with the minor connector of the mesial rest, it would provide reciprocation and prevent lingual migration of the abutment.

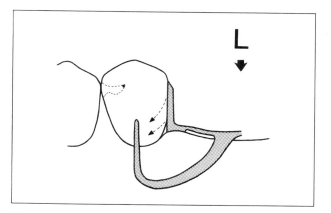

Fig. 3-5   When a functional load *(L)* is placed over a distal extension area, the prosthesis rotates around the rest and the lower portions of the guide plate contact the distal guide surface. This binding must be prevented with a "releasing" design or physiologic relief of the guide plate.

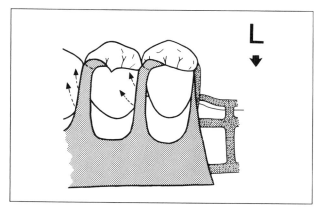

Fig. 3-6   When a functional load *(L)* is placed over a distal extension area, the prosthesis rotates around the primary rest and the minor connectors move upward and mesially.

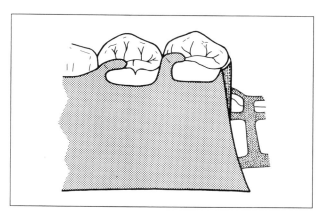

Fig. 3-7a   On a distal extension RPD, plating distal to the terminal rest must end exactly at the survey line shown in Fig. 3-7b.

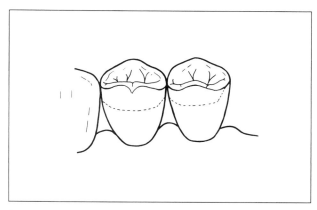

Fig. 3-7b   Survey line *(dotted).*

Research comparing the concepts noted above has been inconclusive. Assuming adequate patient home care and periodic recall and maintenance, excellent clinical success can be expected using any of the three designs if certain conditions are ensured. First, either by initial design or by way of physiologic relief, the guide plate must be prevented from binding against the abutment (Fig. 3-5). Second, the mesial minor connector must have freedom to move between the abutment and the adjacent tooth during function (Fig. 3-6). Third,

metal (e.g., guide plate, plating) located distal to the terminal rest must not be allowed to extend above the height of contour (Figs. 3-7a and b). Fourth, the mesial rest–I-bar–guide plate design should be avoided on mesially inclined terminal abutments because it is extremely difficult to achieve any "releasing" capacity for the guide plate (Fig. 3-8). During function, the guide plate will contact the tooth, preempt the mesial rest, and act as a rest on an inclined plane. Efforts to prevent contact with physiologic relief would create a sig-

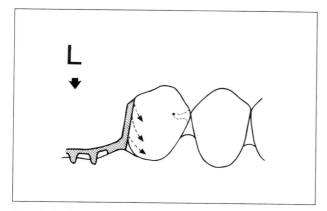

Fig. 3-8 Mesial rest–distal guide plate–I-bar assembly on a mesially inclined terminal abutment for a distal extension RPD. When a functional load (L) is applied, the guide plate binds against the entire length of the guide surface. Physiologic relief would result in the creation of an undesirable space between the occlusal aspects of the guide plate and the abutment tooth.

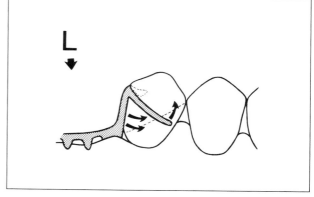

Fig. 3-9 Distal rest–distal guide plate–wrought wire retentive arm assembly on a mesially inclined terminal abutment for a distal extension RPD. Under a functional load (L), the guide plate binds against the distal guide surface. However, physiologic relief can be obtained without opening the contact between the guide plate and the abutment tooth. Although the clasp tip does not release during function, the flexibility of wrought wire decreases the stress transferred to the abutment.

nificant space between the abutment and the prosthesis. In this case, it would be far better to use a distal rest and a wrought wire circumferential clasp (Fig. 3-9). Although the clasp would not release during functional movement, its flexibility would create a stress-breaking effect. Because the distal rest would eliminate any space between the occlusal aspects of the proximal surfaces of the abutment and the artificial tooth, the gingival portion of the guide plate could be relieved without creating an area for food impaction.

Recommendations

Extension RPDs

For the most part, the designs for distal extension RPDs recommended in this text follow the theory espoused by Kratochvil. However, the guide surface preparations are generally more conservative, and there is no concerted effort to eliminate recesses in the gingival third of the proximal surface. When possible, the guide plate contacts the entire length of the prepared guide surface. A foot at the base of the guide plate touches the gingiva and extends 2 to 3 mm over the residual ridge before giving rise to the denture base retentive network.

Guide surfaces should be prepared on all proximal surfaces adjacent to edentulous spaces. They are prepared parallel to the desired path of insertion/dislodgement. The occlusal gingival dimension is generally one half to two thirds the crown length; 3 to 4 mm is more than adequate in most cases. If the natural tooth surfaces are parallel to the path of insertion/dislodgement, no preparation is necessary. A small recess gingival to the guide surface preparation is retained when present. The preparation should follow the natural buccolingual curvature of the proximal tooth surface and extend slightly past the linguoproximal line angle.

When linguoplating is used on posterior teeth, guide surfaces may also be prepared on lingual surfaces. Normally, 2 to 3 mm of length is all that can be expected. No preparation should be done in the gingival third of the tooth.

The guide plate contacts the entire guide surface initially. However, physiologic relief must be provided at the framework try-in (this is especially important when guide plates are located on both sides of a lone-standing abutment). The guide plate should extend far enough lingually so that, to-gether with the minor connector of the mesial rest, it will provide reciprocation and bracing and prevent lingual migration of the tooth. It must not, however, extend above the height of contour. The plate should be approximately 1 mm thick but should taper both occlusally and facially if it does not give rise to a rest or a clasp arm. In areas important to esthetics, guide plates must not extend so far facially that metal will be evident. The lingual margin is thickened to produce an external finish line for the plastic denture base. Such an arrangement will provide bulk for strength and rigidity without compromising placement of the artificial tooth.

Tooth-supported RPDs

Guide surfaces and guide plates for tooth-supported RPDs are similar to those for extension RPDs except that the preparations and corresponding plates are generally longer. Also, because there is no functional movement of the prosthesis, metal can, and usually does, extend above the height of contour. Physiologic relief is unnecessary.

Physiologic relief of the framework

Physiologic relief of guide plates and minor connectors is accomplished at the framework try-in appointment. It should be performed before trays for an altered cast impression, record bases, or completed denture bases are attached. A mixture of chloroform and rouge or one of the commercially available disclosing materials is applied to guide plates and minor connectors. The framework is seated in the mouth and manual pressure is used to place stress on the denture base retentive network. An effort is made to equal or surpass the movement that might be expected when biting forces are applied. The framework is removed from the mouth, and areas of contact are relieved. The process is repeated until functional loads produce no evidence of binding.

Tooth-supported RPDs do not require physiologic relief because they exhibit no functional motion.

Chapter 4

Major Connectors

A major connector is the part of a removable partial denture (RPD) that connects the components on one side of the arch to the components on the other side. It is the main component to which all other elements are directly or indirectly attached.

Major connectors must be rigid, conform to existing anatomic structures without interfering with movable tissues, and avoid food entrapment. Rigidity ensures that stresses applied to one portion of the denture are effectively distributed over the entire supporting area. Rigidity also enables the other components, such as retentive arms, to be effective.

Major connectors must not impinge on movable tissues or gingiva during insertion, removal, or function. *Marginal gingiva must never be used for support of an RPD.* The major connector should, as nearly as possible, blend with existing recesses, crevices, and embrasures. Large, operable, bony prominences or tori should be removed to avoid compromise in the location and design of the connector.

Relief over bony prominences must be provided in the fabrication of the framework. Postinsertion adjustment may result in excessive metal removal and weakening of the connector. The amount of relief depends on *(1)* the location and severity of the prominences, *(2)* the character of the tissue covering the prominences, *(3)* the degree of support provided by the abutments, *(4)* the quality of support offered by the residual ridges, and *(5)* the design of the major connector. A major connector must provide rigidity and, where applicable, support. However, it should not cover teeth or mucosa without a valid reason.

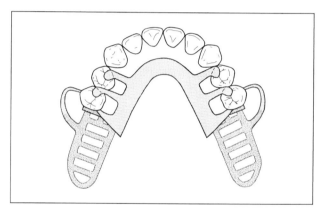

Fig. 4-1 Mandibular RPD framework with lingual bar major connector.

Mandibular major connectors

Lingual bar connector

A lingual bar (Fig. 4-1) is the preferred mandibular major connector except in the presence of a high floor of the mouth, extreme lingual tilt of anterior teeth, or inoperable lingual tori. Properly fabricated, the lingual bar will provide adequate rigidity without compromising plaque control and gingival health.

In cross section, the lingual bar is half pear shaped and at least 4 mm in height. The superior border should be 3 to 4 mm below the gingival margin. Thus, selection of a lingual bar as a major connector requires a distance of 7 to 8 mm from the gingival margin to the floor of the mouth (Fig. 4-2). Intraoral measurements should be made and recorded prior to the formulation of the final de-

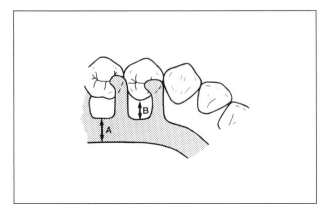

Fig. 4-2 The mandibular lingual bar connector should be at least 4 mm in height (A). The superior border of the bar must be 3 to 4 mm or more below the gingival margin (B).

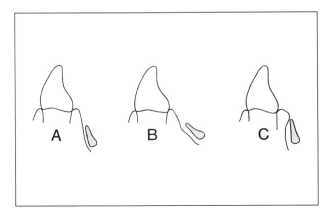

Fig. 4-3 Minimal relief is required beneath a lingual bar if the tissues exhibit a vertical fall (A); relief must be increased if the lingual tissues slope more horizontally (B); only blockout (not relief) is necessary if the lingual tissue is undercut (C).

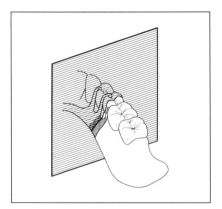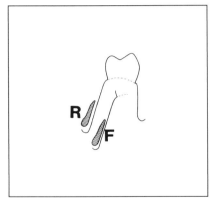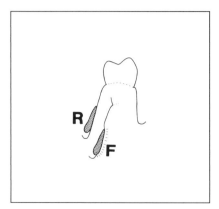

Fig. 4-4a (left) Cross section through a mandibular lingual bar major connector. The shaded area of the bar represents that portion distal to the terminal rest (the area requiring relief).

Fig. 4-4b (middle) Adequate relief beneath the major connector when the RPD is at rest (R) prevents impingement on the lingual tissues during function (F).

Fig. 4-4c (right) Inadequate relief beneath the major connector when the RPD is at rest (R) will result in displacement of and damage to the lingual tissues during function (F).

sign. The patient is instructed to touch the tip of the tongue against the anterior palate. A periodontal probe is placed against the gingiva, lingual to the mandibular anterior teeth, and measurements are made (opposite each tooth) from the floor of the mouth to the gingival margin. These measurements are transferred to the study cast. If less than 7 mm of height is recorded, a linguoplate major connector should be selected. It is extremely important that the location of the floor of the mouth be accurately determined. Postinsertion re-

duction of the inferior border of the metal bar will greatly reduce its strength and rigidity (the inferior border of the bar is the thickest and contributes greatly to the desired rigidity).

The amount of relief needed beneath a lingual bar depends on the contour of the lingual tissues and the anticipated functional motion of the prosthesis. If there is a vertical fall to the lingual tissues, minimal relief is necessary (Fig. 4-3). If the lingual tissues slope more horizontally, 26- to 28-gauge relief is recommended. If the lingual tissue

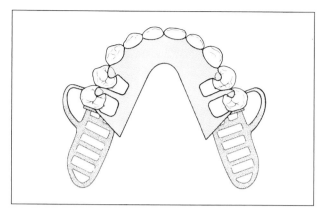

Fig. 4-5 Mandibular RPD framework with a linguoplate major connector.

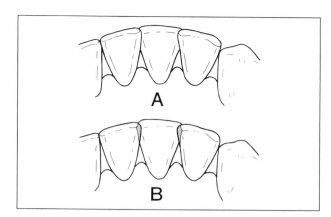

Fig. 4-6 If a linguoplate major connector is selected, the mesio- and distoincisal corners of overlapping anterior teeth (A) should be recontoured to eliminate excessive undercuts below the contact points (B).

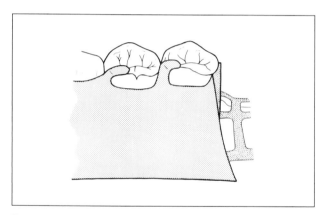

Fig. 4-7a The linguoplate extends posterior to the terminal rest.

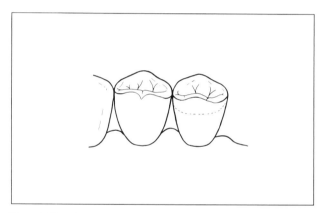

Fig. 4-7b In the case shown in Fig. 4-7a, the metal of the framework must end exactly at the survey line (dotted).

is undercut, the recess must be blocked out. Extra relief is required over bony prominences and in areas posterior to the axis of rotation in distal extension RPDs (Figs. 4-4a to c). Less relief is usually needed in tooth-supported RPDs.

Linguoplate (lingual plate) connector

A linguoplate connector (Fig. 4-5) consists of a lingual bar plus a metal plate extending superiorly above the cingula, but not higher than the middle third of the teeth. The superior border must be scalloped so that it extends to the contacts interproximally. A linguoplate is indicated in the presence of a high lingual frenum or floor of the mouth (or when the same effect is created by extensive recession or periodontal surgery); in the presence of inoperable lingual tori; or when the mandibular natural anterior teeth may need to be replaced in the near future. A linguoplate may also be necessary to provide indirect retention when all of the posterior teeth are missing (rest seats and rests

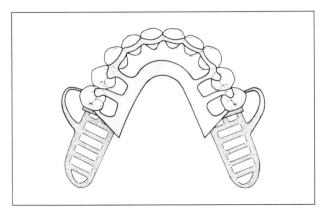

Fig. 4-8 Mandibular RPD framework with a double lingual bar major connector.

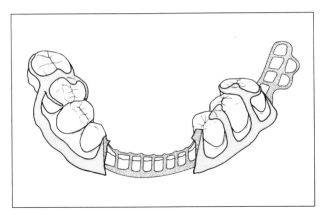

Fig. 4-9 Mandibular RPD framework with a labial bar major connector.

must be provided at least on the canines) or when the patient objects to a lingual bar.

A linguoplate has the disadvantage of covering the teeth and gingivae, thereby complicating oral hygiene and increasing the possibility of caries and periodontal problems.

Overlapping proximal tooth surfaces should be recontoured to avoid interproximal undercuts at the incisal corners (Fig. 4-6). Failure to do so will result in poor adaptation of the plate and impaction of food between the teeth and its superior border. If the plating extends posterior to the terminal rest on a distal extension RPD, the metal must end exactly at the survey line (Figs. 4-7a and b). If it extends above the survey line, it will preempt the planned rest during functional movement. If it ends below the survey line, it will not contact the tooth and will create an area for food collection.

Double lingual bar (lingual bar and Kennedy bar)

The double lingual bar (Fig. 4-8) is composed of a conventional lingual bar and a second narrower bar located between the cingula inferiorly and the contact points superiorly. The double lingual bar has been recommended when indirect retention must be obtained from the mandibular anterior teeth and large interproximal spaces have resulted from periodontal disease or surgery. A linguoplate would provide the required indirect retention but would

be esthetically inferior if the metal were visible through the interproximal areas. Although the double lingual bar may provide a better esthetic result in this case, it does have the potential for creating areas of food impaction and may be irritating to the tongue.

The form and placement of the inferior bar are exactly the same as for the lingual bar major connector. The upper border must clear the gingival margin by 3 to 4 mm. Thus, the double lingual bar cannot be used as a substitute for a conventional lingual bar when a high floor of the mouth exists. The superior bar must have rests in prepared rest seats at least on the canines.

Labial bar connector

The labial bar major connector (Fig. 4-9) is only selected when no other major connector will suffice. It is indicated when the remaining natural teeth are severely lingually inclined (an arrangement often associated with congenital defects or trauma). Recontouring, orthodontic treatment, or restoration with crowns may correct the problem, but when such treatment is impossible or impractical, the labial bar is a possible solution.

The superior border of the labial bar should be at least 3 to 4 mm below the marginal gingiva. Because the labial bar is longer than the lingual bar, it must be heavier to provide the same degree of rigidity.

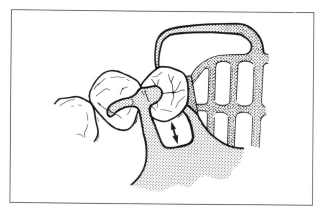

Fig. 4-10 The borders of a maxillary major connector should be located at least 6 mm *(arrow)* from the gingival margin.

Maxillary major connectors

Regardless of type, maxillary major connectors share several important characteristics. Because there are no movable tissues on the palate, the borders of these connectors may be located farther from the gingival margins than could those of mandibular major connectors. Except in cases where linguoplating is used, the border of the connector should be at least 6 mm from the gingival margin (Fig. 4-10). All components of a maxillary major connector should cross the palate at right angles (Fig. 4-11). Curves in the connector should be placed to one side of the midline. Whenever possible, coverage of the anterior palate should be avoided to minimize interference with tongue function and speech. The anterior borders of maxillary major connectors should be hidden in a valley between rugae so that the external surfaces of the connectors are even or nearly even with the crest of the tissue (Fig. 4-12).

The borders of all maxillary major connectors should be beaded (0.5 to 1.0 mm wide and deep). The bead is shallower over the midline suture and fades out as it approaches within 6 mm of the marginal gingiva. The bead maintains positive contact with the soft tissues, increases the rigidity of the connector, provides a finish line for the technician, and creates bulk at the borders of the connector so that the edges may be tapered and made less noticeable to the tongue. Relief for maxillary

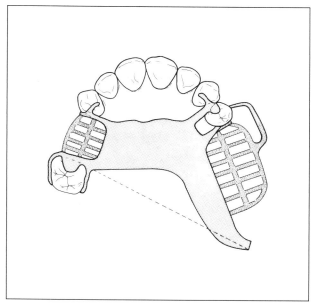

Fig. 4-11 The borders of a maxillary major connector should cross the palate at right angles to the midline (*solid line* is correct, *dotted line* is incorrect).

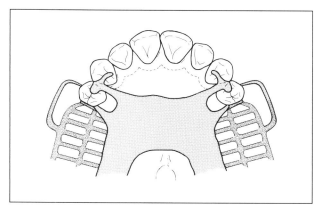

Fig. 4-12 The anterior border of a maxillary major connector should be hidden in a valley between the rugae *(solid line)* and should never be placed forward of the indirect retainers *(dotted line).*

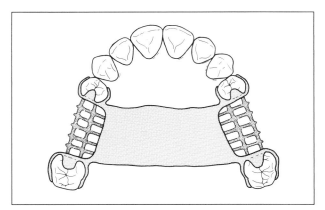

Fig. 4-13 Maxillary RPD framework with a palatal strap major connector.

major connectors is usually provided only over tori and prominent midline sutures.

Much of the dental literature related to the nomenclature and design of maxillary major connectors dates back to the time when gold-based alloys were still being used. Consequently, the term *bar* is often seen. With the advent of the more rigid stellite alloys, palatal bars have been almost universally replaced by palatal straps. The strength of the new alloys allows for the straps to be quite thin, much less bothersome to the tongue, and generally more comfortable. The rigidity provided by single straps is adequate and that of anterior-posterior straps is excellent.

Palatal strap connector

A palatal strap (Fig. 4-13) is a major connector used primarily in tooth-supported (Kennedy Class III) RPDs. The strap is generally as wide as the area bounded by the four principal rests (minimum width of 8 to 10 mm). Although the rigidity provided by a palatal strap is not absolute, it is usually adequate. Fortunately, as the edentulous span increases, the strap becomes wider and rigidity improves accordingly. Because the RPD is tooth-borne, support furnished by the strap is minimal even when the edentulous segments are relatively large. The anterior border of the strap should be located in a valley between rugae, and both borders of the strap should be beaded.

Anterior-posterior palatal strap connector

The anterior-posterior (A-P) palatal strap (Figs. 4-14 to 4-17) is the most versatile of all maxillary major connectors. It may be used for Kennedy Class I, II, III, or IV partially edentulous arches. The thin straps provide excellent rigidity and strength with minimal tissue coverage and little interference with tongue function. Minimal tissue coverage does, however, detract from the support contributed by the major connector.

The anterior, posterior, and lateral straps should be 6 to 8 mm wide. The lateral straps should be positioned symmetrically, and the palatal border of the straps should be located at the junction of the vertical and horizontal portions of the palate. The anterior strap must not be placed forward of the most anterior rests, and the anterior border should be located in a valley between the rugae. When possible, the posterior border of the posterior strap should be located at the junction of the hard and soft palates. For the palatal opening to be of significant benefit, it should be 15 mm or more in anteroposterior dimension. If the opening is less than 15 mm, it would be better to use a wide palatal strap or palatal plate.

Although the single palatal strap is usually used in Class III (tooth-supported) situations, an A-P palatal strap may be indicated when the edentulous segments are large and tissue coverage from a single strap would be excessive. Since support is provided almost entirely by the abutments, loss of support created by selecting an A-P strap is inconsequential. When the A-P palatal strap is used in Class III RPDs, the posterior border of the posterior strap is not necessarily placed at the junction of the hard and soft palates. However, it should be placed as posterior as is consistent with the location of the posterior abutments.

The A-P palatal strap is the major connector of choice in the presence of an inoperable torus that ends posteriorly 6 to 8 mm short of the junction of the hard and soft palates. It is much more rigid than the U-shaped connector.

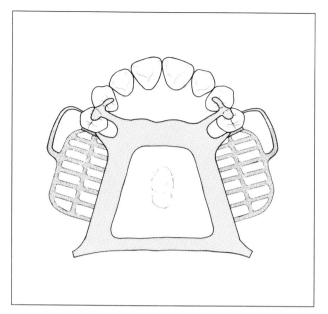

Fig. 4-14 An A-P palatal strap major connector used to circumvent a torus that ends posteriorly 6 to 8 mm or more anterior to the junction of the hard and soft palates.

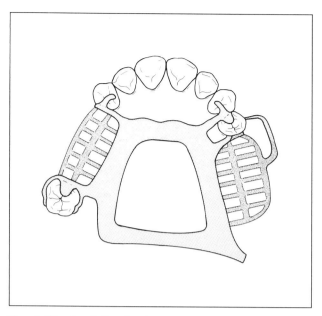

Fig. 4-15 An A-P palatal strap used as the major connector for a Kennedy Class II RPD.

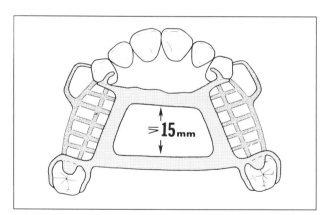

Fig. 4-16 An A-P palatal strap used as the major connector for a Kennedy Class III RPD. The palatal opening should be 15 mm or more in an anteroposterior dimension.

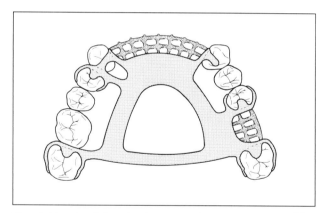

Fig. 4-17 An A-P palatal strap major connector used for a Kennedy Class IV RPD.

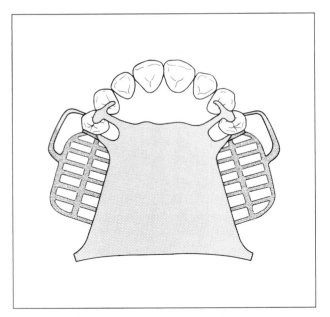

Fig. 4-18   A palatal plate major connector.

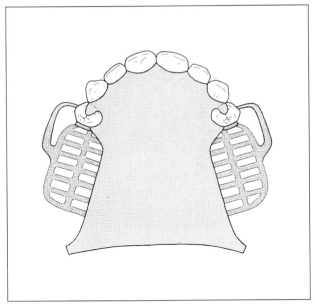

Fig. 4-19   A palatal plate major connector with linguo-plating.

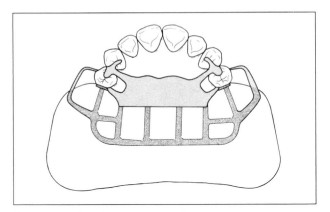

Fig. 4-20   A palatal plate major connector composed partly of metal and partly of plastic.

Palatal plate connector

The palatal plate connector (Fig. 4-18) is primarily indicated in Kennedy Class I arch forms where only the anterior teeth (or anterior teeth plus one or more premolars) remain, the support from the residual ridge is poor, the abutments are periodon-

tally weakened, and/or adequate direct retention is difficult to obtain. Although the palatal plate provides optimal rigidity and support, it cannot be used when a torus is present. Because of the extensive soft tissue coverage, the palatal plate may diminish taste perception, interfere with tongue function, and be uncomfortable to some patients. Its use should be reserved for those cases where maximum palatal support is necessary or where denture style retention (created by intimate contact of the metal plate with the underlying mucosa) is needed to augment the other retentive qualities of the RPD. Linguoplating (Fig. 4-19) may be used to provide indirect retention or to allow for subsequent replacement of natural teeth that have a questionable prognosis. Linguoplating should never be used indiscriminantly, however, and must always be accompanied by adequate rest seats and rests.

The palatal plate connector may be composed entirely of metal or may be part metal and part plastic (Fig. 4-20). Plastic in the posterior portion allows for postinsertion revision of the posterior palatal bead and for relining/rebasing over residual ridges that are still in the process of recontouring.

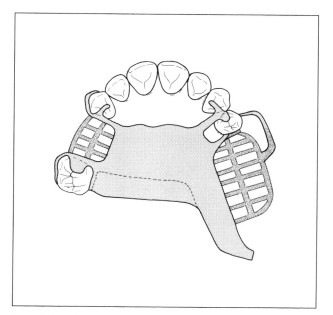

Fig. 4-21 A modified palatal plate major connector. The posterior border may be located at the solid or dotted line, depending on the desirability of plating the molar and the degree of rigidity and support required.

Fig. 4-22 A U-shaped major connector used to circumvent a large, inoperable torus.

Unfortunately, the plastic portion of the palate must be considerably thicker than the metal. In addition, the junction of the metal and the plastic often creates an abrupt change in thickness and may be disturbing to the patient's tongue.

A third type of palatal plate connector, the all-plastic palate, *should be avoided* except where the prosthesis is considered transitional and loss of the remaining teeth is imminent. Plastic palatal connectors are flexible and unhygienic. They are often associated with periodontal damage and papillary hyperplasia.

Regardless of the style of the palatal plate connector, a bead should be placed in the posterior palatal seal area. If the palate is entirely metal, the bead must be placed in the master cast prior to framework fabrication. If the posterior portion is plastic, the bead may be placed any time prior to processing. The dimensions of the bead for a metal palate are approximately 1 mm wide and 1 mm deep. For either a combination or an all-plastic palate, the bead should be slightly deeper to compensate for dimensional change of the plastic during processing. Because the dimensions of the bead are heavily dependent on the character of the

palatal tissue, placement of the bead is the responsibility of the dentist.

Modified palatal plate connector

A modified palatal plate (Fig. 4-21) is a plate-type connector used in Kennedy Class II RPDs. The anterior-posterior dimension of the plate portion is generally determined by the location of the most anterior and the most posterior rests on the tooth-supported side (as is done for the single palatal strap in Kennedy Class III RPDs). The posterior border of the plate may be located anterior to the junction of the hard and soft palates. On the extension side, the connector curves posteriorly (after crossing the midline at a right angle) and continues backward, ending with a butt joint at the entrance to the hamular notch.

The modified palatal plate offers excellent rigidity and good support. Some denture style retention can be expected. In Kennedy Class II RPDs, an A-P palatal strap major connector may be substituted for a modified palatal plate if the abutments are periodontally sound, the residual ridges provide sufficient support, and direct retention is adequate. Under these circumstances, additional denture style retention from the connector is unnecessary.

All borders of the modified palatal plate are beaded. The bead must be discontinued 6 mm from the gingival margin.

U-shaped (horseshoe) palatal connector

The U-shaped connector (Fig. 4-22) often lacks rigidity, particularly at the open ends. Increasing tissue coverage and bulk will improve rigidity but may interfere with tongue function and speech. A U-shaped connector is indicated when a large, inoperable torus extends posteriorly to within 6 to 8 mm or less of the junction of the soft and hard palates or when the patient cannot tolerate contact of the prosthesis with the posterior portion of the palate. If the torus ends 6 to 8 mm or more anterior to the junction of the hard and soft palates, an A-P palatal strap is the connector of choice. It will provide rigidity with less extensive tissue coverage.

Chapter 5

Minor Connectors

Minor connectors are rigid elements that connect primary rests, indirect retainers, clasp assemblies, and denture bases to the major connector.

By rigidly connecting the components of a removable partial denture (RPD), minor connectors contribute significantly to broad stress distribution. When stresses are applied to the artificial replacement teeth, the forces are transferred to the abutment teeth by the major and minor connectors (prosthesis to abutment). In addition, major and minor connectors are instrumental in transferring the effects of retainers, rests, and reciprocating/bracing components around the arch (abutment to prosthesis). If minor connectors are lacking or improperly designed, stresses remain localized in the area where they are generated. Properly designed minor connectors contribute to horizontal stabilization, reciprocation/bracing, and encirclement.

Types/classification

Several different classifications of minor connectors have been suggested. The classifications are usually based on either location or function. Unfortunately, neither method arranges the types of minor connectors in a sequence compatible with the customary design process. Because this text is arranged according to the design sequence, several types of minor connectors are considered in other chapters.

Guide plates are minor connectors located on the proximal surfaces of abutment teeth next to an edentulous space. Guide plates were discussed in detail in chapter 3.

Minor connectors that join the denture base to the major connector are considered in chapter 7.

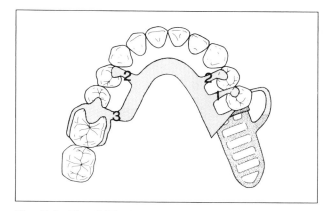

Fig. 5-1 The RPD elements referred to as *minor connectors* in this chapter attach primary rests *(1)*, indirect retainers *(2)*, or clasp assemblies *(3)* to the major connector.

Linguoplating is also sometimes classified as a minor connector. Discussion of linguoplating can be found in chapter 4.

In this chapter, only those minor connectors *not located next to an edentulous space* will be considered. These minor connectors (Fig. 5-1) attach primary rests, indirect retainers, or clasp assemblies to the major connector. For purposes of clarity, these are the only elements that will be referred to as *minor connectors*. The other types of minor connectors will be called by their more descriptive terms; that is, *guide plates, denture base retentive elements,* and *linguoplating.*

Minor connectors should be positioned in interproximal spaces (embrasures). They must be rigid and strong, must not interfere with normal anatomic contours or the opposing occlusion, and should not trap food. Surfaces that are already convex should be avoided whenever possible.

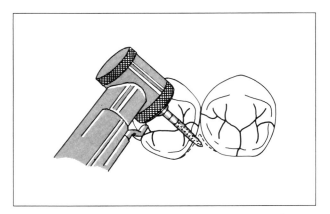

Fig. 5-2 Slight reduction at the junction of the linguo-proximal and occlusal surfaces is occasionally necessary to create the space needed for strength of the minor connector.

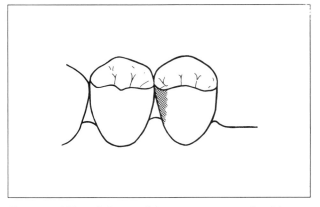

Fig. 5-3 When it is possible to create a small guide surface preparation, the guide surface–minor connector relationship will help to determine a precise path of insertion/dislodgement.

Major and minor connectors should join at a right angle so that the gingival crossing will be abrupt and cover as little of the marginal gingiva as possible. However, the angles created at the junction should be rounded. Whenever possible, 4 to 5 mm of space should be present between adjacent vertical minor connectors.

The space needed for strength of the minor connector, particularly where it joins the rest or clasp assembly, should be created during mouth prepa-

ration (Fig. 5-2). Adequate bulk can be assured by recontouring the embrasure area. Gross undercuts that could potentially act as food traps can also be eliminated.

Occasionally, small guide surfaces can be prepared so that a guide surface–guide plate relationship can be established for a minor connector and its corresponding abutment (Fig. 5-3). This relationship can, in turn, help to determine a precise path of insertion/dislodgement.

Chapter 6

Retention and Retainers

Retention is that quality of a removable partial denture (RPD) which resists the forces of gravity, the adhesiveness of foods, and the forces associated with opening the jaws. The term *retention* refers to resistance to dislodgement of the prosthesis in an *occlusal* direction (Fig. 6-1). Movement of the prosthesis toward the tissues is resisted by rests in tooth-supported RPDs and by rests and basal seat tissues in extension RPDs. The attempted use of mechanical retainers to resist functional forces (those toward the residual ridge) will result in either the deformation of the retainers or the transfer of undesirable torquing forces to the abutments (Fig. 6-2).

The importance of retention, particularly mechanical retention, has often been overestimated. Dentists have frequently been delighted with RPDs that snap into place or exhibit extreme amounts of retention. However, such prostheses are much more prone to failure, either from damage to the abutments or from permanent deformation of the clasps. The ideal amount of retention is that which will retain the RPD against *reasonable* dislodging forces without placing undue strain on the abutment teeth or the components of the clasp assembly.

The need for retention varies greatly among patients. It appears that retention is most necessary for new partial denture wearers and patients with limited adaptive capacity. Many satisfied long-term partial denture patients have prostheses that exhibit little or no mechanical retention. The patients' neuromuscular control and adaptability provide all the retention that is necessary for acceptable partial denture function.

The collection of information and the formulation of judgments about retention must begin early in

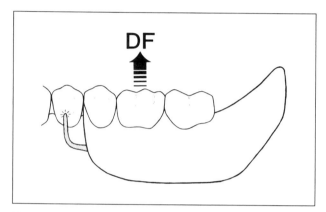

Fig. 6-1 Retention refers to resistance to dislodging forces *(DF)* that pull away from the basal seat tissues.

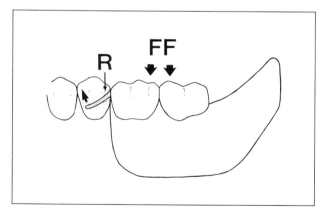

Fig. 6-2 Retainers should not be used to resist tissue-ward (functional) movement of an extension base. Functional forces *(FF)* cause depression of the base and rotation around the rest *(R)*. The accompanying upward movement of the clasp tip has the potential for torquing the abutment.

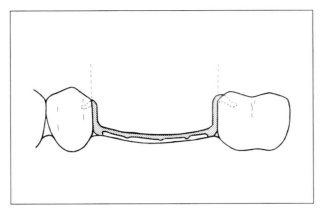

Fig. 6-3a Frictional retention results from guide surface–guide plate contact if the preparations are parallel and the metal is in intimate contact with tooth structure.

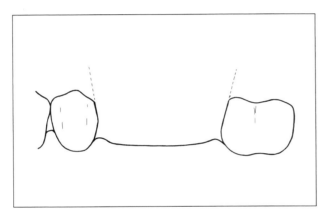

Fig. 6-3b Frictional retention is greatly reduced or eliminated if the guide surface preparations are not parallel.

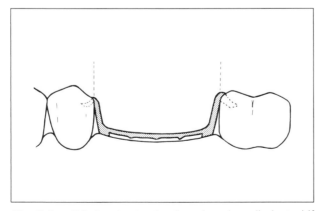

Fig. 6-3c Frictional retention is reduced or eliminated if intimate contact of metal and tooth structure is lost due to excessive laboratory blockout or injudicious relief of the guide plates.

the diagnostic process. If an existing RPD is satisfactory without significant retention (but must be remade for other reasons), it is probably safe to assume that only minimal retention will be needed in the new prosthesis. It would be unwise to crown abutments or undertake extensive restorations simply to increase the retentive areas. Conversely, if the major problem with the RPD is lack of retention, if the patient is a new denture wearer, or if the patient exhibits poor coordination and adaptability, considerable restorative dentistry may be warranted to ensure the ultimate success of the new prosthesis.

Sources of retention

The total inherent retention of an RPD is obtained from *(1)* denture style retention (adhesion, cohesion, and interfacial surface tension), *(2)* frictional retention from guide surface–guide plate contact, and *(3)* mechanical retention from clasps (direct retainers).

Overall denture retention is aided by adhesion, cohesion, and interfacial surface tension if the metal or plastic denture base (or major connector) is closely adapted to the underlying mucosa and if a thin film of saliva exists between the two surfaces. Adhesion is the attraction of unlike molecules, whereas cohesion is the attraction of like molecules. Interfacial surface tension is an attractive force occurring at the surface of a fluid film. All three phenomena are directly proportional to the area covered. Although denture style retention potentially exists anywhere there is initimate contact between tissues and the denture base material, it is of greatest assistance in the maxillary arch when complete palatal coverage is used.

Frictional retention is of substantial benefit when there are multiple guide surface–guide plate contacts. However, if the guide surface preparations are not parallel, if blockout of the master cast is excessive, or if the guide plates are overrelieved, frictional retention is minimal or nonexistent (Figs. 6-3a to c). In addition, on distal extension RPDs where the path of insertion/dislodgement cannot be precisely dictated by only two guide plates, frictional retention decreases dramatically. Clinically, frictional retention is most effective when the abut-

Figs. 6-4a and b Components of a clasp assembly; rest *(R)*; minor connector *(MC)*; guide plate *(GP)*; retentive arm *(RA)*; reciprocating/bracing arm *(RBA)*.

Fig. 6-4a *(left)* I-bar clasp assembly.

Fig. 6-4b *(right)* Circumferential clasp assembly.

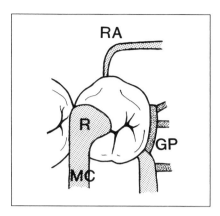

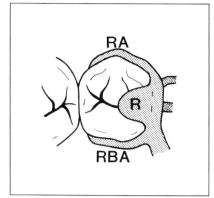

ments receive crowns that have milled parallel proximal and lingual surfaces. Obviously, such an ideal situation is not always possible or practical.

Mechanical retention and mechanical retainers (direct retainers, clasps)

Mechanical or direct retention in an RPD is the retention obtained by the use of attachments or clasps that resist removal from the abutment teeth and displacement in an occlusal direction. Only extracoronal retainers (clasps) will be discussed in this text.

All clasps are part of larger units called *clasp assemblies*. The components of a clasp assembly are *(1)* one or two rests, *(2)* a retentive arm, *(3)* a reciprocating or bracing element, and *(4)* one or more minor connectors (Figs. 6-4a and b). Although rests and minor connectors are considered in detail in other chapters of the text, their action is an integral part of the function of clasp assemblies, and pertinent aspects of their function will be considered here as well.

An ideal clasp assembly should possess the following qualities: *(1)* support, *(2)* bracing action, *(3)* reciprocation, *(4)* retention, and *(5)* greater-than-180° encirclement. In addition, clasp arms should be totally passive when the RPD is fully seated and should activate only when a dislodging force occurs. The clasp should not transfer torquing forces

to the abutment when functional forces (those toward the residual ridge) are applied to the prosthesis. The entire assembly should be compatible with existing tooth and tissue contours and consistent with the esthetic demands of the patient.

Support

The importance of adequate support for a clasp assembly cannot be overemphasized. The term *support* implies resistance to movement of the assembly in a gingival direction. Support is provided almost entirely by rests. Some support is furnished by other rigid metal located above the survey line (e.g., the rigid portions of retentive arms and bracing and reciprocating arms). However, these components usually lie on inclined surfaces and should never be expected to provide primary vertical support.

Bracing and reciprocation

Bracing and reciprocation provide resistance to potentially harmful horizontal components of force. Bracing occurs when the RPD is completely seated. It is produced by rigid portions of clasps, guide plates, and minor connectors (Fig. 6-5). Since the terminal portions of retentive arms must be flexible, they do not contribute significantly to bracing.

Bracing elements, united by *rigid major connectors,* are capable of distributing horizontal forces

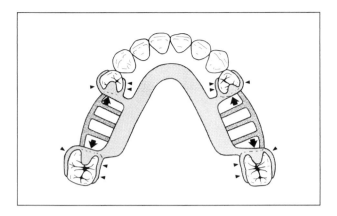

Fig. 6-5 Bracing is produced by rigid portions of clasp arms *(darts)*, minor connectors, and guide plates *(arrows)*. Effective cross-arch bracing also requires a rigid major connector.

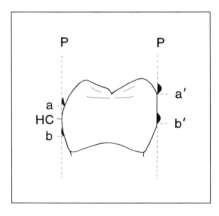

Fig. 6-6 For true reciprocation to occur, the inferior edge of the lingual reciprocating arm must contact the tooth from *a'* to *b'* as the inferior edge of the buccal retentive arm travels from *a* to *b*, over the height of contour *(HC)*. The flattened lingual tooth surface must be parallel to the path of insertion/dislodgement *(P)*.

throughout the partially edentulous arch. If the major connector is improperly designed and flexible, horizontal forces remain localized in the quadrant where they are generated.

Reciprocation is a specialized, dynamic form of bracing. It is the means by which a rigid portion of a framework neutralizes the horizontal forces produced by the retentive clasp arm during insertion and removal of the prosthesis. Effective, or true, reciprocation means that the force applied to the tooth by the retentive arm must be offset by an opposing rigid element from the moment the clasp tip contacts above the survey line until it lies passively in the undercut (Fig. 6-6). Proper timing of the contact is essential. If the clasp arm contacts above the height of contour *before* the opposing rigid elements contact, true reciprocation does not exist and the tooth will be placed under lateral stress.

Reciprocation can be achieved by nonflexible clasp arms, guide plates, and minor connectors that are located on the same tooth as the retentive arm. Although rigid metal or clasp contact in other areas may ensure a particular path of insertion and/or the effectiveness of the retentive arm, it does not produce true reciprocation (Fig. 6-7).

For effective reciprocation to occur, rigid metal must contact the tooth *during the entire time* that the retentive arm is passing over the height of contour. One of the following must be true to produce effective reciprocation: *(1)* a reciprocating arm must pass over a flattened tooth surface (Fig. 6-8), *(2)* a flattened surface of rigid metal must contact the height of contour of a curved tooth surface (Fig. 6-9), or *(3)* a flattened surface of rigid metal must contact a flattened surface of the tooth (Figs. 6-10a and b).

When reciprocation for a clasp is not provided, there is a combination of retentive arm flexure and tooth movement as the clasp tip passes over the

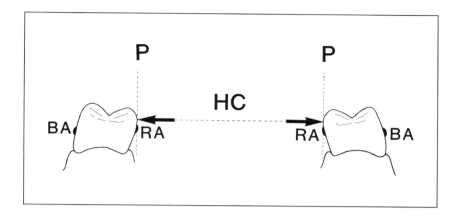

Fig. 6-7 Lingual retentive arms *(RA)* located on opposite sides of the arch and passing over the height of contour *(HC)* at the same time will help to ensure retention, particularly if the path of insertion/dislodgement *(P)* is clearly defined by rigid elements of the prosthesis. However, effective reciprocation does not exist because the buccal arms *(BA)* will not contact the teeth as the retentive arms pass over the height of contour.

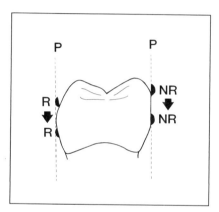

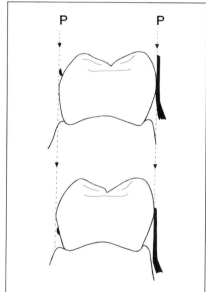

Fig. 6-8 Reciprocation is obtained if a rigid nonretentive arm *(NR)* makes contact with a flattened surface of the tooth as the retentive arm *(R)* passes over the height of contour and into the prescribed undercut. The flattened tooth surface must be parallel to the path of insertion/dislodgement *(P)*.

Fig. 6-9 *(right)* Reciprocation is achieved if a flat surface of rigid metal (e.g., linguoplating) maintains contact with the tooth as the retentive arm passes over the height of contour. The inner surface of the plating must be parallel to the path of insertion/dislodgement *(P)*.

Fig. 6-10a *(left)* Reciprocation can be obtained from contact of a flat surface of rigid metal and a prepared flat tooth surface.

Fig. 6-10b *(right)* The prepared tooth surface must be parallel to the path of insertion/dislodgement so that the metal and the tooth will remain in contact as the retentive arm passes over the height of contour. This form of reciprocation occurs most commonly when guide plates wrap to the lingual surface *(arrow)* or where lingual tooth surfaces have been prepared to receive plating.

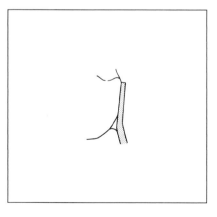

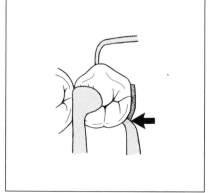

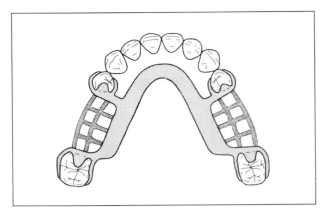

Fig. 6-11a Cast retentive arms are commonly used in tooth-supported RPDs.

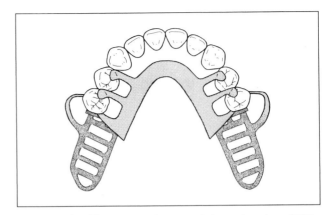

Fig. 6-11b They are also used in extension RPDs where the clasp tips disengage during functional movement.

Figs. 6-12a and b Wrought wire retentive arms *(WW)* are indicated where clasp tips lie in front of the axis of rotation *(AR)*.

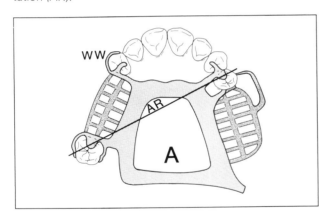

Fig. 6-12a Maxillary unilateral distal extension RPD.

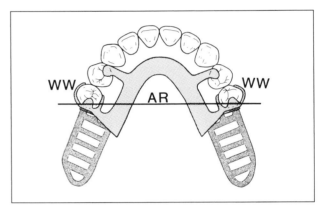

Fig. 6-12b Mandibular bilateral distal extension RPD.

height of contour. The division of these two actions depends on the flexibility of the clasp, the depth of the undercut utilized, and the stability of the abutment.

Clinically, true reciprocation is uncommon because few teeth have natural contours that will allow for proper timing. Maxillary molars are frequently tilted buccally and mandibular molars lingually. It is sometimes difficult to achieve adequate retention, much less reciprocation. Consequently, many rigid clasp assembly elements function for bracing only. This, however, is an important function and should not be minimized. In addition to distributing horizontal forces, effective bracing elements can provide resistance to clasp arms that have become nonpassive because of improper adjustment or accidental bending. They also prevent further movement of tilted abutments.

Mechanical retention

Most of the retention in an RPD is created by mechanical retainers or clasps. Clasps should provide only that amount of retention that is necessary to retain the RPD without placing undue stress on the abutments. The type of clasp used should be the

Figs. 6-13a and b Greater-than-180° encirclement prevents permanent tooth movement. In each case, the opening between the elements of the clasp assembly is smaller than the width of the tooth structure that could potentially move through the opening.

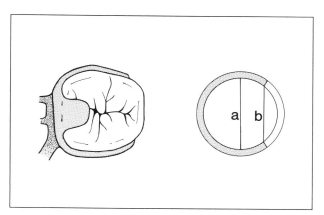

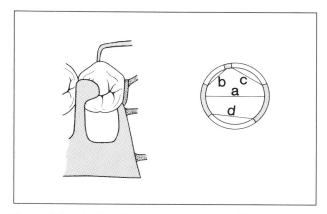

Fig. 6-13a In the circumferential clasp assembly, line *b* is shorter than line *a*.

Fig. 6-13b In the I-bar clasp assembly, lines *b, c,* and *d* are shorter than line *a.*

simplest that will provide the necessary retention. Factors important in the selection of a particular clasp design include *(1)* tooth contour (location of undercut), *(2)* tissue contour, *(3)* flexibility of the arm, *(4)* tooth coverage, *(5)* esthetic requirements, *(6)* the capacity for adjustment, maintenance, and replacement, and *(7)* the ability to provide stabilization (bracing). The amount of retention provided depends on the angle of convergence of the retentive tip and the tooth, the depth of undercut used, and the flexibility of the retentive arm.

Clasp retention is based on the resistance of metal to deformation and is therefore proportional to the flexibility of the arm. Retentive arm flexibility is dependent on the shape, bulk, and stiffness of the metal. As the flexibility of the arm increases, the depth of undercut that can be used also increases. Conversely, a more rigid retentive arm can provide adequate retention by utilizing a relatively smaller undercut. A flexible arm in a minimal undercut may not provide adequate retention, and a rigid arm in an excessive undercut may result in abutment tooth movement and/or permanent deformation of the arm. There must be a harmonious balance between the flexibility of the arm, the retention required, the available undercut, and the health of the abutment. To ensure proper flexibility, a retentive arm should exhibit uniformly tapering thickness and width. Its thickness should be

approximately one half as great at the tip as at the origin.

Retentive arms may be cast metal or wrought wire. Cast metal arms have a crystalline structure and tend to be more rigid. The retentive tips of cast arms are usually placed in 0.01-in. undercuts. A 0.02-in. undercut may be used if the arm is long and slender, if true reciprocation exists, and if the arm releases during function. Wrought wire arms, by virtue of their round shape and fibrous internal structure, exhibit greater overall flexibility and are capable of flexing in any spatial plane. The tips of wrought wire arms are most commonly placed in 0.02-in. recesses. However, smaller-diameter wire may be placed into a 0.03-in. undercut, while larger arms will usually create adequate retention if located in 0.01-in. recesses. If the tip of the arm does not release during functional movement of the prosthesis, the use of a smaller-diameter wire and a smaller undercut is recommended.

Cast retentive arms are usually selected when the RPD is tooth supported, when the retentive tip releases during functional movement, or when minimal undercut is being utilized (Figs. 6-11a and b). Wrought wire clasps are indicated for extension RPDs when the retentive tips of the clasps are placed forward of the axis of rotation (Figs. 6-12a and b). Here, the greater flexibility of the wrought wire will decrease the transmission of torquing forces to the abutment. Wrought wire clasps are also occasionally indicated for tooth-supported RPDs when utilization of a deeper undercut will decrease the amount of visible metal and thus improve the esthetic quality of the prosthesis.

Greater-than-180° encirclement

Encirclement of an abutment prevents permanent tooth movement. The RPD must contact tooth structure at at least three points (Figs. 6-13a and b). The contacts may be made by guide plates, minor connectors, reciprocating or bracing arms, and retentive tips. In addition, many authorities feel that a proximal contact between an abutment and an adjacent tooth will suffice as a component of encirclement.

It is important to remember that the action of retentive arms is potentially harmful. Therefore, it is best to reduce the dependence on mechanical retention by creating (1) good vertical support from rests, (2) true reciprocation whenever possible, (3) guide surface–guide plate contact ensuring a definite path of insertion/dislodgement, (4) rigid major and minor connectors and bracing elements, and (5) maximum extension of denture bases in areas supported by the residual ridge.

Importance of guide surfaces, guide plates, and the path of insertion/dislodgement

As noted previously, guide surfaces and guide plates have the potential to contribute directly to retention via frictional resistance. They also make an extremely important contribution to the effectiveness of mechanical retainers. The interaction of multiple guide surfaces and guide plates determines the path of insertion/dislodgement, and retentive recesses or undercuts exist only in relation to that path. If there is no distinct path of insertion/dislodgement, the quality of mechanical retention is unknown and may be nonexistent. If the clasp can escape the recess without flexing, no retention occurs.

Merely tilting the surveying table does not create retentive areas or retention. Rigid metal against parallel tooth surfaces must be present in the mouth. If mechanical retention is to occur, the

number and location of the guide surface–guide plate contacts must dictate a specific path of removal or the clasps must be located so that they will be activated under all random dislodging forces (Fig. 6-14) (also see chapter 3 and chapter 9).

The axis of rotation and retainer selection

In tooth-supported RPDs, all functional forces (those toward the basal seat) should be transferred to teeth by rests. A tooth-supported RPD does not exhibit functional motion and, therefore, has no axis of rotation. From a mechanical standpoint, any available undercut may be utilized and any clasp selected. The choice of retainer depends on the location of the available undercut, the ability to provide adequate reciprocation and/or bracing, the ability to minimize disruption of normal tooth and tissue contours, and esthetic requirements.

Location of undercut, reciprocation and bracing, hygiene, and esthetics are also important in selecting retainers for extension RPDs. In addition, one must carefully consider the action or movement of the retentive arms as the extension base moves toward the tissue.

When a functional force is exerted on a distal extension base, the base moves toward the tissue and the prosthesis rotates around a line (axis of rotation) that connects the most posterior point on each side of the arch where rigid metal rests on tooth structure (Figs. 6-15a and b). Portions of the RPD anterior or forward of the axis of rotation will move in an occlusal direction. The tissueward movement of the denture base and upward movement of the anterior portion of the RPD cannot be and should not be prevented by mechanical retainers. Attempts to do so will result in the transfer of torquing forces to the abutment (Fig. 6-16). Ideally, the retentive tips of the clasps should either remain in passive contact with the abutment or should disengage from the tooth and move into a deeper undercut (Fig. 6-17). If retentive tips of clasps must be placed forward of the axis of rotation, the design of the clasp should provide for a marked increase in flexibility. Wrought wire clasps are usually indicated (see Figs. 6-12a and b). The gauge of wrought wire selected depends on (1) the relationship of the clasp to the axis of rotation, (2)

Fig. 6-14 In extension RPDs, there are insufficient guide surface–guide plate contacts to ensure a distinct path of insertion/dislodgement. The tip of the I-bar retainer on the canine must be placed forward of the greatest mesiodistal curvature of the facial surface (and in the prescribed undercut) so that the arm must flex to escape the recess. If the tip of the clasp is placed behind the greatest mesiodistal curvature, a random dislodging force could possibly move the assembly very slightly distally and the clasp could escape the undercut without flexing. If a guide surface–guide plate relationship could be established on the mesial surface of the canine, it would be possible to place the retentive tip at the greatest mesiodistal curvature.

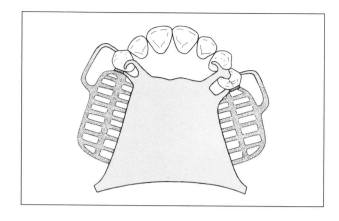

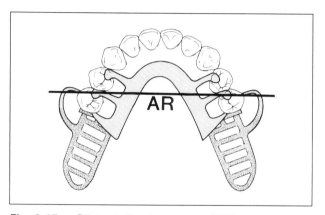

Fig. 6-15a Bilateral distal extension RPD.

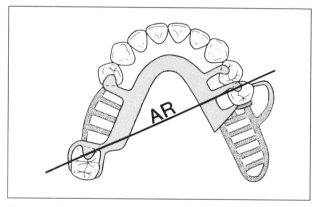

Fig. 6-15b Unilateral distal extension RPD. The axis of rotation (AR) passes through the most posterior points where rigid metal contacts tooth structure above the height of contour.

the periodontal status of the abutment, (3) the amount of undercut engaged, and (4) the support offered by the residual ridges in the extension areas. Since it is so difficult to accurately estimate the flexibility of clasps and the capacity for abutments to withstand stress, it is far safer if the retentive arm disengages during functional movement of the extension base.

Indirect retention and indirect retainers

An indirect retainer is defined as a part of an RPD that assists the direct retainers (clasps) in prevent-

ing dislodgement of distal extension denture bases by functioning through lever action on the opposite side of the fulcrum line.

Indirect retainers are rests that are located anterior to the retentive arms on distal extension RPDs (Figs. 6-18a and b). Indirect retainers function when dislodging forces attempt to move the denture away from the basal seat tissues. By preventing downward movement of the anterior portion of the RPD, the indirect retainers force the direct retainers to activate when movement away from the basal seat is attempted by the extension base (Fig. 6-19). The more anterior the location of the indirect retainer, the greater the efficiency and retention of the direct retainer. Anterior placement of the rests increases the length of the segment of the lever

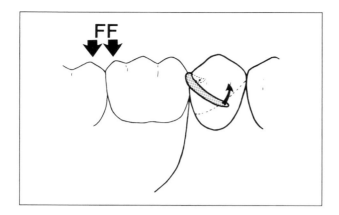

Fig. 6-16 On distal extension RPDs, a clasp tip placed in an undercut forward of the axis of rotation has the potential for torquing the abutment when functional forces *(FF)* are applied to the extension base.

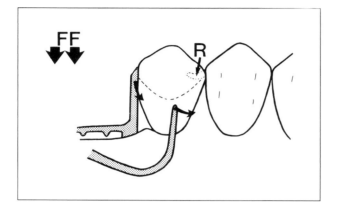

Fig. 6-17 When an I-bar clasp assembly functions properly, the retentive tip moves downward and forward into a deeper undercut (releasing from the abutment) when functional forces *(FF)* are applied to the extension base. Note that the distal guide plate also moves slightly downward and forward. At the time of the framework try-in, the gingival aspect of the guide plate must be physiologically relieved to eliminate binding of the metal against the abutment. Otherwise, the guide plate will preempt the action of the planned rest *(R)* and the retentive tip will move upward, engaging the abutment.

arm between the resistance (clasp) and the fulcrum (indirect retainer) (Fig. 6-20). In addition to their primary function, indirect retainers act as vertical stops for the anterior portion of the RPD, thus preventing food from forcing the major connector onto the underlying soft tissues.

Although the benefit from an indirect retainer increases as the location is moved forward, the periodontal support and morphology of the teeth and the occlusal or incisal clearance must also be considered. For mandibular distal extension RPDs, indirect retainers are usually placed in the mesio-occlusal fossa of first premolars or the cingula or incisal edges of canines. On maxillary distal extension RPDs, occlusal clearance is often a problem, and esthetic considerations usually contraindicate incisal rests. Consequently, indirect retainers are

most commonly placed on the cingula of the canines or the mesio-occlusal fossa of the first premolars when the occlusion permits. Although anterior linguoplating may produce indirect retention, it should never be used for that purpose unless the plating is accompanied by adequate rest seats and rests at least on the canines.

Suprabulge mechanical retainers

Suprabulge mechanical retainers originate from a point at or above the height of contour—usually from a rest, minor connector, or guide plate—and angle downward across the clinical crown where the tip is located in a prescribed undercut.

Figs. 6-18a and b Indirect retainers *(arrows)* are rests located anterior to the retentive tips on distal extension RPDs.

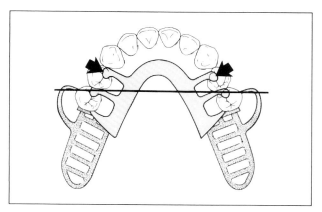

Fig. 6-18a Bilateral distal extension RPD.

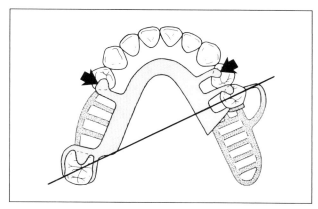

Fig. 6-18b Unilateral distal extension RPD. The left indirect retainer is more effective than the right because it lies farther anterior to a line connecting the tips of the two retentive arms.

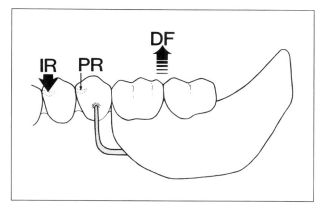

Fig. 6-19 An indirect retainer *(IR)* prevents downward movement of the anterior portion of the RPD and enhances the effectiveness of the direct retainer in resisting upward dislodging forces *(DF)* on the extension base. Because the primary rest *(PR)* is forward of the retentive tip, it also acts somewhat as an indirect retainer. However, it is so close to the tip that its benefit is very limited.

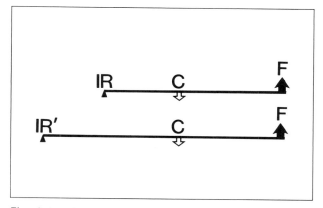

Fig. 6-20 Diagrammatic representation of a dislodging force *(F)*, a clasp *(C)*, and an indirect retainer *(IR)*. If the indirect retainer is moved forward to *IR'*, the effectiveness of the clasp is improved because $IR'-C$ / $C-F$ $> IR-C$ / $C-F$.

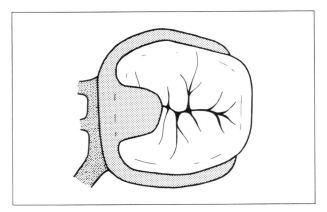

Fig. 6-21 A circumferential clasp assembly. Either arm may be retentive, but the other must be reciprocating/bracing.

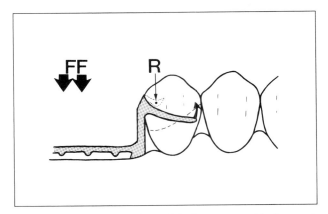

Fig. 6-22 If a circumferential clasp assembly is used, functional forces *(FF)* applied over an extension base will cause the prosthesis to rotate around the rest *(R)*. The tip of the retentive arm will move upward and apply torquing forces to the abutment.

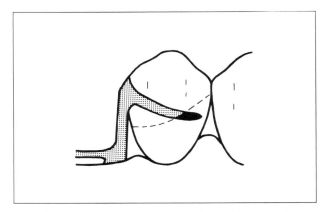

Fig. 6-23 Bending of a circumferential clasp to increase retention must be limited to the terminal portion of the arm. Inward bending of the portion of the arm above the height of contour *(dotted survey line)* will prevent seating.

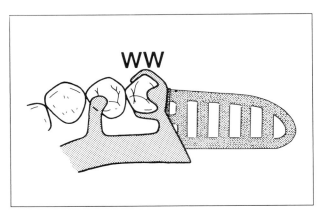

Fig. 6-24 A combination clasp assembly for a mandibular distal extension RPD. The buccal retentive arm is wrought wire *(WW)*, and the lingual reciprocating/bracing arm is cast.

Circumferential clasp

A circumferential clasp (Fig. 6-21) is a suprabulge clasp in which both the buccal and lingual arms originate from a common source. The undercut engaged is on the opposite side of the tooth (mesiodistal) from the point of origin. Usually, one arm is retentive and the other is reciprocating/bracing. If both arms are retentive, both must be flexible, and some reciprocation/bracing is lost. Cast circumferential clasps are ideally suited for tooth-sup-

ported RPDs because of the potential for excellent retention and reciprocation/bracing. They are not usually indicated for extension RPDs because the retentive tip lies forward of the axis of rotation and has the potential for applying torquing forces to the abutment (Fig. 6-22).

Disadvantages of the circumferential clasp include the amount of tooth structure covered, the display of metal, and the disruption of normal food deflection patterns necessary for stimulation of the gingivae. A cast circumferential clasp is also difficult to adjust. The half-round form prevents edge-wise adjustment. In addition, bending the clasp to increase retention must be accomplished *exactly* at the correct location (Fig. 6-23). Any bending of the arm prior to the point where the arm crosses the height of contour will prevent seating of the clasp assembly because the originating portion of the arm lies above the survey line.

A combination clasp (Fig. 6-24) is a circumferential clasp assembly composed of a wrought wire retentive arm and a cast reciprocating/bracing arm. The combination clasp is most commonly used for extension RPDs when *(1)* a tissue undercut below the terminal abutment precludes the use of a bar clasp (Fig. 6-25a), *(2)* the mesial tilt of the terminal abutment would cause the guide plate to preempt the mesial rest in an I-bar clasp assembly (Fig. 6-25b), or *(3)* a retainer is placed on a tooth that lies in front of the axis of rotation (e.g., in a Class II RPD with a modification space) (Fig. 6-25c).

Wrought wire arms may occasionally be se-lected for esthetic reasons. Their increased flexibility allows the clasp tips to be placed in deeper undercuts and closer to the gingivae. Wrought wire arms also allow for greater adjustability. Because of their round form, they can be adjusted in any spatial plane (Fig. 6-26). Because of their fibrous structure, considerably more adjustment is possible before failure (breakage) occurs. Wrought wire arms do have the disadvantages of requiring an additional laboratory procedure and increasing the potential for permanent deformation by the patient.

The rest–proximal plate–Akers (RPA) clasp assembly represents a hybrid of rest–proximal plate–I-bar (RPI) clasp and conventional circumferential clasp assemblies (Fig. 6-27a). It consists of a mesial rest, a proximal plate, and a circumferential retentive arm originating from the proximal plate. The retentive arm may be either cast or wrought wire. The RPA clasp has been recommended for extension RPDs when the tissue undercut below the abutment contraindicates the use of a bar clasp. However, very specific circumstances must exist if the retainer is to disengage during function. The contour of the abutment must be such that the occlusal border of the originating portion of the arm will lie exactly on the survey line (Fig. 6-27b). The portion of the tooth below the survey line (except at the tip) must be blocked out. The rigid portion of the arm must not lie above the survey line

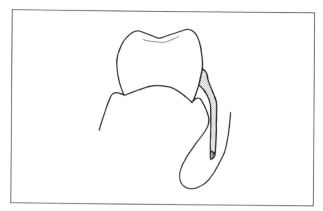

Fig. 6-25a A combination clasp is most commonly used for distal extension RPDs when a tissue undercut below the abutment precludes the use of a bar clasp.

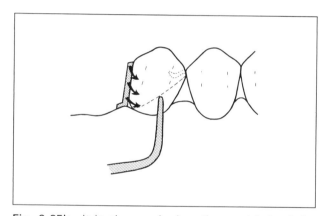

Fig. 6-25b It is also used when the mesial tilt of the abutment tooth would cause the guide plate to preempt the mesial rest in an I-bar clasp assembly.

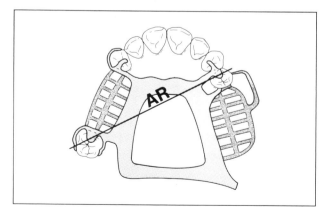

Fig. 6-25c And it is used when the retainer is located on a tooth that lies bodily in front of the axis of rotation *(AR)*.

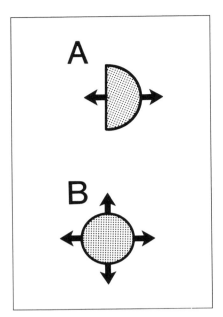

Fig. 6-26 *(left)* A half-round cast clasp *(A)* can only be adjusted buccolingually. Edgewise adjustment is difficult if not impossible. Wrought wire arms *(B)* can be adjusted in any spatial plane.

Fig. 6-27a *(below)* Occlusal view of an RPA clasp assembly.

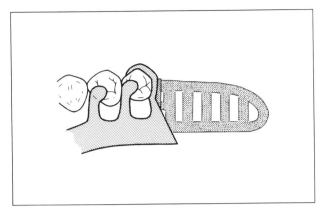

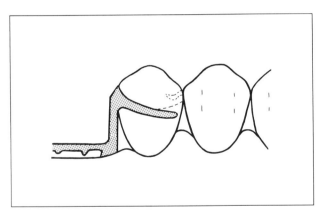

Fig. 6-27b The originating portion of the arm must lie exactly on the survey line.

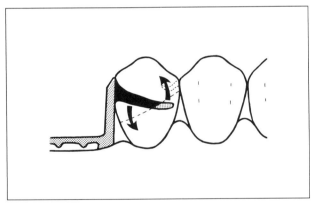

Fig. 6-27c If it does not, it will preempt the mesial rest.

or it will act as a rest on an inclined plane, preempt the planned mesial rest, and cause the retentive tip to lie forward of the axis of rotation (Fig. 6-27c). In such a case, the clasp tip no longer releases during function and has the potential for applying torquing forces to the abutment. The RPA clasp should also be avoided when the terminal abutment inclines mesially. During function, the distal guide plate would bind against the terminal abutment and preempt the mesial rest. Relieving the guide plate would create a space between the plate and the abutment. If the terminal abutment has a mesial inclination or if the rigid portion of the RPA assembly cannot be placed exactly at the survey line, it would be preferable to select a combination clasp assembly composed of a distal rest (to create a definite vertical stop), a cast lingual arm (to provide for bracing/reciprocation), and a wrought wire retentive arm (to provide flexibility and stress relief to the abutment).

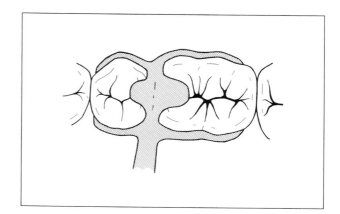

Fig. 6-28 A typical embrasure clasp assembly.

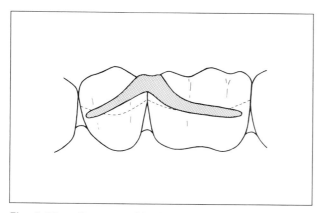

Fig. 6-29a Because of hygiene problems with the configuration in Fig. 6-29b, circumferential retentive arms are almost always preferred.

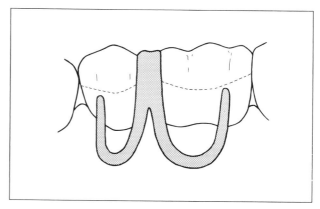

Fig. 6-29b Double I-bars used as retentive arms for an embrasure clasp.

Embrasure clasp

An embrasure clasp (Fig. 6-28) is used when no edentulous space exists at the clasp assembly site. It approaches the retentive area by passing through an embrasure.

The retentive arms of embrasure clasps are almost always of the suprabulge type (Fig. 6-29a). Although double or single infrabulge clasps (Fig. 6-29b) have been used, they tend to create food repositories and are therefore not the retainers of choice. Except in rare cases, embrasure clasps are cast. The limited space available across the occlusal surface is seldom adequate for the passage of wrought wire clasps.

Embrasure clasps may be used in Class II, III, or IV RPDs. In a Class II RPD, the anterior reten-

tive arm lies forward of the axis of rotation and should be omitted, should engage a minimal undercut, or should be located entirely above the survey line so that it functions only for bracing (Fig. 6-30).

There are several potential problems when embrasure clasps are used. The most common is breakage (Fig. 6-31), and the cause is usually inadequate occlusal clearance and concomitant lack of metal thickness. The problem can be avoided by adequate rest seat preparation *and* by careful preparation where the clasp assembly enters and exits the rest area (Fig. 6-32). Wedging of the abutments can also occur if rest seat preparations are omitted or inadequate. The rest seat preparations must be deeper toward the center of the occlusal surface than at the marginal ridges (Fig. 6-33).

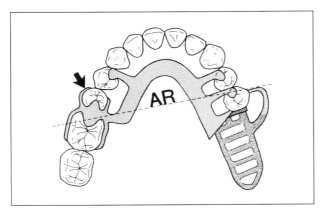

Fig. 6-30 In this Class II RPD, the anterior retentive arm of the embrasure clasp (arrow) lies in front of the axis of rotation (AR) and should be omitted, should engage a minimal undercut, or should be located entirely above the survey line.

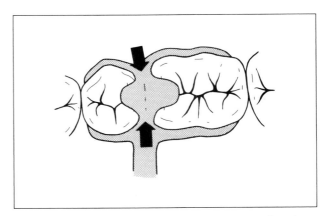

Fig. 6-31 The embrasure clasp is prone to breakage where the buccal and lingual clasp arms join the rest area (arrows).

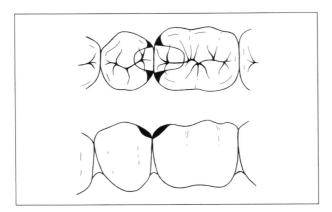

Fig. 6-32 The incidence of breakage is greatly reduced if buccal and lingual access preparations (shaded) are added to the normal rest seat preparations.

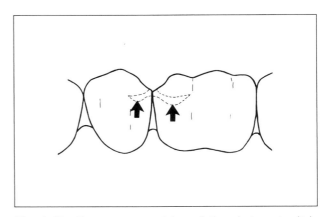

Fig. 6-33 To prevent wedging of the abutments, it is essential that rest preparations for embrasure clasps be deeper at the center (arrows) than at the marginal ridges.

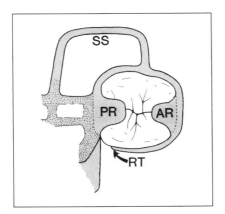

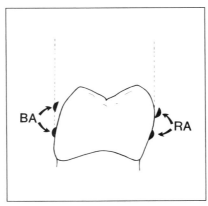

Fig. 6-34 (left) A ring clasp on a mesiolingually tilted mandibular right molar. Primary rest (PR); auxiliary rest (AR); support strut (SS); retentive tip (RT).

Fig. 6-35 (right) True reciprocation in a ring clasp is rare because the buccal arm (BA) does not contact the tooth as the retentive arm (RA) passes over the height of contour.

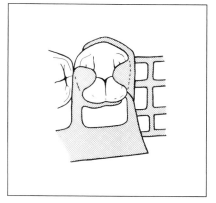 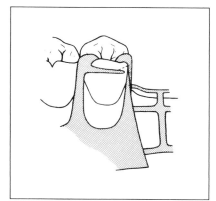 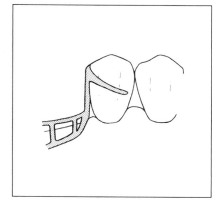

Fig. 6-36a Occlusal view of a half-and-half clasp on a mandibular right second premolar.

Fig. 6-36b Lingual view.

Fig. 6-36c Facial view.

Ring clasp

A ring clasp arises from the junction of the guide plate and rest, encircles the entire abutment, and engages an undercut near the point of origin but on the opposite side of the tooth (Fig. 6-34). A ring clasp is most commonly used to engage a mesiolingual undercut on a tilted mandibular molar. It may also be used on a buccally tilted maxillary molar. It is seldom, if ever, the retainer of choice for premolars or anterior teeth.

The clasp assembly for a ring-type retainer should incorporate a support strut and an auxiliary distal rest. The rest assists in preventing further tipping of the abutment. The rest and strut combine to ensure rigidity for reciprocation and/or bracing. The improved rigidity also decreases the potential for accidental deformation of the retentive arm.

Although the originating portion of a ring clasp may provide bracing, it rarely produces true reciprocation because of the tilt of the abutment. The originating portion of the clasp does not contact the tooth as the retentive tip passes over the height of contour (Fig. 6-35).

The ring clasp covers considerable tooth structure and is, therefore, a poor retainer in a caries-prone individual. It has been suggested that abutments that are to receive ring clasps be crowned to reduce caries susceptibility. However, if the tooth is to receive a crown, it would be more logical to create a distobuccal or distolingual undercut appropriate for a simple circumferential clasp.

Half-and-half clasp

The half-and-half clasp (Figs. 6-36a to c) consists of a cast buccal circumferential clasp arm originating from the guide plate and a cast lingual circumferential arm originating from the minor connector. The half-and-half clasp is primarily indicated for lingually inclined premolars. The buccal arm provides for bracing only (true reciprocation is impossible because of the lingual tilt of the abutment). The lingual arm utilizes an undercut adjacent to the edentulous space for retention.

In tooth-supported RPDs, no functional motion occurs, and rests for half-and-half clasps may be located in the mesial fossa, distal fossa, or both.

When a half-and-half clasp is selected for a distal extension RPD, a distal rest should be used. A mesial rest is usually used in conjunction with the distal rest unless it interferes with the opposing occlusion. If the mesial rest is omitted, a mesial rest on the first premolar or a cingulum or incisal rest on the canine must be included to provide indirect retention (Fig. 6-37). Because the retentive tip of the lingual arm lies very close to the axis of rotation (which passes through the distal rest), only slight movement of the tip occurs during functional movement, and torquing forces on the abutment are minimal (Figs. 6-38a and b). Nonretentive portions of the lingual arm and the buccal bracing arm will move occlusally, away from the abutment. If the distal rest is omitted, the rigid portion of the bracing arm will preempt the remaining mesial rest and will act as a rest on an inclined surface.

61

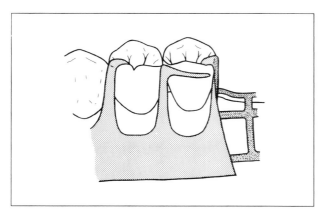

Fig. 6-37 If the opposing occlusion interferes with placement of a rest in the mesial fossa of the second premolar or distal fossa of the first premolar, indirect retention must be achieved by placing a rest in the mesial fossa of the first premolar or the lingual or incisal aspect of the canine.

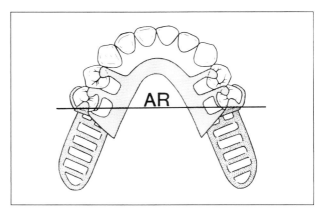

Fig. 6-38a In a distal extension RPD, the axis of rotation (AR) passes through the distal rests.

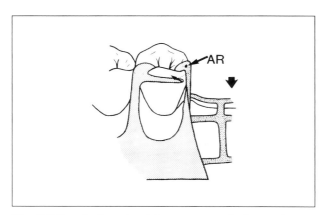

Fig. 6-38b As functional forces are applied over the endentulous area, the RPD rotates around the axis of rotation (AR) and the retentive tip of the lingual arm moves very slightly mesio-occlusally. The amount of movement is minimal because the tip is very close to the axis.

As previously stated, the half-and-half clasp is most commonly used on lingually tilted premolars where the lingual undercut is adjacent to the edentulous space. If a buccal undercut is present, a conventional circumferential or bar clasp is preferred. Obviously, if linguoplating is necessary, a half-and-half clasp cannot be utilized. A buccal undercut would have to be created by recontouring or crowning the abutment.

Reverse-action (hairpin) clasp

A reverse-action, or hairpin, clasp (Fig. 6-39) is a suprabulge retainer that engages an undercut next to the edentulous space (adjacent to the origin of the arm). It is most commonly utilized on mesially tilted mandibular molars where the tip of the clasp lies in a mesiobuccal undercut. Ideally, only the lower portion of the arm is flexible. A rigid lingual arm provides reciprocation/bracing. Because the reverse-action clasp covers extensive tooth structure, the abutment is prone to caries. The reverse-action clasp is generally considered a "last choice" retainer, even for mesially tilted molars. The preferred solution would be a modified T-bar clasp engaging a mesiobuccal undercut or an I-bar engaging a mesiolingual undercut.

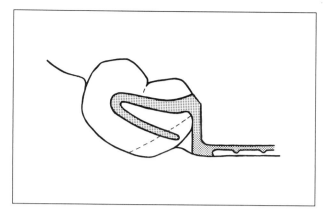

Fig. 6-39 A reverse-action clasp on a mandibular right molar abutment for a tooth-supported RPD.

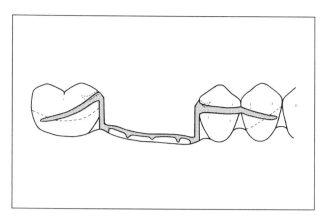

Fig. 6-40 An extended arm clasp used on a mandibular tooth-supported RPD.

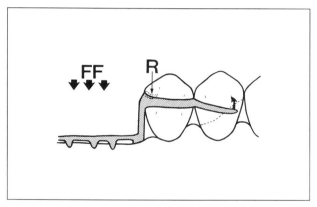

Fig. 6-41a An extended arm clasp should not be used for extension RPDs because functional forces (FF) will cause rotation around the rest (R) and upward movement of the clasp tip.

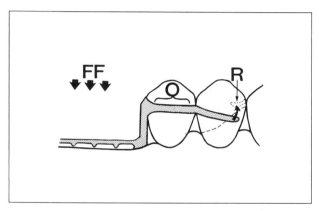

Fig. 6-41b Moving the rest (R) forward complicates the situation even more. Because the originating portion (O) of the arm lies above the height of contour, it will act as a rest on an inclined surface. The movement of the retentive tip is still upward.

Extended arm clasp

The extended arm clasp (Fig. 6-40) is a rarely used mechanical retainer. It is not appropriate for distal extension RPDs because the retentive tip lies forward of the axis of rotation (Fig. 6-41a). Even if the terminal rest is moved anteriorly, the originating portion of the clasp will be on an inclined surface above the survey line and thus preempt the planned rest (Fig. 6-41b).

An extended arm clasp is indicated only when (1) the RPD is tooth supported, (2) the tooth next to the edentulous space has no buccal undercut,

(3) the tooth next to the edentulous space has no usable lingual undercut (e.g., if linguoplating must be used), (4) the occlusion in the area of the embrasure will not permit passage of a clasp arm to an undercut on the second tooth from the edentulous space, and (5) the second tooth from the edentulous space has a buccal undercut available. Its use has been suggested where increased splinting and stabilization are desired. Undesirable aspects of the extended arm clasp include the amount of tooth structure covered by metal and the propensity for distortion or breakage of the arm.

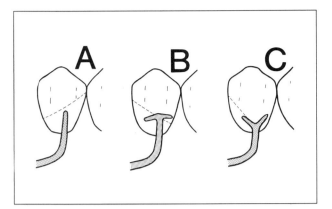

Fig. 6-42 Infrabulge retainers. I form *(A)*; T form *(B)*; Y form *(C)*.

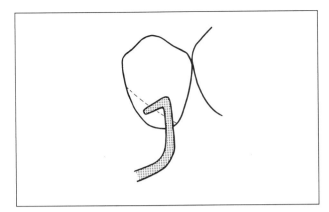

Fig. 6-43 Modified T form of infrabulge retainer.

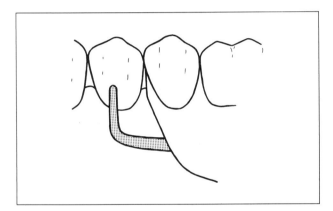

Fig. 6-44 Infrabulge retainer on a completed RPD. The horizontal portion of the bar is parallel to and approximately 3 mm below the gingival margin. The vertical portion of the arm crosses the gingival margin at a right angle.

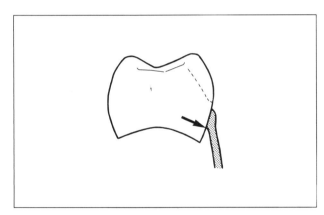

Fig. 6-45 The I-bar terminates in a "foot" that lies entirely below the height of contour. The gingival extent of the foot *(arrow)* contacts the tooth at the specified degree of undercut.

Infrabulge mechanical retainers

An infrabulge retainer (bar clasp) is a retainer that emanates from the denture base or denture base retentive network and approaches an available undercut from a gingival direction. The most common infrabulge retainers are the I, T, and Y forms (Fig. 6-42). The Y and T forms of infrabulge retainers usually have only one tip in an undercut. The second tip does not provide retention and produces only minimal bracing because the arm as a whole is not rigid. Because the second tip serves no particular function and unnecessarily covers tooth structure, it is often omitted, creating a modified T- or modified Y-bar clasp (Fig. 6-43).

Infrabulge retainers should exit the denture base, travel parallel to and 3 mm or more below the gingival margin, and turn occlusally to cross the margin at a right angle (Fig. 6-44). The foot of the tip (approximately the terminal 2 mm) rests in the specified undercut, usually in the gingival third of the tooth (Fig. 6-45). The approach arm must not impinge on the gingiva (30-gauge relief is recommended). The arm should exhibit uniform taper and may engage a 0.01-in. or 0.02-in. undercut, depending on the flexibility of the arm and the functional motion exhibited by the prosthesis.

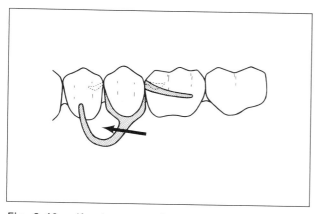

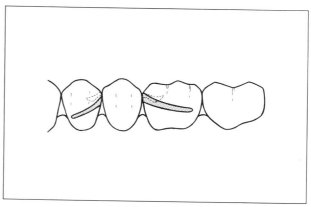

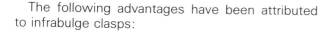

Fig. 6-46a   If only one tooth is missing in a tooth-supported segment, an infrabulge clasp tends to create an unhygienic area *(arrow)*.

Fig. 6-46b   A circumferential clasp is a better solution.

The following advantages have been attributed to infrabulge clasps:

1. Minimal tooth contact and minimal distortion of normal tooth contours, leading to improved tissue stimulation and oral hygiene and decreased caries and periodontal problems
2. Improved esthetics if the approach portion of the arm is not visible as it crosses the gingiva
3. Increased retention because of tripping action (except with the T form, which approaches the undercut from above or from the side)
4. Decreased torquing forces applied to terminal abutments in extension RPDs
5. Improved adjustability because the location of the bend is less critical than for circumferential clasps

Possible disadvantages of infrabulge clasps include the following:

1. They cannot be used in the presence of soft tissue undercuts, a shallow vestibule, or high frenal attachments.
2. Bracing action provided by bar clasps is considerably less than that provided by cast circumferential clasps.
3. The bar clasp will not totally disengage in certain distal extension cases (where the undercut is located on the distofacial surface of the terminal abutment.
4. Appearance may be adversely affected if the

smile line is high enough to expose the approach arm as it crosses the gingiva.
5. They may not be retentive unless rigid elements determine a specific path of insertion/dislodgement.

Infrabulge retainers for tooth-supported RPDs

In theory, infrabulge retainers may be used to engage a facial undercut on any abutment bordering a tooth-supported area. However, if only one tooth is missing, the descending and ascending portions of the arm lie so close together that food repositories are created and oral hygiene suffers (Fig. 6-46a). In addition, the increased curvature of the arm reduces flexibility somewhat. When possible, circumferential clasps are preferred in such cases (Fig. 6-46b). When two or more teeth are missing, the span is usually wide enough to permit the use of infrabulge clasps without compromising oral hygiene (Fig. 6-47).

A facial bar clasp is accompanied by a lingual reciprocating or bracing arm if the rest is placed next to the edentulous space (Fig. 6-48a). However, if the rest is placed on the portion of the occlusal surface away from the edentulous space, the combination of the guide plate and minor connector will provide the necessary reciprocation/bracing, and no lingual arm will be necessary (Fig. 6-48b).

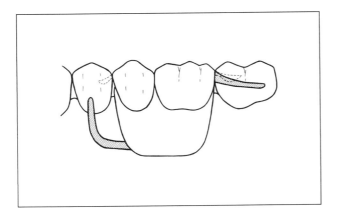

Fig. 6-47 If two or more teeth are missing, the food collection problem associated with an infrabulge clasp improves somewhat because there is no descending portion to the I-bar. However, a circumferential clasp is still the preferred retainer unless the undercut is located at the center of the facial surface or adjacent to the edentulous area.

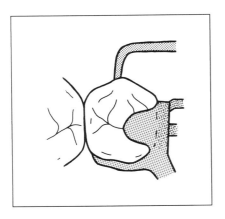 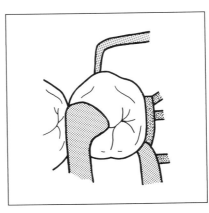

Fig. 6-48a *(left)* If the rest for a bar clasp is located next to the edentulous space, as is usually the case for tooth-supported segments, a lingual reciprocating/bracing arm is used.

Fig. 6-48b *(right)* If the rest is placed away from the edentulous space, the guide plate is extended slightly to the lingual surface so that it will combine with the mesial minor connector to provide reciprocation/bracing.

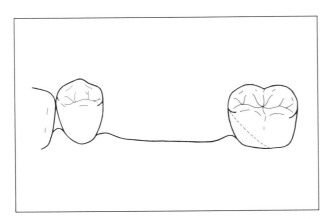

Fig. 6-49a Mandibular partially edentulous segment in which the only retentive recess on the molar abutment is located at the mesiolingual aspect.

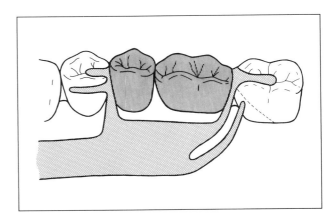

Fig. 6-49b RPD with lingual I-bar retainer.

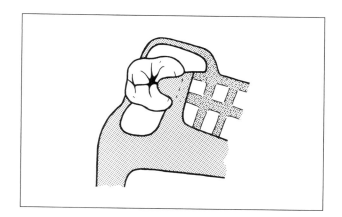

Fig. 6-50 RII clasp assembly on a maxillary molar abutment for a tooth-supported segment.

Tilted molars, particularly mandibular molars, present a difficult clasping problem. Frequently, the only undercut available is located on the mesiolingual aspect (Fig. 6-49a). Although a ring clasp can be used, it covers considerable tooth structure in an area prone to plaque accumulation. Another possible solution is the utilization of a mesiolingual I-bar emanating from the inferior distal border of the major connector (Fig. 6-49b). Because any stress created by the I-bar is opposed by the natural mesiolingual drift of the abutment, a buccal arm may not be necessary. However, if additional bracing is desired, a buccal arm should be included. Because of the tilt of the abutment, it is impossible for the buccal arm to provide true reciprocation.

The RII clasp assembly (Fig. 6-50) consists of a rest, a lingual I-bar (usually rigid), and a buccal I-bar (usually flexible and retentive). The assembly is most commonly used on molar abutments of maxillary tooth-supported segments. The lingual I-bar is located at the distolingual line angle and provides for bracing. The buccal retentive I-bar is usually located at the distal portion of the facial surface. The RII assembly is purported to be more hygienic than the more conventional circumferential clasp assembly.

Infrabulge retainers for distal extension RPDs

One of the major attributes of infrabulge clasps (particularly I-bars) is their potential for disengaging during functional movements of extension RPDs. For the I-bar system to function ideally, the axis of rotation must pass through a mesially located rest, and the tip of the I-bar must be placed in an undercut located at or in front of the greatest mesiodistal curvature of the facial surface of the abutment but behind the axis of rotation (Fig. 6-51). No rigid metal distal to the mesial rest may lie above the survey line or it will preempt the planned mesial rest. The guide plate cannot be allowed to bind against the guide surface. During functional movement, rotation *must* occur around the mesial rest if the clasp tip is to disengage.

The mechanics related to the use of bar clasps for terminal abutments when the only available undercut is on the distobuccal surface are considerably more complicated. A distal rest, circumferential lingual bracing arm, and modified T-bar (Fig. 6-52) or a mesial rest, distal guide plate, and modified T-bar (Fig. 6-53) may be used. Both designs represent a compromise because in each instance, the retentive tip moves toward the buccal bulge of the abutment and does not totally disengage during functional movement of the extension base. However, the design with the mesial rest seems to be preferable since the retentive tip moves downward and forward rather than upward and forward.

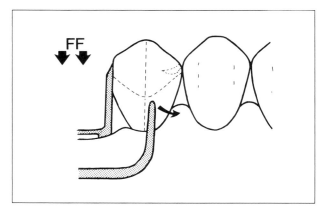

Fig. 6-51 For the I-bar to release *(arrow)* when functional forces *(FF)* are applied, the retentive tip must be placed at or in front of the greatest mesiodistal curvature of the facial surface but behind the rotational axis that passes through the rest. In addition, the guide plate must not bind against the distal surface of the abutment.

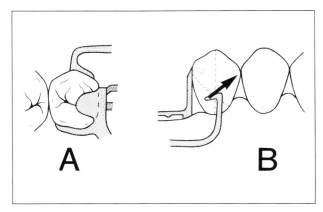

Fig. 6-52 Distal rest and modified T-bar clasp on a terminal abutment for a mandibular distal extension RPD *(A)*. During function, the retentive tip moves occlusally and mesially *(B)*.

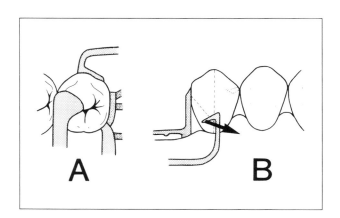

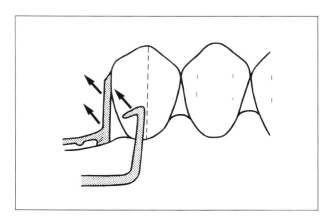

Fig. 6-53 Mesial rest and modified T-bar clasp on a terminal abutment for a mandibular distal extension RPD *(A)*. During function, the retentive tip moves gingivally and mesially *(B)*.

Fig. 6-54 On distal extension RPDs, the approach arm of a modified T-bar clasp must lie mesial to the greatest mesiodistal curvature unless a guide surface–guide plate relationship can be established for the mesial minor connector. If the approach arm is positioned behind the mesiodistal height of contour, the retentive tip may be able to escape the undercut by moving upward and backward. Such movement is possible because the guide surface–guide plate contact does not establish a precise path of insertion/dislodgement.

Whenever an infrabulge clasp is used to engage a distobuccal undercut, the approach arm must lie in front of the greatest mesiodistal curvature (Fig. 6-54). If it does not, there is the possibility that the retentive tip could escape the undercut by moving occlusally and distally, because the distal guide plates do not dictate a specific path of dislodgement. Under such circumstances, no retention would occur.

A small guide surface may be prepared on the mesiolingual surface of the terminal abutment so that it will contact the minor connector leading to the mesial rest. If precisely done, it may limit distal movement, and the I-bar may be placed at the greatest mesiodistal curvature of the facial surface. However, if laboratory procedures are not done accurately, the restriction on disto-occlusal movement may be lost and retention may be nonexistent.

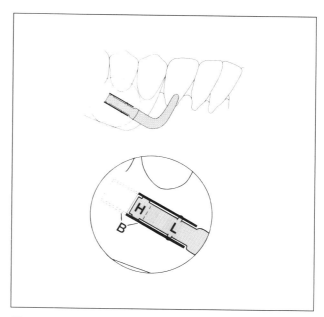

Fig. 6-55 An Oddo hinge in combination with an I-bar on a mandibular canine. Hinge *(H)*; latch *(L)*; retentive box or housing *(B)*.

Specialized retainers

Oddo hinge clasp

The Oddo hinge clasp modification (Fig. 6-55) is primarily indicated when anterior abutments have more than average labial inclination and, thus, a height of contour very near the incisal edge. The hinge is opened, the prosthesis seated, and the hinge closed. The tip of the bar clasp can be located in a much greater undercut than normal. The retentive tip is located in the gingival third of the tooth, and the body of the arm is hidden in the labial vestibule. Relatively simple adjustments in the housing will compensate for minor wear. The entire assembly can be replaced without remaking the RPD.

Rigid metal retention

A rigid metal portion of a partial denture framework may be used to provide retention in certain situations. During insertion, a segment of rigid metal is first placed into an undercut. Then the framework is rotated to place and secured by direct re-

tainers. This form of retention is usually restricted to tooth-supported partial dentures. *Rotational path of insertion* and *dual path of insertion* are terms often used to describe frameworks that employ rigid metal retention. Rigid metal retention can be used to eliminate selected clasps and to utilize undercuts on the mesio- and distoproximal surfaces of abutments.

Types

The three basic types of rotational paths that can be used with rigid metal retainers are anterior to posterior, posterior to anterior, and lateral. Jacobson and Krol (1982) reduced these situations to two functional categories associated with placement of the prosthesis. Category I describes all prostheses in which the rest associated with the rigid metal retainer seats first, and the remainder of the framework rotates to place with the rest acting as a pivot point.

Category I includes all tooth-supported partial dentures replacing bilaterally missing posterior

Figs. 6-56a and b Rigid metal used to engage undercuts on tilted mandibular molars. The path of insertion is posterior to anterior, with the points of rotation being the most distal aspects of the posterior rests.

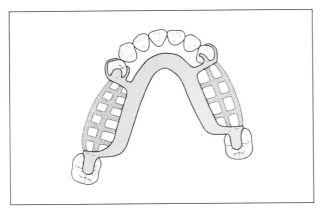

Fig. 6-56a   Occlusal view.

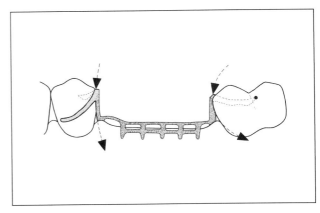

Fig. 6-56b   Buccal view.

Figs. 6-57a and b Rigid metal retention used to engage distal undercuts on maxillary canines. The path of insertion is anterior to posterior, and the rotation points are at the mesial aspects of the anterior rests. Because the arc of the rigid metal traverses the body of the canine, it might seem that the path described would be an impossiblity. However, since the guide plate (and rigid metal retention) is located on the mesiolingual surface, the facial portion of the tooth does not prevent insertion. In addition, a small amount of linear posterior to anterior movement assists in positioning the rigid metal into the undercut.

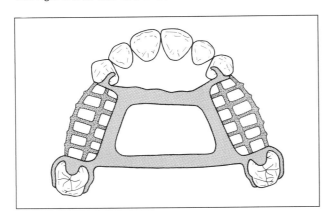

Fig. 6-57a   Occlusal view.

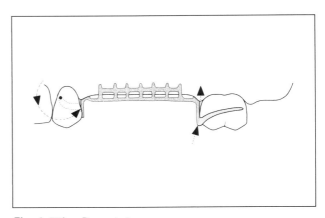

Fig. 6-57b   Buccal view.

teeth. Rigid metal may be placed in mesial undercuts of mesially inclined molars or distal undercuts of anterior teeth or premolars. In the first case (Figs. 6-56a and b), the path of insertion is posterior to anterior, with points of rotation around the most distal portions of the posterior occlusal rests. The anterior segment of the framework is retained by conventional direct retainers. In the second

case (Figs. 6-57a and b), the partial denture seats anterior to posterior, with rotation points at the most mesial portions of the anterior rests. Category I partial dentures have a single axis of rotation through the rest during insertion and are often called *rotational path partial dentures.*

Category II (Figs. 6-58a and b) describes prostheses in which rigid metal slides straight into the un-

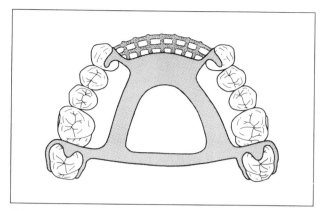

Fig. 6-58a In the maxillary Class IV partial denture shown, rigid metal is used to provide retention on the mesiolingual aspects of the canines.

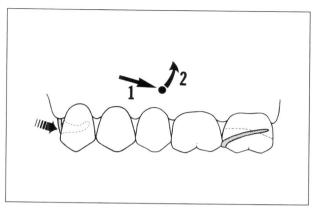

Fig. 6-58b The initial path of insertion is nearly parallel to the occlusal plane *(1)*. When the rigid metal contacts the canines, the posterior portion of the prosthesis is rotated to place *(2)*.

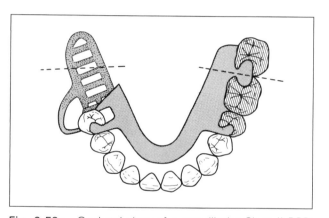

Fig. 6-59a Occlusal view of a mandibular Class II RPD utilizing a Hart-Dunn attachment between the first molar pontic and the second molar abutment.

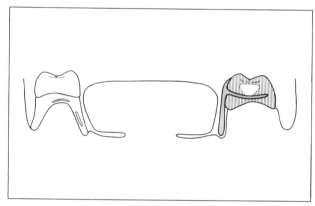

Fig. 6-59b Cross section of the completed RPD at the level of the retentive arm.

dercuts; then the remainder of the framework is rotated to place. Partial dentures in this category usually replace three or more adjacent anterior teeth. The seating of this type of framework requires two distinct paths of movement. First is the straight path of movement of the rigid metal retainers into the mesial undercuts of the anterior teeth. Second is the rotational movement during the final seating of the framework. Rotation occurs at the contact point between the rigid metal and the mesial undercuts of the anterior teeth. These partial dentures seat anterior to posterior. The term *dual*

path may be used to describe the two distinct movements.

Category II also includes tooth-supported partial dentures that utilize a lateral path of insertion. The mechanics of lateral path partial dentures are identical to those of anterior-posterior path partial dentures replacing anterior teeth.

The Hart-Dunn attachment (Mann, 1958) may be used on unilateral distal extension partial dentures in which the dentulous side has been restored with a fixed partial denture (Figs. 6-59a and b). A wrought wire arm is placed under the pontic

71

for retention; then the extension side is rotated to place and retained by a conventional clasp system. The Hart-Dunn attachment is helpful in avoiding problems associated with tight interdigitation of the teeth on the dentulous side of the arch since it avoids crossing the occlusal surface with the originating portion of a clasp assembly. Also, the wrought wire clasp is able to rotate under the fixed partial denture so that torquing forces to the abutments are minimized.

Sectional partial dentures may also utilize rigid metal retention. The prosthesis is fabricated in two distinct parts. Each section has an independent straight path of insertion that allows placement of rigid metal in opposing undercuts. The sections are then joined by a pin, latch, or magnet to prevent separation.

Clinical application

Several clinical situations favor a partial denture design using rigid metal retention. The first is a patient with a high lip line in whom anterior clasps will create an undesirable display of metal. Such conditions may exist in maxillary partial dentures replacing three or more anterior teeth. These partial dentures use an anterior-posterior path of insertion. Success depends on adequate undercuts on the mesial surfaces of the anterior abutments. Esthetic considerations may also be important in maxillary tooth-supported dentures replacing posterior teeth if the canines or first premolars are anterior abutments. Here, the path of insertion is still anterior-posterior, but the crucial undercut is on the distal aspect of the anterior abutment.

Another situation occurs in tooth-supported partial dentures replacing posterior teeth in which the only available undercuts on the posterior abutments are located on the mesial surfaces of mesially tilted molars. It is difficult to design adequate conventional clasp assemblies for these teeth. Recesses for clasp tips may be inaccessible, or clasp assemblies may be bulky and unhygienic. The use of rigid metal retention will circumvent both problems. A posterior-anterior path of insertion is used, and conventional clasps are placed on the anterior abutments.

Clinically, the difference between Class I (rotational path) and Class II (dual path) partial dentures is not very distinct. It appears likely that in both, insertion and removal are characterized by a combination of the movements described for each. The division of the two types of movement, straight and rotational, varies slightly according to the contour and position of the abutment teeth, the anatomy of the residual ridges, and supporting structures surrounding the abutment teeth. Regardless of classification, the crucial factor is that, by creating or allowing a nonlinear path of insertion/dislodgement, a rigid portion of the partial denture framework may be located in an undercut and provide retention.

Chapter 7

Denture Base Retentive Elements

Denture base retentive elements (or networks) are minor connectors that join the denture base to the major connector. The three most common types are *(1)* open latticework, *(2)* mesh, and *(3)* metal bases. Denture base retentive elements must be rigid so that they effectively transfer forces from the denture base to the natural teeth and vice versa. This is a prime consideration in the concept of broad stress distribution. These elements must be strong enough to resist breakage but not so bulky that they interfere with the arrangement of the artificial teeth.

Open latticework

Open latticework (Fig. 7-1) is the preferred type of denture base retentive element for extension partial dentures and for tooth-supported segments where there is adequate vertical space. The attachment to the plastic denture base is stronger than that provided by mesh because there is a greater bulk of resin through the larger openings. The attachment is also stronger than that provided by nailheads, beads, or wire loops on metal bases.

The components of the open latticework are completely embedded in the denture base plastic. The struts meet the major connector at a butt joint. When vertical space is limited, struts may interfere with the setting of teeth. In such cases, a longitudinal strut should not be placed over the crest of the ridge, and cross struts should be located between the planned positions of replacement teeth whenever possible. If a cast infrabulge (bar) clasp is used, it should be an extension of a main cross strut.

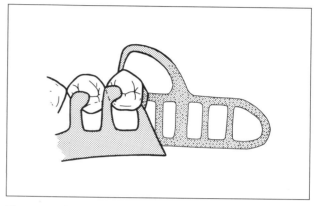

Fig. 7-1 Open latticework is the preferred type of denture base retentive element because the attachment to the plastic is stronger than with mesh. The latticework for a mandibular distal extension RPD should extend approximately two thirds of the distance to the retromolar pad.

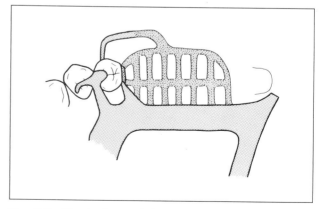

Fig. 7-2 The latticework for a maxillary distal extension RPD should extend at least two thirds of the distance to the hamular notch. The center longitudinal strut may be omitted if it interferes with positioning of the denture teeth.

73

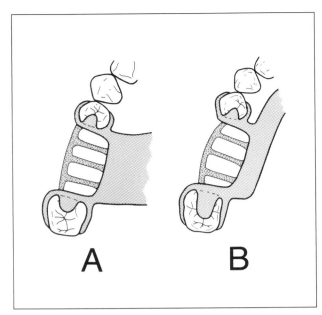

Fig. 7-3 Latticework for tooth-supported segments consists of one buccal longitudinal strut and one or more cross struts, depending on the mesiodistal span of the segment. Retention on the lingual aspect is created by an undercut in the metal at the external finish line. Maxillary tooth-supported segment (A); mandibular tooth-supported segment (B).

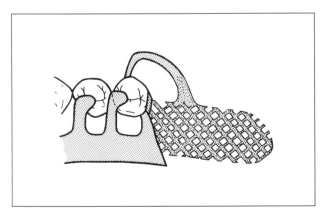

Fig. 7-4 Mesh is preferred over open latticework when vertical space is restricted. It covers approximately the same area as latticework but is generally much thinner.

For a mandibular extension removable partial denture (RPD), the latticework should extend approximately two thirds of the distance to the retromolar pad. There are usually longitudinal struts on each side of the residual ridge. The lingual longitudinal element should be placed at least 3 mm above the lower border of the major connector so that the retentive network will not be exposed by postinsertion adjustment of the denture border.

On a maxillary distal extension RPD (Fig. 7-2), the latticework should extend posteriorly at least two thirds of the distance to the hamular notch. Retention on the palatal side is formed by an undercut in the external finish line of the major connector.

The latticework for both maxillary and mandibular tooth-supported segments (Fig. 7-3) is similar to that for maxillary extension bases. Retention is created on the buccal aspect by a longitudinal strut and on the lingual aspect by the junction with the major connector.

Mesh

Mesh (Fig. 7-4) is basically a thin sheet of metal perforated with many small holes. It covers approximately the same portion of the residual ridge as outlined by the struts for open latticework. The small projections of plastic extending through the mesh tend to be weaker than those created by the open latticework. Retentive mesh is primarily indicated where there is limited vertical space, that is, where the bulk and height of the struts of the open latticework would interfere with the arrangement of teeth. Mesh is not routinely recommended because of the inferior strength factor.

Metal denture bases

Metal bases (Fig. 7-5) are most commonly used for posterior tooth-supported segments where the residual ridge is well-healed and the available vertical space is so limited that an acrylic resin base would be thin and weak. Because relining is not possible, metal bases are generally not indicated for extension RPDs.

Denture teeth can be joined to a metal base by denture base plastic in combination with bead, nailhead, or wire loop retention. However, the attachment is not quite as strong as that provided by open latticework. Replacement teeth can also be added to metal bases with processed, heat-cured, or light-activated resins without intervening denture base plastic. Although tube teeth could conceivably be used, they will be very prone to fracture and/or loss if the vertical space is limited.

No relief is placed under metal bases, and there is no internal finish line. There may or may not be an external finish line, depending on the method of tooth replacement.

Finish lines

Finish lines occur where the acrylic resin of the denture base meets the metal of the framework. The junction of the two materials should form a butt joint. There is an internal and an external finish line at each junction. They should be offset so that the metal is not weakened.

The internal finish line (Fig. 7-6) is located on the tissue surface side of the framework. It is formed by the 24- to 26-gauge relief wax placed on the master cast prior to duplication. The internal finish line is normally placed farther from the abutment tooth or residual ridge than the external finish line.

The external finish line (Fig. 7-7) is located on the polished surface of the RPD. It is the finish line that is drawn on the cast during the design process. A slight undercut in the metal that forms the finish line helps to improve the mechanical retention between the base and the framework.

For a mandibular distal extension RPD, the external finish line begins at the distolingual aspect of the terminal tooth and angles posteriorly as it progresses toward the floor of the mouth. The lingual finish line for a mandibular tooth-supported RPD should be located just far enough lingually to allow for setting of the artificial teeth. If it is placed too far lingually (and thus inferiorly), the major connector will be weakened.

For maxillary RPDs, the palatal finish line should be located so that it allows for proper positioning of the artificial teeth while still maintaining normal tissue contours and a smooth transition from metal to plastic.

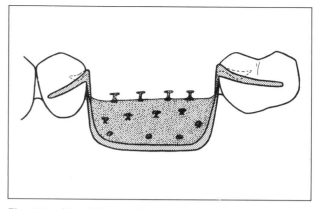

Fig. 7-5 Metal denture bases are most commonly used over well-healed posterior residual ridges where vertical space is a problem. Attachment of the metal and the denture base plastic can be achieved with nailheads, beads, or wire loops.

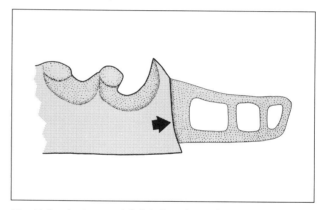

Fig. 7-6 An internal finish line *(arrow)* is located on the tissue side of the RPD at the junction of the major connector and the denture base.

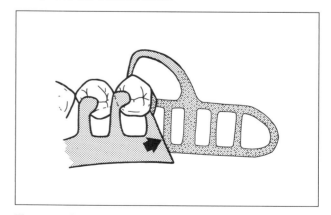

Fig. 7-7 An external finish line *(arrow)* is located on the external surface of the RPD. It is the finish line that is drawn on the cast during the design process.

Replacement Teeth

Because the primary subject of this text is partial denture framework design, the following discussion will emphasize those types of replacement teeth that must be incorporated into the framework during fabrication.

Materials used for replacement teeth include acrylic resin (plastic), porcelain, gold, and stellite alloys. Plastic is by far the most commonly utilized. Because plastic teeth chemically bond to the denture base resin, their length and shape can be dramatically altered without loss of retention. Porcelain teeth, on the other hand, are dependent on mechanical means for attachment to the denture base. Extensive recontouring may result in loss of the diatoric holes or pins necessary for retention. In addition, porcelain teeth are quite abrasive, particularly if the glaze is broken. Thus, they should not be used to oppose natural teeth or gold restorations. Gold is occasionally used to fabricate occlusal surfaces for posterior plastic teeth, especially if the opposing occlusion is also restored with gold. However, the cost is prohibitive for many patients.

The vast majority of replacement teeth for removable partial dentures (RPDs) are attached to the prosthesis by way of a retentive network and an acrylic resin denture base. The advantages of this technique are (1) the availability of a large number of teeth of various shapes, sizes, and shades, (2) the flexibility in positioning teeth, (3) the ability to compensate for extensive residual ridge loss, (4) the ability to perform an altered cast procedure for extension RPDs, (5) the ability to utilize the framework for record making and subsequently for accurate mounting of casts and arrangement of teeth, and (6) the capacity to reline/rebase the prosthesis when residual ridge resorption occurs.

In addition, the occlusion can be accurately developed in a wide variety of materials (porcelain, plastic, metal). The resulting prosthesis will achieve maximum utilization of the support offered by the residual ridge and will be relatively easy to repair.

The retentive network/resin base combination is the safest and best technique if (1) the prosthesis is an extension RPD, (2) the residual ridge is still in the process of recontouring, (3) there has been significant residual ridge loss, (4) there are multiple missing teeth, or (5) the spacing is unusual. When there are small tooth-supported segments exhibiting limited vertical space between the residual ridge and the opposing teeth, or when there is a history of repeated fracture or extensive wear of the artificial teeth, the selection of commercially available facings, custom-made facings, tube teeth, or metal teeth is preferred if the residual ridges are well-healed and exhibit minimal resorption. However, with any of these replacements, an esthetic try-in is often complicated or time-consuming, and relining procedures are impossible. Each of these types of replacement teeth must be incorporated into the design and specified on the work authorization form. Information regarding shade, shape, and position of artificial teeth must be provided. If multiple replacements are needed or unusual configurations are anticipated, facings or denture teeth can be arranged on a record base and subsequently placed in the mouth for patient approval. The laboratory can then fabricate an index of the arrangement so that it can be reproduced in the prosthesis.

Metal backings are always used with prefabricated facings and are usually used with custom-made facings. Metal backings should be used if

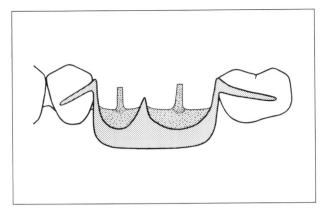

Fig. 8-1a Mandibular tooth-supported RPD before attachment of tube teeth.

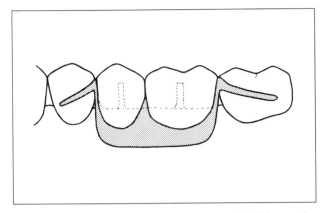

Fig. 8-1b After attachment of tube teeth. When tube teeth are used for anterior replacements, the facial aspect of the tooth is almost always butted against the residual ridge so that metal will not be visible.

the replacement teeth will occlude with the opposing teeth to prevent extrusion or provide occlusal guidance, or if there has been rapid wear or frequent breakage of previous replacement teeth. When metal backings are indicated, precise planning for the occlusion is necessary. The laboratory must be provided with casts that are mounted on an articulator, related with an accurate record, or marked with orientation lines.

Tube teeth

Tube teeth (Figs. 8-1a and b) are modified denture teeth and are probably the most commonly used form of replacement other than the denture tooth/ retentive network/denture base combination. They can be used for anterior or posterior replacements in tooth-supported segments where the residual ridge is well-healed.

Tube teeth are relatively easy to fabricate and can make use of the vast selection of shades and molds available for denture teeth. The esthetic result is usually excellent and can be enhanced further by butting the facial aspect of the tooth to the ridge so that a metal collar will not be evident.

Tube teeth are custom shaped to fit the framework and are incorporated into the framework fabrication process. Thus, the shade for tube teeth must be determined prior to framework fabrication and subsequently provided to the laboratory.

A denture tooth of the appropriate shade and approximate size is selected. The tooth is contoured so that it will conform to the edentulous space. A vertical channel is made, entering from the gingival end of the tooth. The framework is waxed on the refractory cast and the tube tooth is positioned in the wax-up. A "post" corresponding to the vertical channel in the tooth is incorporated into the wax pattern. When the wax pattern is complete, the tube tooth is removed and the framework is cast. Following finishing and polishing, the tube tooth is attached to the framework with cement or autopolymerizing resin.

Tube teeth are especially useful when one or two teeth are being replaced. They are not usually indicated for large edentulous segments because the tissue surface cannot be relined. They are contraindicated for anterior areas where extensive residual ridge loss would necessitate unnaturally long teeth.

Tube teeth are not particularly strong and are prone to fracture under heavy occlusal forces. Replacement is difficult if not impossible. Posterior tube teeth cannot be protected by a metal occlusal surface because they are placed on the framework in a vertical direction. Posterior tube teeth should be avoided where occlusal forces will be great and where vertical space is restricted. Similarly, anterior tube teeth cannot be protected by a metal backing. Thus, they should not be used where anterior guidance will be provided by the replacement tooth or teeth or where vertical space is limited.

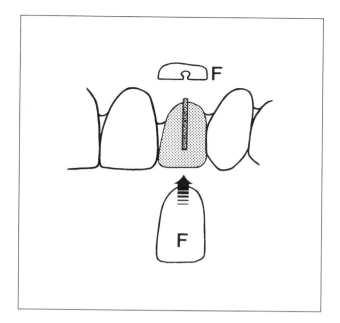

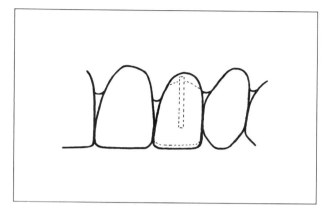

Fig. 8-2a *(left)* A slotted facing *(F)* used to replace a maxillary lateral incisor. The facing is inserted on the backing in a vertical direction and is retained by the relationship of the slot and the rail and by a luting medium.

Fig. 8-2b *(below)* The backing supports the facing but is not visible when the RPD is inserted in the mouth.

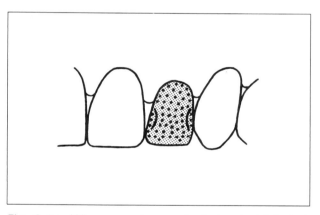

Fig. 8-3a When a custom-made facing is fabricated, loops or beads are usually used to form the attachment.

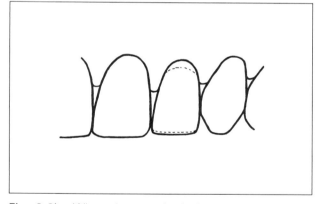

Fig. 8-3b When the prosthesis is seated, the entire metal substructure is hidden by the facing.

Commercially available facings

Prefabricated facings may be of the slotted (Figs. 8-2a and b) or pin type. They are almost always used to replace anterior teeth and must be protected by a metal backing. Because of the backing, the facings are strong, require very little interocclusal space, and can usually be replaced. The major disadvantages to prefabricated facings relate to esthetics. Quite frequently, the metal backing alters the expected shade and destroys the depth of color and translucency normally seen in natural teeth. In addition, esthetics may suffer if more than one tooth is replaced. Although the appearance of the facings may be improved by custom shaping, replacement then becomes more difficult if not impossible.

Custom facings

The new cross-linked acrylic resin copolymers are satisfactory in hardness and wear resistance for

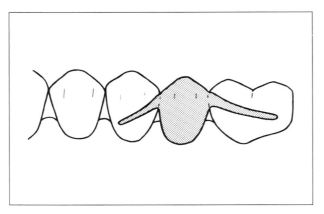

Fig. 8-4 Metal teeth are indicated only when the mesiodistal space is small and when esthetics are not important. Here, a metal tooth is used to replace a mandibular first molar where the mesiodistal space has been reduced by mesial drifting of the second molar.

most patients. In addition, in the hands of a skilled technician, gingivoincisal blending of shade can approach that of denture teeth. Because they are directly attached to the framework, custom facings are particularly advantageous where vertical space is limited. An initial opaque layer blocks the effect of the metal on the shade. Both body and surface staining are possible. Because the technician has considerable control over contour, the replacement tooth/teeth can be adapted to various sizes and shapes of edentulous spaces. The framework is fabricated with recesses in the wax pattern for the artificial teeth. Retention is provided by undercuts, beads, and/or wire loops (Figs. 8-3a and b). The attachment is considerably stronger than that for cemented prefabricated facings. However, custom facings should still be protected by a metal backing. When used for posterior teeth, the occlusal surface may or may not be protected by metal, depending on the occlusal pattern and prior history of wear and/or fracture.

Custom facings may be fabricated utilizing conventional processing techniques or with heat- or light-activated methods.

Processed acrylic resins

The packing and processing of tooth-colored methyl methacrylate facings has been almost entirely replaced by the use of heat- and light-activated materials. The former technique is difficult and time-consuming and produces unpredictable results relative to shade and translucency.

Heat-activated acrylic resins

The heat-activated materials are supplied as powder and liquid. An opaque layer is first placed on the metal. Then body and incisal portions are formed in layers and cured under pressure at approximately 250°F. Custom staining can be incorporated into the body of the material or added to the surface after contouring is completed. The final finish is obtained by polishing with abrasives of decreasing coarseness.

Light-activated resins.

The light-activated materials are usually microfilled BIS-GMA resins. The opaque layer is autopolymerizing. Curing of the body and incisal layers is activated by white light (under vacuum). The body can be semi-cured and easily cut back prior to building the incisal layer. Custom staining can be incorporated into the body portion or added to the surface.

Metal teeth

All-metal teeth (Fig. 8-4) are indicated for posterior edentulous spaces where there is restricted interarch space or where drifting has decreased the anteroposterior width of the edentulous space. They are primarily used as space maintainers to prevent further drifting. Resin facings may be used but are seldom necessary.

Chapter 9

Mouth Preparation

Following emergency treatment and possibly initial periodontal treatment, diagnostic information has been collected and used to develop a treatment plan and a tentative removable partial denture (RPD) design. It is assumed that the necessary procedures in the areas of occlusion, periodontics, endodontics, orthodontics, oral surgery, operative dentistry, and fixed prosthodontics have now been accomplished. Contours of any new crowns should be consistent with the tentative design. Guide surfaces, rest seats, and retentive recesses should have been incorporated into the crowns with the aid of a surveyor. Phase I of mouth preparation is now complete.

If any major changes (e.g., unplanned extractions) have occurred or if crowns have been placed since the tentative design was formulated, new study casts should be made and surveyed. The tentative design must be reviewed, corrected, and placed on the new cast. Areas for tooth modification are drawn in red and the framework outlined in blue. The result is considered the final design and will be used as a road map for Phase II of mouth preparation.

Phase II consists of alteration of tooth contours to (1) produce distinct guide surfaces, (2) reduce interferences, (3) provide improved clasp location, (4) provide access for the minor connectors between the rests and major connector, (5) create adequate rest seats, and (6) prepare retentive recesses if none exist naturally. It is strongly recommended that the modifications in tooth contours be performed first on the study cast. In addition, the prepared diagnostic cast should be in the office on the surveyor when intraoral alterations are accomplished.

Preparing guide surfaces

Guide surfaces must be considered with respect to the axis of rotation of the RPD and the consequent movement of the denture during function. The relationship of guide surfaces and guide plates was discussed in detail in chapter 3.

It is important to remember that mouth preparations for guiding surfaces must duplicate those planned during the surveying and design process, or the desired action will not be produced.

All tooth surfaces do not necessarily need to be altered. If they are parallel to the desired path of insertion/dislodgement, there is no need to change the natural contours.

Guide surfaces should be prepared before rest seats so that the guide surface preparations will not reduce the extent of the rest seats. If the order is reversed, the center of the rest seat may be too near the marginal ridge, and the marginal ridge will be sharp and excessively lowered.

Guide surfaces for guide plates

Guide surfaces for guide plates are prepared with a cylindrical diamond stone or carbide bur. They should be parallel to the path of insertion/dislodgement and parallel to each other (Fig. 9-1). They bound each edentulous space and are more effective in providing cross-arch bracing if widely separated.

The occlusogingival length of the proximal guide surface preparation varies slightly depending on whether the RPD is tooth supported or tooth and tissue supported (an extension). Generally, guide surface preparations for extension RPDs are

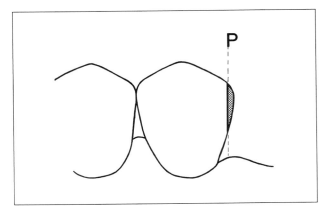

Fig. 9-1 A proximal guide surface preparation should be parallel to the path of insertion/dislodgement *(P)*. The shaded area represents the tooth structure to be removed.

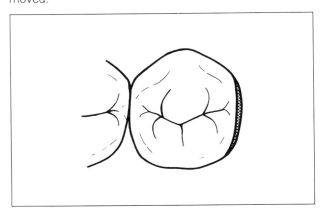

Fig. 9-2 Occlusal view of proximal guide surface preparation. The preparation curves buccolingually to follow the normal tooth contour.

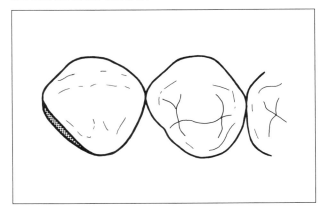

Fig. 9-3 Guide surface preparations on anterior teeth are usually restricted to the linguoproximal aspect so that the mesiodistal width of the facial surface is not decreased.

shorter, leaving a small space below the gingival extent of the preparation. The space, in conjunction with physiologic relief, prevents the guide plate from binding against the abutment during functional movements of the extension base (those toward the residual ridge). The occlusogingival dimension is usually one half to two thirds the crown length; 3 to 4 mm is more than adequate in most cases.

The proximal preparations should curve buccolingually to follow the natural tooth contour (Fig. 9-2). They should extend slightly past the linguoproximal line angle if the corresponding guide plate is expected to provide reciprocation. If a retentive or reciprocating/bracing arm is to emanate from the guide plate, the guide surface should not form a sharp linguoproximal line angle, or strength will be lost at the junction of the two elements.

Great care must be exercised to avoid ditching the cervical portion of the tooth. If the abutment tilts so that a parallel guide surface cannot be prepared without ditching the tooth, the path of insertion/dislodgement or the type of clasp assembly will have to be changed, or the abutment will need to be crowned.

Guide surface preparations for anterior teeth are usually restricted to the linguoproximal aspect (Fig. 9-3). The mesiodistal width of the abutments should not be reduced unless space is needed for an artificial replacement (see "Guide surfaces for esthetics," following).

Guide surfaces for minor connectors

It is sometimes possible to create small guide surfaces in areas where minor connectors pass between teeth to connect major connectors and rests (Fig. 9-4). In tooth-supported RPDs, there are usually so many other, larger areas of guide surface–rigid metal contact that the contribution of guide surfaces for minor connectors is relatively insignificant. On some extension RPDs, however, minor connectors contacting parallel surfaces can contribute substantially to the action of clasps by preventing distal movement of the prosthesis. When a mesial rest–distal guide plate–I-bar clasp assembly is selected, the two guide plates do not dictate a definite path of insertion/dislodgement. Retention can be assured by placing the tip of the I-bar in front of the greatest mesiodistal curvature of the facial surface. If it is possible to prepare a mesiolingual guide surface, distal displacement of the prosthesis will be prevented, and the I-bar can be placed at the greatest mesiodistal curvature.

Guide surfaces for lingual plating and reciprocating/bracing elements

Creation of lingual guide surfaces is frequently advantageous, particularly on mandibular posterior teeth where the height of contour is very close to the occlusal aspect of the tooth. The preparation of flat surfaces allows for true reciprocation by plating or rigid lingual arms (Fig. 9-5). In addition, the surface provides an *area* (rather than a line) to which the technician may wax and finish the metal. Lingual guide surfaces are usually quite short; 2 to 3 mm is all that can be expected. Again, great care must be exercised in order that the tooth is not ditched in the gingival third.

Guide surfaces for esthetics

Although guide surfaces for anterior teeth are usually restricted to the linguoproximal aspect they may occasionally be utilized to increase space where drifting prevents placement of an artificial tooth or teeth consistent with adjacent natural teeth (Figs. 9-6a and b). Because the reduction is so critical, it is best done on the study cast first. If an appropriate artificial tooth or facing is not available or if a heat- or light-cured facing is to be used, a wax diagnostic tooth can be fabricated.

Reducing interferences

The lingual surfaces of lingually inclined mandibular premolars may interfere with the placement of the major connector. If these surfaces are not reduced, the lingual bar will be located medially in the floor of the mouth when the prosthesis is fully seated (Fig. 9-7). If the lingual aspects of the teeth are reduced parallel to the path of insertion/dislodgement, guide surfaces may be prepared concomitantly.

Overlapping proximal surfaces, particularly on mandibular anterior teeth, create interferences if a linguoplate major connector must be used. These teeth should be recontoured to avoid interproximal

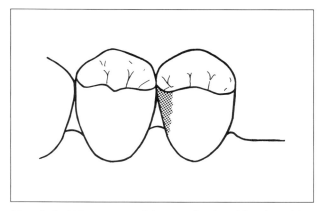

Fig. 9-4 When a mesial rest–distal guide plate–I-bar clasp assembly is used on the terminal abutment for a distal extension RPD, a small guide surface should be prepared on the mesiolingual aspect whenever possible.

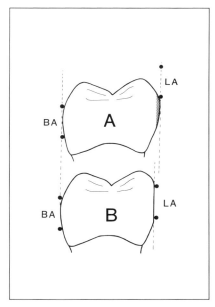

Fig. 9-5 Diagrammatic representation of recontouring to produce reciprocation. True reciprocation does not exist *(A)* because the rigid lingual arm *(LA)* is not in contact with the tooth as the buccal arm *(BA)* passes over the height of contour. The lingual arm thus functions for bracing only. However, if the shaded area is removed *(B)*, a guide surface parallel to the path of insertion/dislodgement is created, and the lingual arm contacts the tooth during the entire time the buccal retentive arm is traversing the height of contour. The lingual arm now provides both bracing *and* reciprocation.

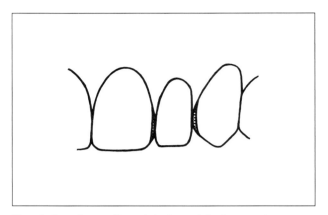

Fig. 9-6a A maxillary left lateral incisor replacement tooth would be narrow and unesthetic unless the central incisor and canine were recontoured by removing the shaded areas.

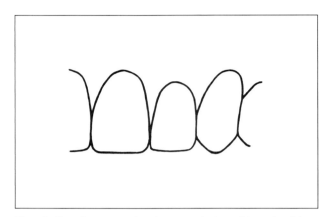

Fig. 9-6b A more pleasing result is achieved with a wider lateral incisor.

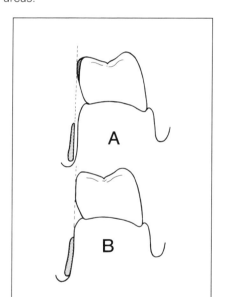

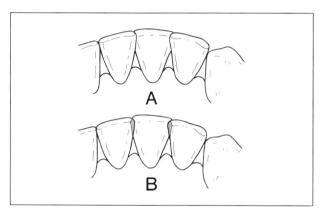

Fig. 9-8 When a linguoplate major connector is selected, the mesio- and distoincisal corners of overlapping anterior teeth (A) should be recontoured to eliminate excessive undercuts below the contact points (B).

Fig. 9-7 A lingually inclined mandibular posterior tooth may cause the lingual bar to be located too far medially in the floor of the mouth (A). If the shaded area is removed, the lingual bar can be positioned farther laterally, eliminating the space between the major connector and the tissues (B).

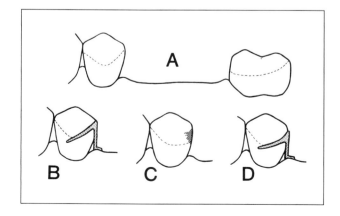

Fig. 9-9 (right) Buccal view of a mandibular tooth-supported segment (A). Because of the location of the height of contour on the distobuccal aspect, the origin of a circumferential clasp arm would be very near the occlusal surface and might interfere with the opposing occlusion (B). The shaded area has been removed, lowering the height of contour (C). The origin of the clasp arm may now be located farther gingivally (D).

undercuts at the incisal corners (Fig. 9-8). Failure to do so will result in poor adaptation of the plate and impaction of food between its superior border and the teeth.

Recontouring to improve clasp location

All reciprocating and bracing clasp arms and the originating portions of suprabulge-type retentive arms must be located above the height of contour. On posterior teeth, the height of contour is often very close to the occlusal surface, creating the possibility of the arms' interfering with the opposing occlusion (Fig. 9-9). For first premolars and anterior teeth, particularly in the maxillary arch, the problem is compounded by esthetic considerations. The originating portion of a circumferential clasp would be very near the incisal edge and would be objectionable to most patients. With judicious recontouring, the height of contour can be moved gingivally so that the originating portion of the clasp would be less noticeable.

Recontouring is also beneficial when lingual I-bars are the retainers of choice for molar abutments on Class II or Class III mandibular RPDs (Fig. 9-10). Because of drifting and tilting, the mesiolingual undercut is frequently large and the survey line very near the occlusal surface. Placement of the I-bar on an unmodified tooth will cause the approach portion of the arm to lie medially in the floor of the mouth, where it will act as a food repository and may be irritating to the tongue. Careful reshaping will lower the height of contour, decrease the retentive recess, and allow the approach arm to lie closer to the lingual aspect of the residual ridge.

Providing access for minor connectors

Slight modifications in the linguoproximal areas where minor connectors join rests will provide the space necessary for bulk and strength of metal (Fig. 9-11). The recontouring will also allow positioning of the minor connectors so that they will not interfere with the opposing occlusion or be noticeable to the tongue.

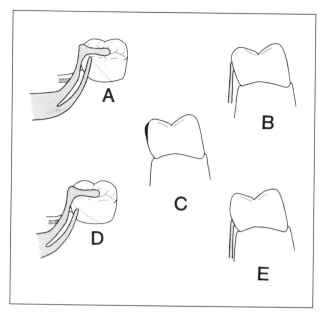

Fig. 9-10 A mesiolingual I-bar retentive arm on a mandibular right molar. Due to the mesiolingual tilt of the tooth, the tip of the I-bar is very close to the occlusal surface *(A)* and the approach portion of the arm is located medially in the floor of the mouth *(B)*. If the shaded area *(C)* is removed, the tip of the I-bar can be located more gingivally *(D)*, and the approach arm nearer the tissues *(E)*.

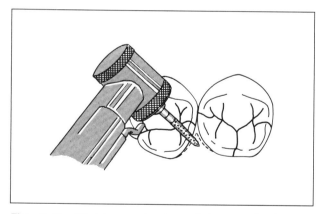

Fig. 9-11 Slight recontouring of interproximal areas where minor connectors will be located will allow for bulk and strength at the junction of the rest and minor connector.

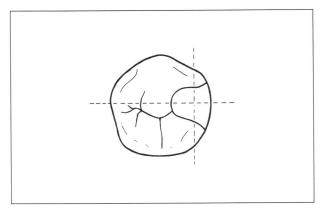

Fig. 9-12a Occlusal view of a rest seat preparation.

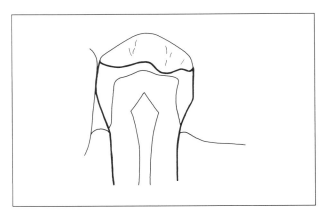

Fig. 9-12b Mesiodistal section through the preparation.

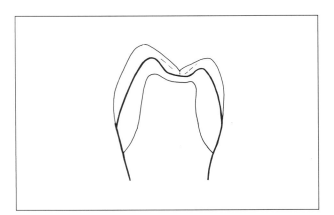

Fig. 9-12c Buccolingual section through the preparation.

Creating rest seats

A rest seat is that portion of a tooth or restoration prepared to receive a metallic occlusal, incisal, or lingual rest of an RPD (see chapter 2).

Rest seats are usually prepared totally in enamel. If the enamel is penetrated during preparation, a restoration should ordinarily be placed. However, in patients who have a low caries rate in spite of longstanding dentin exposure, restorations may not be necessary. Highly polished preparations, impeccable oral hygiene, and periodic fluoride treatments should eliminate caries under rests.

Occlusal rest seats

An occlusal rest seat is prepared with a No. 4 or No. 6 round carbide bur or diamond stone. It should be spoon-shaped with no sharp edges, line angles, or vertical walls (Figs. 9-12a to c). It must allow for slight functional movement of the metal rest within the recess without torquing the abutment. This is particularly important in extension RPDs because support from the abutments is more rigid than that provided by the residual ridge.

The width of the prepared recess for an occlusal rest should be approximately one half the distance between the buccal and lingual cusp tips. The mesiodistal extent of the preparation is dictated by the morphology of the occlusal surface and the axial inclination of the tooth. When the abutment has a normal mesiodistal inclination, the rest seat is prepared so that the deepest portion coincides with the nearest naturally occurring fossa (Fig. 9-13,A). If, however, the abutment exhibits tilting (e.g., on mandibular molars), extension to the center of the tooth is preferred (Fig. 9-13,B). Functional forces will be transmitted in a more axial direction, and the possibility of further tilting will be minimized. The marginal ridge should be reduced 1.0 to 1.5 mm, and the center portion of the seat should be approximately 0.5 mm deeper than the common plane of the rest. The proximo-occlusal line angle at the marginal ridge must be contoured to eliminate a sharp line angle (Fig. 9-14).

Occasionally, tipping of a mandibular molar abutment results in a lack of occlusion with the opposing maxillary teeth, and an overlay rest is indicated. Part or all of the occlusal surface may be

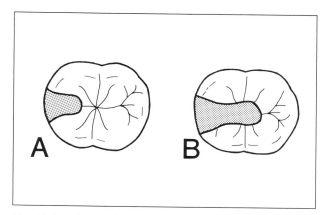

Fig. 9-13 An occlusal rest on a mandibular right first molar. Conventional outline form *(A)*; outline form extended to the central fossa *(B)*.

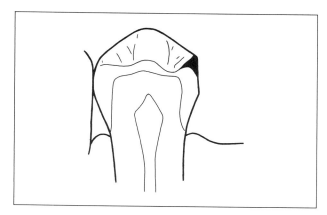

Fig. 9-14 A distal rest seat preparation on a mandibular right second premolar. The marginal ridge is reduced by 1.0 to 1.5 mm, and the proximo-occlusal line angle is rounded *(shaded area)*.

Figs. 9-15a and b Modification of rest seat preparations to accommodate an embrasure clasp. Shaded areas denote additional tooth structure to be removed.

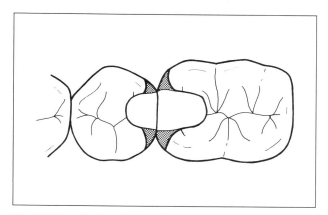

Fig. 9-15a Occlusal view.

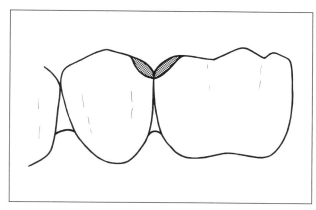

Fig. 9-15b Facial view.

restored by the rest. Deep grooves and pits should be minimized by recontouring the enamel. In addition, the use of pit and fissure sealants may be warranted.

The use of embrasure clasps requires slight modification of rest preparations, particularly when an opposing cusp passes tightly through the embrasure in lateral excursions (Figs. 9-15a and b). Buccal and lingual extensions of the rest seat will provide space for clasp arms that will maintain a 1.0- to 1.5-mm thickness without interfering with the opposing occlusion.

Cingulum rest seats

Cingulum rest seats are prepared with a small round carbide bur or diamond stone and a tapered round-ended or flame-shaped diamond stone (Fig. 9-16). They are most commonly located on maxillary and mandibular canines. Because the lingual surfaces of these teeth tend to be rather steeply sloped, a very distinct recess is necessary to prevent the creation of lateral stresses during function (Fig. 9-17). Cingulum rest seats should be semilunar in shape and 1.0 to 1.5 mm deep over the cen-

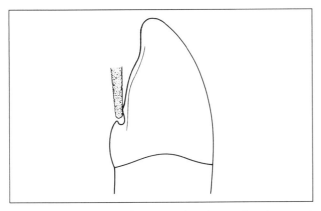

Fig. 9-16 After initial preparation for a cingulum rest seat is made with a small round bur or diamond stone, the lip of tooth structure above the groove is blended into the lingual surface with a tapered diamond. In some cases, the entire preparation may be completed with a tapered, round-ended rotary instrument.

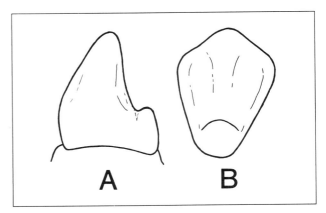

Fig. 9-17 A cingulum rest preparation on a mandibular canine. Proximal view (A); lingual view (B).

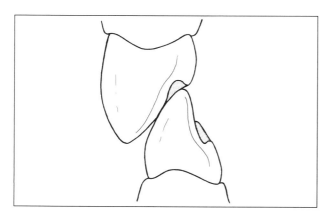

Fig. 9-18 Cingulum rests in place on maxillary and mandibular canines. Because of the occlusal relationship, the maxillary rest must be entirely contained within the rest seat. The mandibular canine rest can be thickened buccolingually as long as it blends with the tooth contours.

ter of the cingulum. Cingulum rests are preferred over incisal rests because they provide for better esthetics, create less leverage on the abutment teeth by loading at a more apical level, and are less bothersome to the tongue.

Maxillary canines generally exhibit a more pronounced cingulum than mandibular canines. However, when the mandibular anterior teeth articulate precisely with the lingual surfaces of the maxillary canines, the rest seat must be larger and deeper so that the entire rest will lie within the rest preparation and still have sufficient mass for strength (Fig. 9-18). A rest seat for a mandibular canine must provide a definite stop, but because there is no opposing occlusion involved, it does not need to be so deep that the entire rest lies within the confines of the recess. Strength can be achieved by thickening the rest buccolingually. If the surface contour of the rest blends into the anatomic form of the tooth, the added bulk will not be unduly disturbing to the tongue.

Sometimes the lingual slope of a canine, particularly a mandibular canine, is so steep that an adequate vertical stop cannot be prepared without penetrating the enamel (Fig. 9-19). In such cases, three options exist: (1) place a small amalgam restoration in the base of the preparation where the dentin has been exposed (Fig. 9-20), (2) place a lingual pin inlay (Fig. 9-21), or (3) fabricate a three-quarter crown (Fig. 9-22). A cingulum rest seat is incorporated into the casting of the pin inlay or three-quarter crown.

Infrequently, partially edentulous configurations dictate that cingulum rests be placed on central or lateral incisors. In these instances, multiple rests may be used to assist in distributing functional stresses over a wider area.

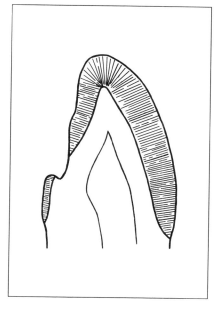

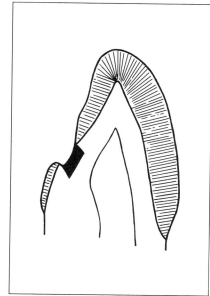

Fig. 9-19 *(left)* A mandibular canine exhibiting a severe slope to the lingual surface. The lingual rest seat preparation has penetrated the enamel.

Fig. 9-20 *(right)* When the preparation exposes dentin, an amalgam restoration may be placed in the base of the rest seat.

Fig. 9-21 *(below)* A lingual pin inlay on a mandibular canine used to create an adequate cingulum rest seat. Proximal view *(A)*; lingual view *(B)*.

Fig. 9-22 *(right)* A three-quarter crown on a mandibular canine used to create an adequate cingulum rest seat.

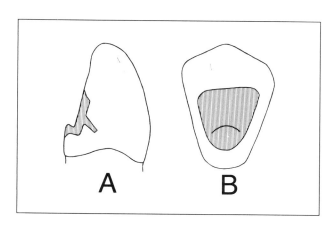

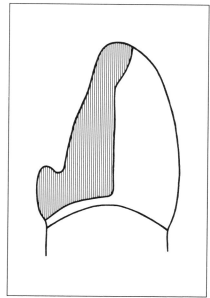

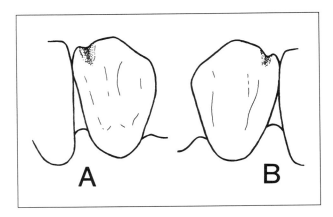

Fig. 9-23 An incisal rest preparation on a mandibular right canine. Lingual view *(A)*; facial view *(B)*.

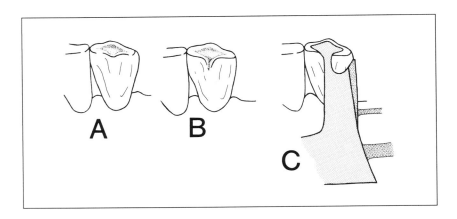

Fig. 9-24 A mandibular right canine exhibiting abrasion and erosion of the incisal edge *(A)*; Prepared groove from the lingual surface to the incisal recess *(B)*; incisal rest seated on the abutment *(C)*.

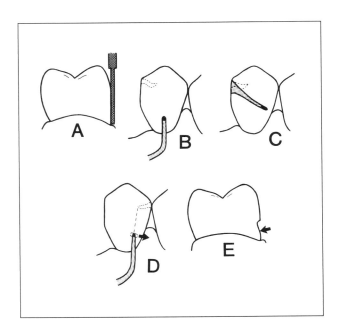

Fig. 9-25 Retentive recesses may be created in enamel when the surface of the tooth is parallel or nearly parallel to the path of insertion/dislodgement *(A)*. If the RPD is tooth supported, the retentive area may be a dimple for an I-bar *(B)* or a groove for a circumferential clasp *(C)*. For extension RPDs, the recess should be a groove along the path the tip will follow during functional movements *(D)*. Because the gingival portion of the recess *(E, arrow)* does not contribute to retention, it should blend smoothly into the surrounding tooth structure.

Incisal rest seats

Incisal rest seats are prepared with a tapered diamond stone or carbide bur. They may be used on any anterior tooth that does not have sufficient lingual contour for the preparation of a cingulum rest. However, incisal rests are seldom used on maxillary anterior teeth because of their undesirable appearance and because the corresponding minor connector often interferes with the occlusion.

An incisal rest seat is a rounded trough or groove preparation that extends over the incisal edge of the tooth (Fig. 9-23). The center of the recess must be lower than the approximating mesial and distal tooth structure. Placement in wear facets or over large proximal restorations should be avoided. The preparation should be 1.0 to 1.5 mm deep and 1.5 mm wide and must be located 1 to 2 mm medial to the mesial or distal corner of the tooth.

Older patients sometimes exhibit a combination of wear and erosion on the incisal edges of mandibular anterior teeth. The resulting recesses can often be modified and used for incisal rest seats (Fig. 9-24). Sharp enamel edges are rounded and access is achieved by preparing a groove from the lingual surface into the incisal recess. Because the rest will lie on a flat or concave surface, there is no need for extension onto the facial surface of the tooth.

Preparing retentive recesses

If adequate undercuts for retention are not present, they may be created by recontouring. However, the area to be modified must be *almost parallel* to the path of insertion/dislodgement. The lip of the groove toward the occlusal surface provides the retention. If the surface of the tooth varies more than a few degrees from parallel, the preparation would have to be excessively deep to provide effective retention. It would almost certainly penetrate the enamel.

The retentive recess created should be consis-tent with the type of retentive arm planned and the functional motion that will be exhibited by the RPD (Fig. 9-25). For tooth-supported RPDs (which exhibit no functional motion) and I-bar retentive arms, a dimple may be used. However, if circumferential clasps are selected, a groove is a better choice. The groove should lie directly under the arm when the RPD is fully seated. It should blend with the tooth structure at its origin and termination. The gingival lip of the groove should be removed (it is not responsible for providing retention).

For extension RPDs with I-bar retentive arms, the recess created should be a groove that imitates the path the retentive tip will follow during functional movements of the RPD. This groove should also blend with the natural tooth structure at its origin, termination, and gingival aspect.

Evaluation of preparations

Proper mouth preparation is vital to the success of RPDs. Without it, the best design is doomed to failure. Every precaution should be taken to ensure that mouth preparation is performed accurately. Rest preparations can be evaluated with soft, nonsticky wax. The wax is pressed into the recess, removed, and inspected for proper form. Occlusal clearance can be estimated by having the patient close the teeth together and move into lateral excursions while the wax is in place. A more precise evaluation of all preparations (especially guiding surfaces) can be achieved by analyzing a cast made from an alginate impression and poured in quick-set plaster. Remember, a path of insertion/dislodgement does not exist simply because it is planned on a diagnostic cast. Parallelism or near parallelism of guiding surfaces must be achieved *in the mouth*.

When all mouth preparations are acceptable, areas of tooth alteration must be polished with rubber points and flour of pumice and treated with topical fluoride. Fluoride application should be repeated at future recall appointments.

PART II
ATLAS

USE OF THE ATLAS IN THE DESIGN PROCESS

The atlas portion of the text is intended to provide a baseline from which the design process can be expanded. Partially edentulous arches are arranged in chapters according to the Kennedy classification. At the beginning of each chapter is a key that further subdivides the classification according to specific characteristics. At the end of the smallest subdivision is a case number that represents the location of design information relating to the specific (or a very similar) partially edentulous arch.

Each case begins with an illustration of the partially edentulous arch and an "ideal" framework design. These are followed by a discussion of design concepts and possible variations. Referencing between cases is used to decrease repetition and thereby increase the number of cases that can be considered.

Obviously, every partially edentulous situation cannot be discussed. Rare combinations of remaining teeth and mirror images of designs considered were deleted to make the number of designs manageable. Some extrapolation will be required when uncommon situations are encountered. The selection of cases was based initially on an analysis of over 5,000 partially edentulous arches for which RPDs were fabricated. The frequency of occurrence was used to develop the key, and additional cases were added to improve continuity of design patterns.

Mandibular Class I Designs

The mandibular Class I is the most common type of removable partial denture. In our study of 3,000 partially edentulous mandibular arches for which RPDs were fabricated, approximately 50% were Class I. Considering frequency of occurrence, the 45 cases discussed in chapter 10 cover slightly over 98% of these partially edentulous arches (or their mirror images).

Because a distal extension RPD is seldom fabricated to replace second or third molars, only those situations where at least all the molars are missing will be considered.

Case reference guide	
Without modification space	
Symmetrical	
All anterior teeth are present	10.1 to 10.3
Canines are missing	10.4
Asymmetrical	
All anterior teeth are present	10.5 to 10.7
Some or all of anterior teeth are missing	10.8 to 10.12
With modification space	
With posterior modification space(s) only	
Symmetrical	10.13
Asymmetrical	10.14 to 10.16
With anterior modification space(s) only	
Symmetrical	
Two teeth in space	10.17 to 10.19
Four teeth in space	10.20 to 10.22
Six teeth in space	10.23
Asymmetrical	
One tooth in space	10.24 to 10.29
Two teeth in space	10.30 to 10.33
Three teeth in space	10.34 to 10.35
Four teeth in space	10.36 to 10.38
Five teeth in space	10.39
Six teeth in space	10.40
With anterior and posterior modification spaces	
One tooth in anterior space	10.41
Two teeth in anterior space	10.42
Three teeth in anterior space	10.43
Four teeth in anterior space	10.44
Five teeth in anterior space	10.45

Case 10.1

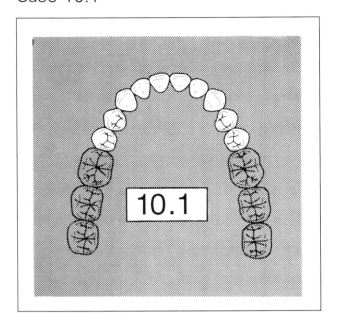

10.1

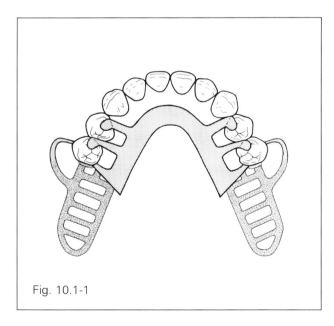

Fig. 10.1-1

Rests

The variations in rest location considered in Figs. 10.1-2 through 10.1-4 primarily apply to the preferred mesial rest, I-bar, distal guide plate design. However, rest location, particularly that of primary rests, is intimately related to the selection of retentive arms, and is discussed further in that section.

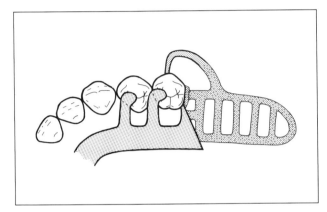

Fig. 10.1-2 On distal extension RPDs, the primary rest is usually placed on the mesio-occlusal aspect of the tooth adjacent to the edentulous space. The indirect retainer would normally be placed on the mesio-occlusal aspect of the first premolar because this location creates an excellent vertical stop yet seldom interferes with the opposing occlusion. In the rare instance when the indirect retainer cannot be placed in this position, it may be moved to the cingulum or incisal edge of the canine.

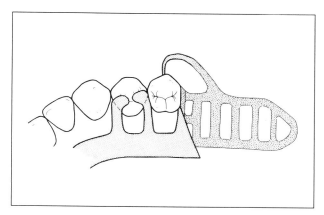

Fig. 10.1-3 If the terminal abutment exhibits significant loss of supporting bone or if the mesio-occlusal fossa is unavailable because of tight interdigitation with an opposing cusp tip, the rest may be moved to the disto-occlusal fossa of the next tooth forward. The indirect retainer may remain on the mesio-occlusal aspect of the first premolar or may be placed on the cingulum or incisal edge of the canine.

Guide plates

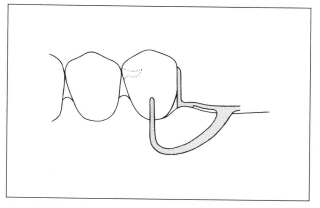

Fig. 10.1-5 Guide surface–guide plate contacts should be parallel to the path of insertion/dislodgement. The occlusogingival dimension of the contact should be one half to two thirds the crown length. A small recess gingival to the guide surface is retained if present.

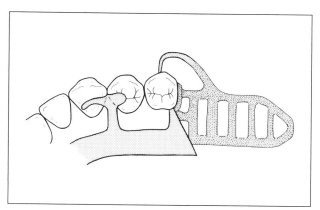

Fig. 10.1-4 If the disto-occlusal fossa of the first premolar is also blocked by the opposing occlusion, the primary rest may be placed in the mesio-occlusal fossa. Although this rest will also function as an indirect retainer, a cingulum or incisal rest is usually added on the canine. It will (1) help to dissipate vertical forces, (2) improve the efficiency of indirect retention (because it lies farther forward of the retentive tip), and (3) provide bracing when the RPD is fully seated. Because there is now no minor connector between the premolars, the guide surface/guide plate relationship on the distal aspect of the second premolar must extend around the distolingual line angle to create reciprocation and/or bracing and, in combination with the proximal tooth contact, provide 180° encirclement. If necessary, the premolars may also be plated. However, the plating must not extend above the height of contour or the plating will preempt the planned rest.

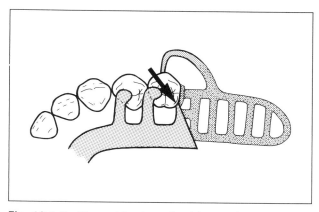

Fig. 10.1-6 The guide plate should curve buccolingually and extend beyond the distolingual line angle *(arrow)* to provide 180° encirclement, bracing, and possibly reciprocation. However, it must not extend above the height of contour, or it will preempt the planned rest.

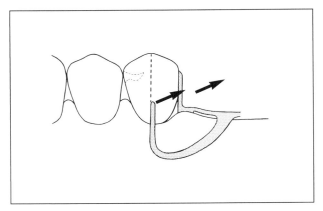

Fig. 10.1-7a In the partially edentulous situation under consideration, the two guide plates do not establish a definite path of insertion/dislodgement. A random dislodging force could cause the RPD to move upward and posteriorly.

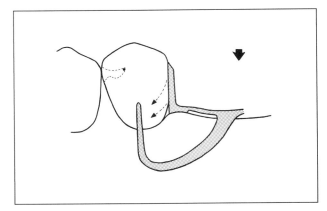

Fig. 10.1-8 When a functional force is applied to the extension area, the lower portion of the guide plate may bind against the abutment and must be physiologically relieved at the framework try-in.

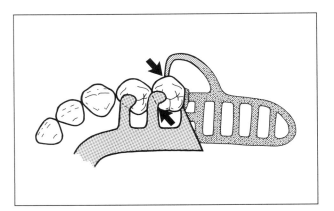

Fig. 10.1-7b If the retentive tip is placed in front of the greatest mesiodistal curvature of the facial surface and/or if a small guide surface–minor connector contact can be established at the mesiolingual aspect of the abutment, the RPD will resist random dislodging forces and exhibit retention.

Major connector

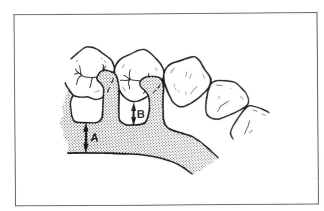

Fig. 10.1-9 The superior-inferior height of a lingual bar should be no less than 4 mm *(A)*. The superior border of the lingual bar must be at least 3 mm below the gingival margin *(B)*.

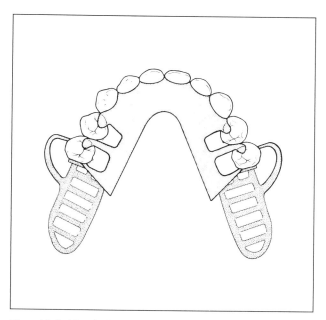

Fig. 10.1-10 A linguoplate should be selected if (1) there is less than 7 mm of vertical space between the gingival margin and the floor of the mouth, (2) the anterior teeth exhibit extreme lingual tilting, (3) the anterior teeth have a questionable prognosis, or (4) inoperable lingual tori restrict the placement of the inferior border of the major connector.

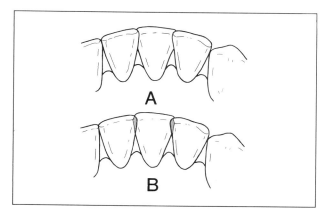

Fig. 10.1-11 When a linguoplate is selected, the mesial and distal incisal corners of overlapping anterior teeth (A) should be recontoured to eliminate excessive undercuts below the contact points (B).

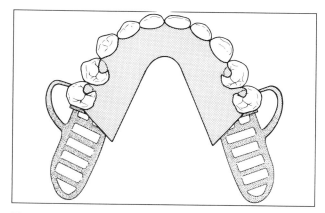

Fig. 10.1-12 Linguoplating may extend posteriorly to include the premolars if (1) the lingual vestibule is shallow, (2) inoperable tori are present, or (3) severe lingual tooth or tissue undercuts interfere with positioning of the lingual bar.

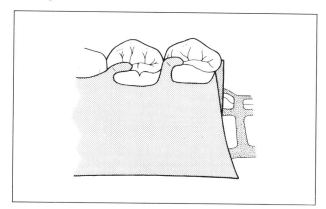

Fig. 10.1-13a Lingual view of the linguoplate extending posterior to the terminal rest.

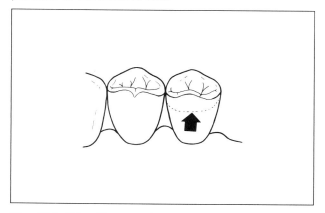

Fig. 10.1-13b The metal must end exactly at the survey line (arrow). If the plating extends above the height of contour, it will preempt the mesial rest during tissue-ward movement of the extension base.

Minor connectors

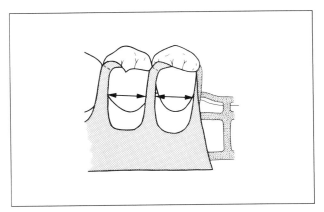

Fig. 10.1-14 Minor connectors that join rests to major connectors should be positioned in embrasures and form right angles at the junctions with the major connector. Whenever possible, at least 4 mm of space *(arrows)* should be present between adjacent vertical minor connectors.

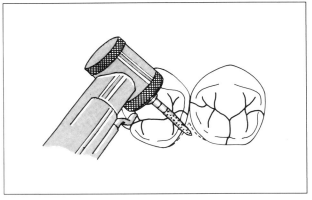

Fig. 10.1-15a If the occlusion limits access where the rest and minor connector join, the occlusolingual aspect of the embrasure area should be enlarged.

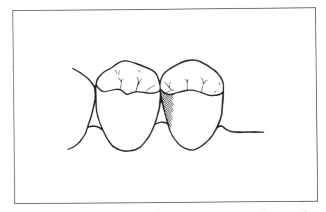

Fig. 10.1-15b A small guide surface preparation on the mesiolingual aspect of the primary abutment may produce guide surface–minor connector contact and aid in determining a precise path of insertion/dislodgement.

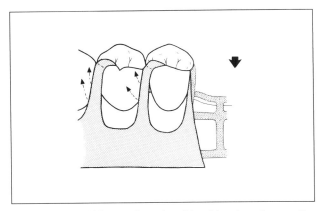

Fig. 10.1-16 When a functional load is placed on a distal extension area, the prosthesis rotates around the primary rest and the minor connectors move upward and mesially. The mesial aspects of the minor connectors should be physiologically relieved at the framework try-in.

Retentive arms

Ideally, the tips of retentive arms should release during functional movement of the extension base. If this is not possible, stressbreaking should be achieved with flexible arms (wrought wire or long, tapered bar clasps). When the contours of the abutments preclude both of these options, consider placing a crown on the abutment—depending on existing or needed restorations and the compromise in clasping that would be necessary if the crown were not fabricated.

Preference for clasp assemblies for terminal abutments on distal extension RPDs is generally as follows: *(1)* I-bar with mesial rest, *(2)* modified T-bar with mesial rest, *(3)* combination clasp with distal rest, and *(4)* half-and-half clasp with distal rest or circumferential embrasure clasp with mesial rest.

Infrabulge clasps are contraindicated when there is a large tissue undercut below the abutment, when a high frenal attachment or shallow vestibule interferes with the approach arm, when periodontal considerations preclude crossing the gingival margin with a clasp arm, or when esthetics are compromised by visibility of a bar clasp crossing gingival tissue.

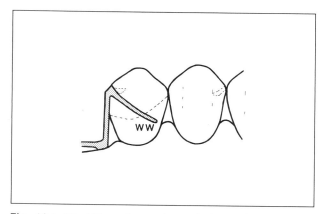

Fig. 10.1-18 When the undercut is located on the mesiofacial surface and a bar clasp is contraindicated, the combination of a *wrought wire (WW)* retentive arm and a cast lingual bracing arm should be selected. A distal rest is used because the originating portion of the arm lies above the height of contour and would preempt a mesial rest. Although the clasp will not release during functional movements of the extension base, it will flex and provide some stress relief for the abutment. A distal rest and a wrought wire circumferential clasp are also preferred if the abutment inclines mesially. Here, the entire guide plate lies above the height of contour and will preempt the mesial rest. Relieving the guide plate would result in a space between it and the occlusal aspect of the proximal tooth surface. If a distal rest is used, only the lower portion of the guide plate is relieved.

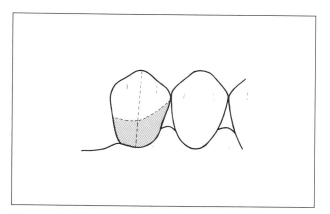

Fig. 10.1-17a When the undercut is located on the mesiofacial surface, the preferred clasp assembly is composed of an I-bar, a mesial rest, and a distal guide plate.

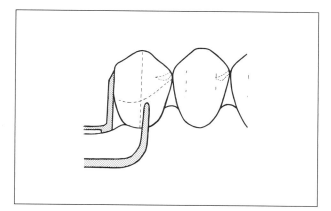

Fig. 10.1-17b In order to ensure retention, the I-bar should be placed just in front of the greatest mesiodistal curvature of the facial surface.

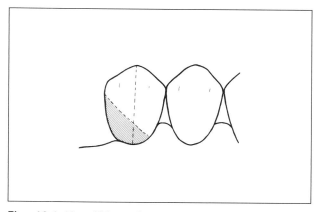

Fig. 10.1-19a When the undercut is located on the distofacial surface, the preferred clasp assembly is composed of a modified T-bar, a mesial rest, and a distal guide plate.

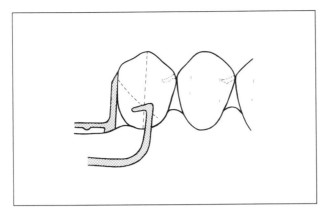

Fig. 10.1-19b The vertical portion of the bar clasp should be located just in front of the greatest mesiodistal portion of the facial surface.

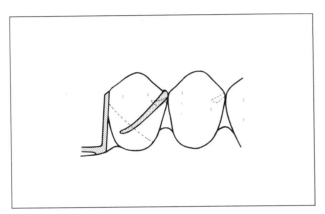

Fig. 10.1-20 When the undercut is located on the distofacial surface and a bar clasp is contraindicated, a circumferential embrasure clasp may be used with a mesial rest. Although the mechanics of the situation are not ideal with either a mesial or a distal rest, the mesial rest is preferred because the tendency for the originating portion of the arm to push the tooth lingually during functional movements of the extension base is resisted by the minor connector and the lingual portion of the distal guide plate. With a distal rest, the retentive tip would move upward and forward, torquing the abutment.

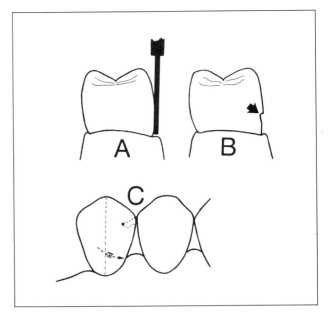

Fig. 10.1-21 If the facial surface exhibits no undercut but is parallel or nearly parallel to the path of insertion/dislodgement (A), an undercut for an I-bar may be created in the enamel (B, arrow). The retentive groove should be located just ahead of the greatest mesiodistal curvature of the facial surface and should duplicate the path the I-bar will follow during functional movements of the extension base (C). When a bar clasp is contraindicated, a mesiofacial undercut may be created and engaged by a wrought wire circumferential clasp. Because the originating portion of the arm will be above the height of contour (and act like a rest), the primary rest should be placed in the distal fossa.

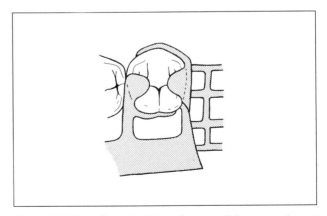

Fig. 10.1-22a If the facial surface exhibits no undercut and is not close to being parallel to the path of insertion/dislodgement, a lingual undercut is almost always present. A half-and-half clasp assembly, composed of mesial and distal rests, a facial bracing arm, and a lingual retentive arm, may be used.

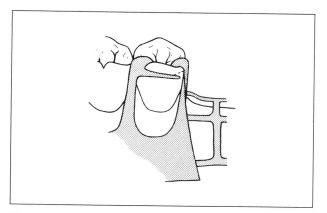

Fig. 10.1-22b The lingual retentive arm originates from the minor connector and engages a distolingual undercut.

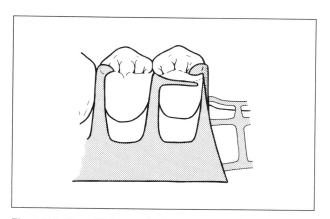

Fig. 10.1-22c If the occlusion prevents placement of a mesial rest on the second premolar, it may be moved forward. Although an additional minor connector is required, the effectiveness of the indirect retainer improves.

Denture base retentive elements/replacement teeth

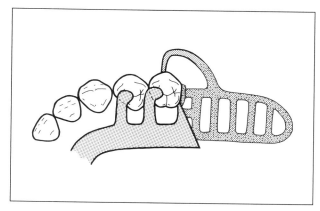

Fig. 10.1-23 Open latticework is the preferred type of denture base retentive element because the attachment of the plastic is stronger. The latticework for a mandibular distal extension RPD should extend approximately two thirds of the distance to the retromolar pad.

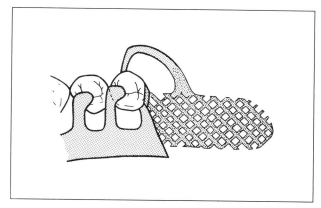

Fig. 10.1-24 Mesh is preferred over latticework when vertical space is limited. It covers approximately the same area as latticework but is generally much thinner. When vertical space is severely restricted, a metal base may be used. However, adjustment is difficult and relining is impossible.

Case 10.2

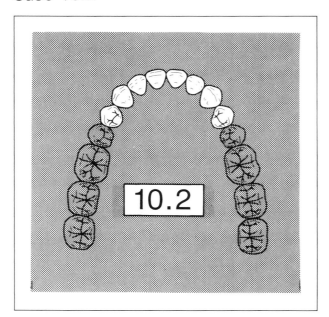

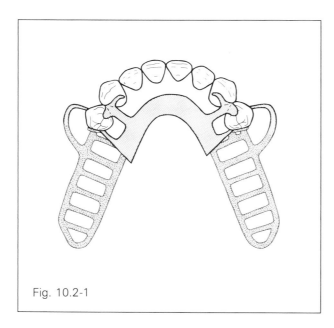

Fig. 10.2-1

Rests

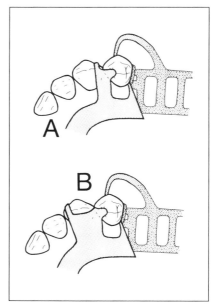

Fig. 10.2-2 The primary rest is almost always placed on the mesio-occlusal fossa of the first premolar. The opposing occlusion seldom interferes with this location. A cingulum rest on the canine is the indirect retainer of choice because it applies stresses at a more gingival level and is superior esthetically. However, a distoincisal (A) or mesioincisal (B) indirect retainer should be selected if the lingual surface of the tooth slopes severely and does not exhibit a definite cingulum. The mesial location slightly improves the efficiency of the indirect retainer but is also more visible. The lingual surface of the canine is usually plated when a mesioincisal rest is used. Uncovering the lingual surface creates a small opening that tends to act as a repository for food and plaque. When the slope of the lingual surface is excessively steep and esthetic considerations preclude the use of an incisal rest, a restoration should be placed to create a definite cingulum rest seat.

Guide plates

Refer to case 10.1.

Major connector

The considerations and options for the major connector are essentially the same as those described for case 10.1. However, there is a slightly greater tendency to use linguoplating for indirect retention.

When plating is selected, cingulum or incisal rest seats and rests should be placed at least on the canines.

Major connectors

Refer to case 10.1.

Retentive arms

The clasp assembly options for the first premolars of case 10.2 are essentially the same as those for the second premolars of case 10.1.

Denture base retentive elements/replacement teeth

Refer to case 10.1.

Case 10.3

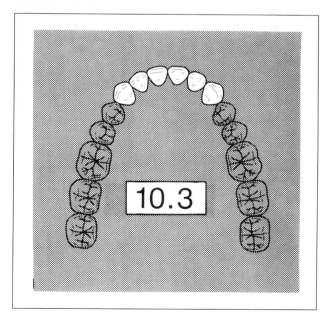

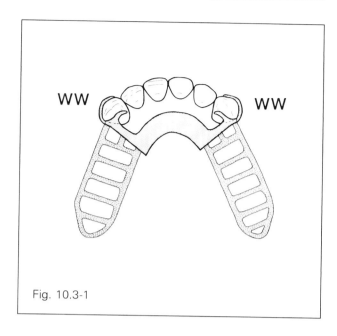

Fig. 10.3-1

Rests

Because the rests on the canines are primary rests, it is imperative that adequate rest seats be prepared. If the slopes of the lingual surfaces are too steep for cingulum rest seats, and incisal rests are contraindicated because of esthetic demands, restorations should be placed to produce the required cingulum rest seats.

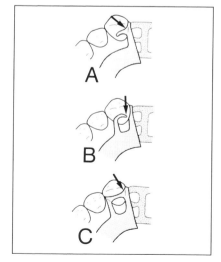

Fig. 10.3-2 A cingulum rest may originate from the distal guide plate (A), or a mesial minor connector (B), or may take the form of a strap connecting the guide plate

and the minor connector (C). It is important to realize, however, that the axis of rotation will pass through the most distal portion of the rests *(arrows)* regardless of their points of origin. Because each functions as a distal rest, the form shown in (A) is generally preferred because it is more hygienic.

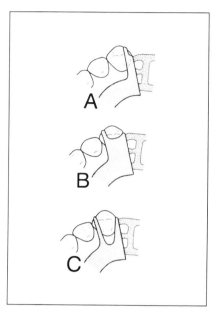

Fig. 10.3-3 Incisal rests may be selected if the lingual surface of the canine is not conducive to placement of a cingulum rest and if metal display is not an important consideration. Distoincisal rest (A); mesioincisal rest with plating on the canine (B); mesioincisal rest without plating on the canine (C). Note that in B, the axis of rotation would pass through the most posterior portion of the plating. Thus, the mesioincisal rest would be preempted during functional motion of the extension base. Only the incisal rest in C would truly function as a mesial rest. Unfortunately, this design would also create a small opening that would be prone to food and plaque accumulation.

Guide plates

When only the anterior teeth remain, the contact of guide surfaces and guide plates seldom, if ever, establish a definite path of insertion/dislodgement, even if mesial minor connectors or linguoplating are used. Guide surfaces are generally so limited in size and number that there is insufficient contact with guide plates to establish a distinct path.

Major connector

It is very difficult to select an "ideal" major connector for this case. A lingual bar is open and may be more hygienic, but it provides no indirect retention. A linguoplate provides indirect retention but may reduce gingival stimulation and promote plaque accumulation.

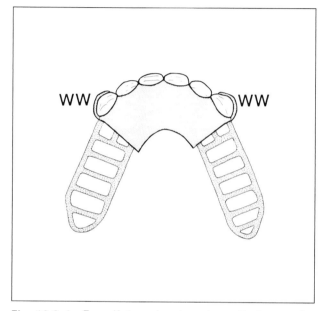

Fig. 10.3-4 Even if there is adequate vertical space for a lingual bar, a linquoplate is frequently selected when only the anterior teeth remain. Although there is some question as to whether a linguoplate can actually stabilize periodontally weakened teeth, it most certainly provides indirect retention and bracing and creates the possibility of adding artificial teeth to the RPD if one or more of the natural teeth are subsequently lost. Rest seats must always be prepared on the canines and, whenever tooth contours permit, should also be placed on the incisors.

Minor connectors

Refer to case 10.1.

Retentive arms

Because almost all vertical stops on anterior teeth are functionally distal rests, retentive tips will not release during tissueward movement of the extension bases. Instead, they will move upward and engage the teeth. In order to limit torquing stresses, circumferential wrought wire or long, tapered bar clasps should be selected to increase retentive arm flexibility. In addition, functional movement of the extension bases should be minimized by periodic relining or rebasing.

Because tissue undercuts below the canines often preclude the use of bar clasps, a wrought wire circumferential clasp is more commonly selected when a mesiofacial undercut is present. If the only available undercut is located on the distofacial surface, a modified T-bar may be used unless an infrabulge clasp is contraindicated, in which case the tooth would need to be altered by recontouring or placing a restoration to create a mesiofacial undercut for a wrought wire circumferential clasp.

Figs. 10.3-5a to c Wrought wire circumferential and cast I-bar retentive arms may be used to engage mesiofacial undercuts on mandibular canines. Because it is almost impossible for guide surface/guide plate contacts to dictate a precise path of insertion/dislodgement, tips of retentive arms must be placed just in front of the greatest mesiodistal curvature of the facial surface.

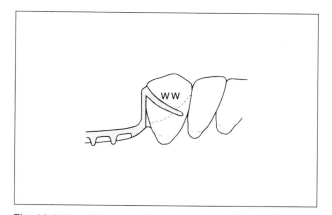

Fig. 10.3-5a   Wrought wire circumferential retentive arm.

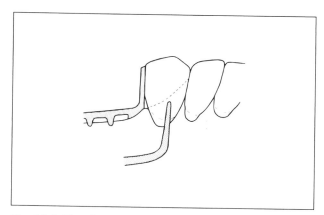

Fig. 10.3-5b   Cast I-bar retentive arm.

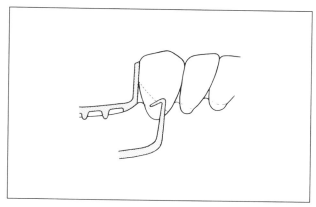

Fig. 10.3-5c   If a modified T-bar is used to engage a distofacial undercut, the approach arm should be located just mesially to the greatest mesiodistal curvature.

Denture base retentive elements/replacement teeth

Refer to case 10.1.

Case 10.4

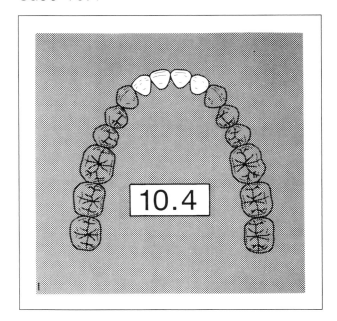

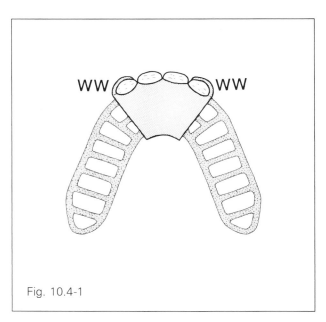

Fig. 10.4-1

With the exceptions noted below, the design principles for case 10.4 are essentially the same as those for case 10.3. However, when only the incisors remain, the long-term prognosis is poor except possibly in the unusual situation where the periodontal support is exceptionally favorable. A fixed splint may improve the prognosis, but should not be considered a panacea for periodontally weakened teeth. Joining together hopeless teeth results in a hopeless splint. If the teeth are relatively sound and cast restorations are fabricated, definite rest seats should be included on all four teeth.

Philosophically, the RPD should be considered "a complete denture with a few teeth remaining." If the prognosis of the remaining teeth is questionable, a complete overdenture should be considered.

Rests

Rest seats under the linguoplating must be prepared on the lateral incisors and should be prepared on all four teeth if possible.

Guide plates

Refer to case 10.3.

Major connector

A linguoplate major connector is almost always used. The double lingual bar may be indicated if large interproximal spaces make the plating visible from the labial aspect. However, sufficient vertical height for a lingual bar (7 to 8 mm) must be present between the marginal gingiva and the floor of the mouth. If less than 7 mm is present, a linguoplate must be selected regardless of esthetic shortcomings.

Minor connectors

Refer to case 10.1.

Retentive arms

Retentive arms should be flexible and engage minimal undercuts (small-diameter wrought wire is usually preferred). Periodic relining or rebasing for maximum residual ridge support is essential.

Denture base retentive elements/replacement teeth

Refer to case 10.1.

Case 10.5

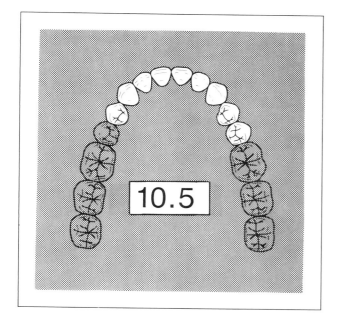

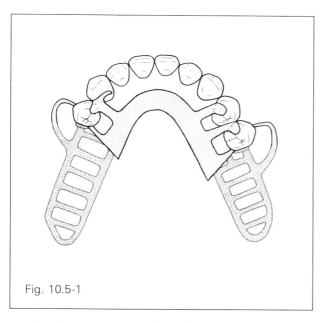

Fig. 10.5-1

For design concepts and variations, refer to case 10.1 for the right side and case 10.2 for the left side.

Case 10.6

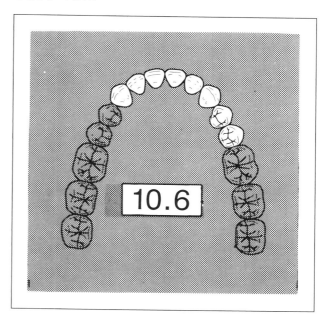

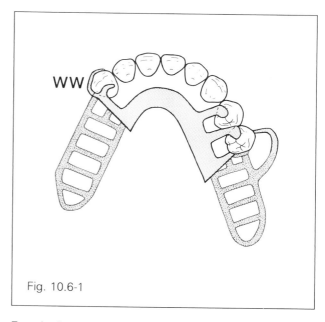

Fig. 10.6-1

For design concepts and variations, refer to case 10.1 for the right side and case 10.3 for the left side.

Case 10.7

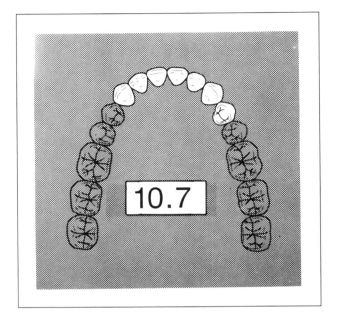

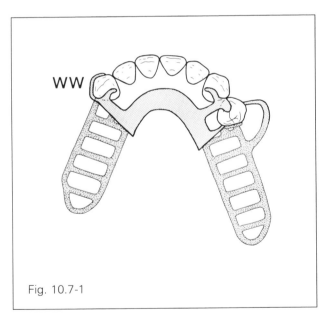

Fig. 10.7-1

For design concepts and variations, refer to case 10.2 for the right side and case 10.3 for the left side.

Case 10.8

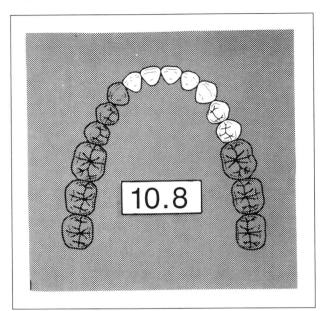

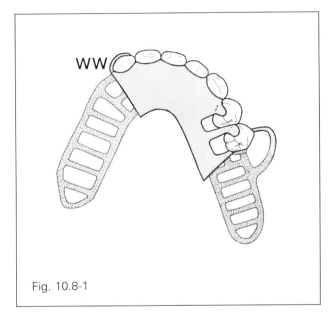

Fig. 10.8-1

For design concepts and variations other than those discussed below, refer to case 10.1 for the right side and case 10.4 for the left side.

Rests

An indirect retainer is usually located in the mesial fossa of the first premolar because it provides a good vertical stop yet seldom interferes with the opposing occlusion. However, the rest on the premolar may be omitted if an acceptable rest seat and rest can be placed on the canine.

On the left side, a rest preparation must be provided under the linguoplating *at least* on the lateral incisor. A restoration may need to be placed to create an acceptable rest seat.

Major connector

A lingual bar major connector may be selected in the rare instance when the periodontal support for the lateral incisor is exceptionally good. In this instance, the rest seat on the lateral incisor must be ideally shaped; a restoration will often be required.

Case 10.9

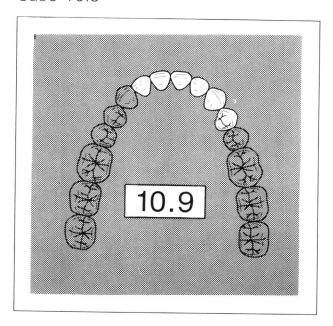

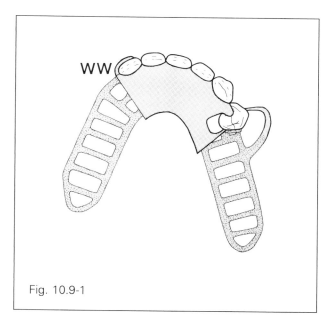

Fig. 10.9-1

For design concepts and variations, refer to case 10.2 for the right side and cases 10.8 and 10.4 for the left side.

Case 10.10

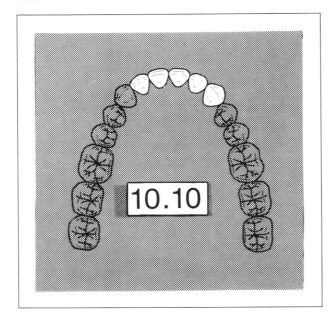

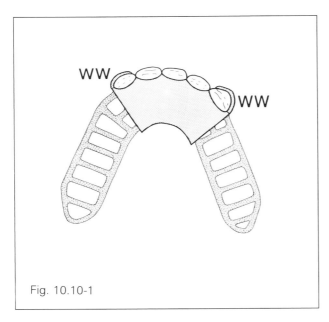

Fig. 10.10-1

For design concepts and variations refer to case 10.3 for the right side and cases 10.8 and 10.4 for the left side.

Case 10.11

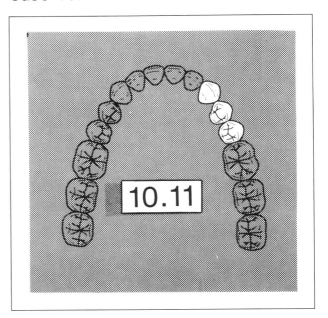

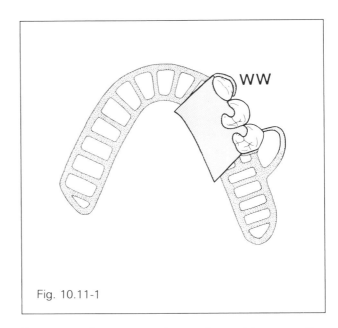

Fig. 10.11-1

Because only three teeth remain, and because the teeth are adjacent to each other, this RPD should almost be regarded as a complete denture. If the teeth have a questionable periodontal prognosis, a complete overdenture should be considered.

Rests

A rest seat must be included beneath the plating on the canine.

Guide plates

Guide surface–guide plate contacts must allow for extensive functional movement without torquing the abutments. Thus, physiologic relief at the framework try-in is extremely important.

Major connector

Linguoplating would almost always be used on the remaining teeth.

Minor connectors

If linguoplating is not used, refer to case 10.1.

Retentive arms

Because of the extensive functional movements possible, there are several choices for the design of clasp arms. It seems reasonable that the retentive arms should not rigidly engage the abutments. Thus the I-bar in Fig. 10.11-1 should be long, tapered, and flexible. The wrought wire clasp should be of small diameter. Another option would be to use cast labial circumferential arms on both the canine and the premolar. Such arms would be located completely above the height of contour and would provide stabilization in the horizontal plane, but no retention. The patient would control the prosthesis with cheeks, lips, and tongue, just as he or she would control a complete denture.

Denture base retentive elements/replacement teeth

Refer to case 10.1.

Case 10.12

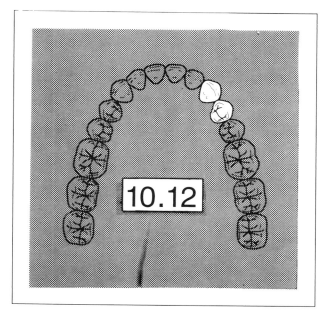

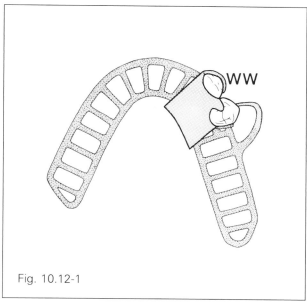

Fig. 10.12-1

The design considerations for case 10.12 are the same as those for case 10.11. With only two teeth remaining, the tendency to select a complete overdenture is even greater. An RPD should be planned only if the periodontal status of the remaining teeth is exceptionally good, or if the RPD is considered transitional to facilitate patient adaptation to a removable prosthesis.

Case 10.13

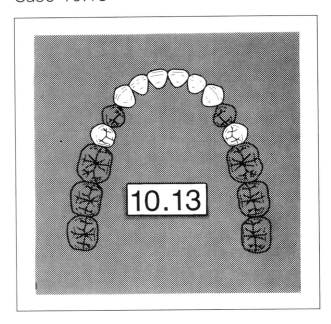

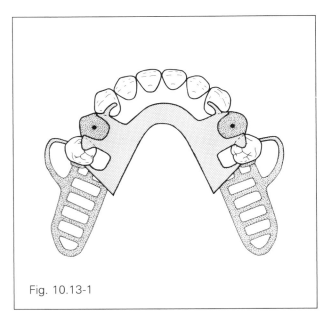

Fig. 10.13-1

Rests

The location of rests on the second premolars depends on the type of retentive arms selected, and is discussed in case 10.1. Either cingulum or incisal rests may be placed on the canines (refer to Figs. 10.3-2 and 10.3-3).

Guide plates

With the first premolars missing, six guide surface–guide plate contact areas exist, and a definite path of insertion/dislodgement can be established. However, "locking" of the lone-standing abutments between the mesial and distal guide plates will transfer torquing forces during functional movements of the extension bases and must be prevented by physiologically relieving the guide plates at the framework try-in.

Major connector

Refer to case 10.1.

Minor connectors

Refer to case 10.1.

Retentive arms

The options and rationale for clasp assemblies on the premolars are the same as those described for case 10.1. However, because the mesial guide plates prevent distal displacement, it is not essential that bar clasps be positioned anteriorly to the greatest mesiodistal curvature of the facial surface.

Denture base retentive elements/replacement teeth

In addition to the tube teeth shown in Fig. 10.13-1, the first premolars may be replaced by heat-cured or light-activated resin, or by denture teeth attached via denture base and retentive network. The last option is more commonly selected when there is an incompletely healed residual ridge, when there is a defect in the contour of the residual ridge, or when the space is wider than that of a normal premolar. Refer also to case 10.1.

Case 10.14

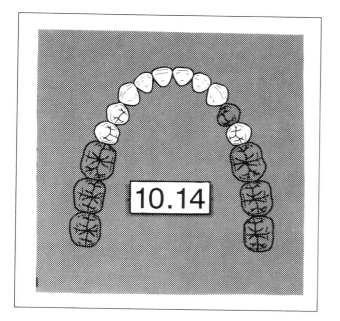

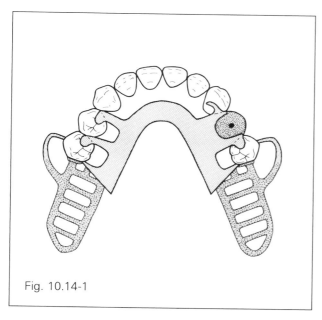

Fig. 10.14-1

For design concepts and variations, refer to case 10.13 for the right side and case 10.1 for the left side.

Case 10.15

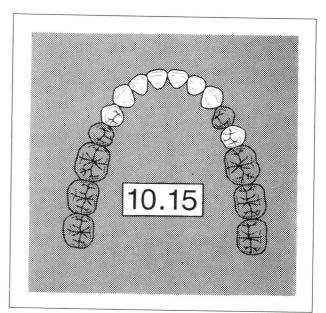

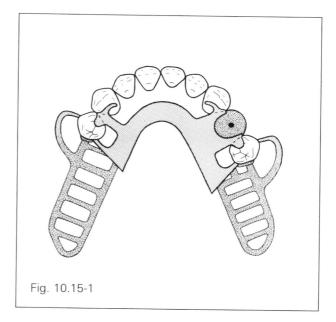

Fig. 10.15-1

For design concepts and variations, refer to case 10.13 for the right side and case 10.2 for the left side.

Case 10.16

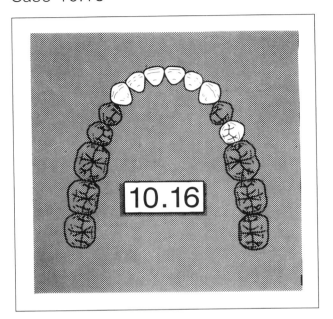

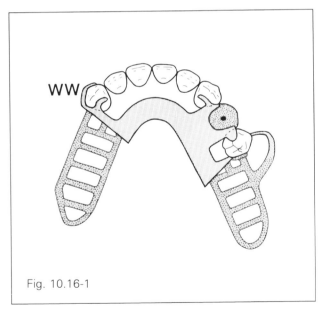

Fig. 10.16-1

Case 10.17

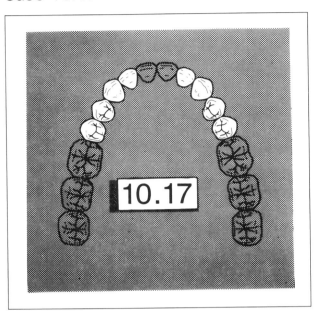

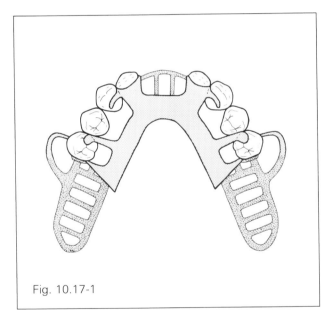

Fig. 10.17-1

For design concepts and variations, refer to case 10.13 for the right side and case 10.3 for the left side.

The design for case 10.17 is essentially the same as that for case 10.1, with a two-tooth anterior modification space. Changes necessitated by the modification space are considered below. Refer to case 10.1 for discussion of the other aspects of the design.

Rests

Because it is frequently difficult to prepare rest seats on the lateral incisors, vertical stops for the anterior segment are usually placed on the canines. In the rare instance when the lateral incisors have exceptionally good bone support and prominent cinguli, rests may be placed on the lateral incisors rather than on the canines.

Because the anterior rests are very effective indirect retainers, mesial rests on the first premolars can be omitted.

Guide plates

Guide plates on the lateral incisors must be located on the mesiolingual surfaces so that they will not be visible or interfere with placement of the central incisors.

Retentive arms

The options for clasp assemblies on the second premolars are the same as in case 10.1. Clasps on the lateral incisors or canines would be unesthetic, and would lie in front of the axis of rotation. They should ordinarily be omitted.

Denture base retentive elements/replacement teeth

The central incisors would most commonly be replaced by denture teeth via retentive network and denture base. However, if the residual ridge is well-healed and exhibits little resorption, and if the width of the space is appropriate for the two missing teeth, acceptable alternatives are facings, tube teeth, or heat-cured or light-activated resins.

Case 10.18

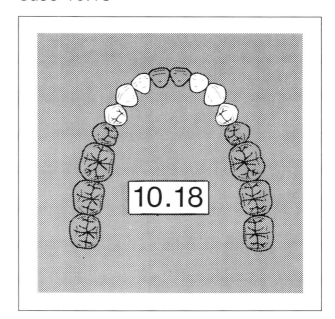

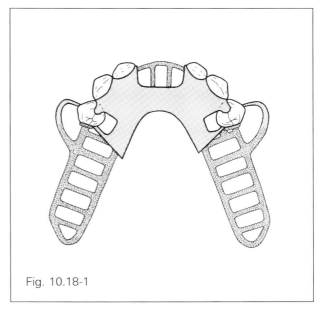

Fig. 10.18-1

For design concepts and variations, refer to case 10.17 for the anterior segment and case 10.2 for the remainder of the design.

Case 10.19

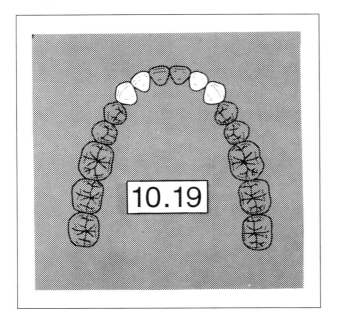

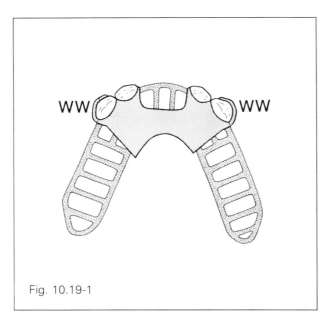

Fig. 10.19-1

Case 10.20

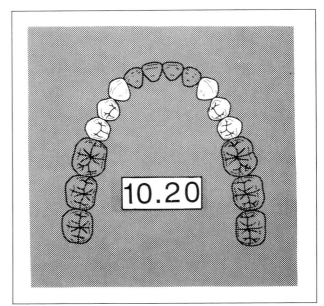

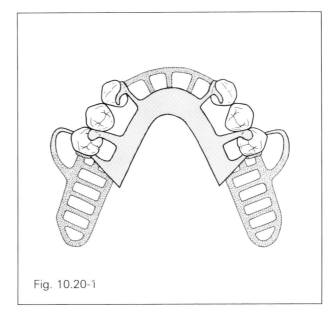

Fig. 10.20-1

For design concepts and variations, refer to case 10.17 for the anterior segment and case 10.3 for the remainder of the design.

The design for case 10.20 is essentially the same as that for case 10.1, with a four-tooth anterior modification space. Changes necessitated by the modification space are discussed below. Refer to case 10.1 for other aspects of the design.

Rests

Because the rests on the canines are very effective indirect retainers, rests on the first premolars are unnecessary.

Figs. 10.20-2a and b Mesial or distal incisal rests on the canines are indicated if steep lingual slopes preclude the use of cingulum rests.

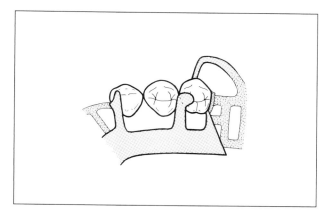

Fig. 10.20-2a

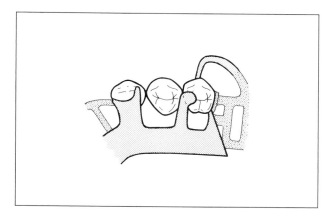

Fig. 10.20-2b

Guide plates

The anterior guide plates should be located on the linguoproximal surfaces of the canines so that they will not be visible or interfere with placement of the denture teeth.

Retentive arms

The options for clasp assemblies for the second premolars are the same as in case 10.1. Clasps on the canines would lie in front of the axis of rotation, may be esthetically displeasing, and should ordinarily be omitted. If retentive arms are placed on the canines, they should be flexible and engage minimal undercuts.

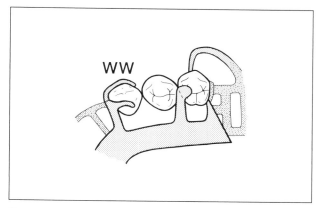

Fig. 10.20-3a Wrought wire circumferential clasp engaging a distofacial undercut. Such clasps often create a significant compromise in the overall esthetic value of the RPD.

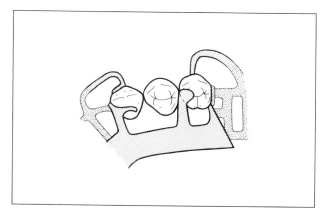

Fig. 10.20-3b Modified T-bar clasp engaging a mesiofacial undercut. The use of bar clasps on canines is often contraindicated by tissue undercuts. In addition, the length of bar clasps in this location may not be great enough to ensure sufficient flexibility.

Denture base retentive elements/replacement teeth

With all four incisors missing, replacement is almost always accomplished with denture teeth, retentive network, and denture base. Prefabricated, heat-cured, or light-activated resin facings should only be considered if the residual ridge is well-healed and exhibits very little resorption. In addition, because modification of the tooth arrangement by the dentist at or subsequent to the try-in is nearly impossible, the width of the space must be almost perfectly suited to the width of the four replacement teeth.

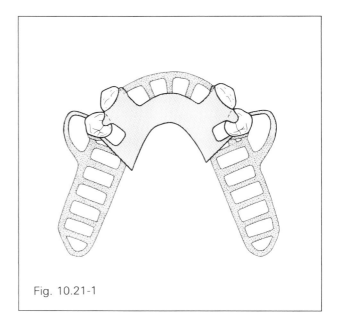

Fig. 10.21-1

For design concepts and variations, refer to case 10.20 for the anterior segment and case 10.2 for the remainder of the design.

Case 10.21

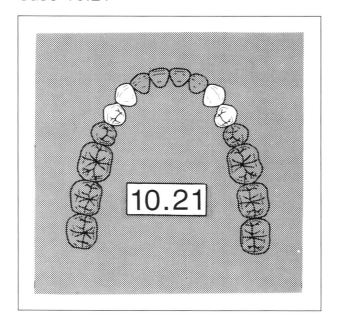

Case 10.22

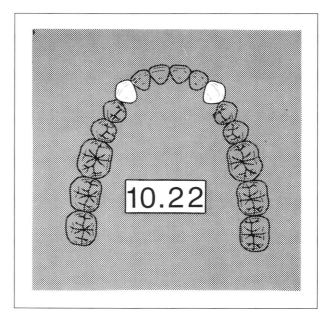

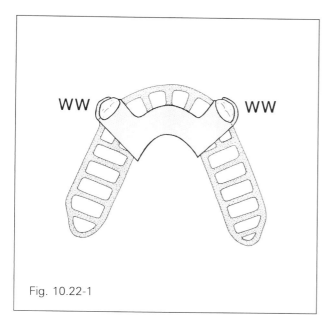

Fig. 10.22-1

With only the two canines remaining, a complete overdenture should receive serious consideration, particularly if the periodontal status is compromised. An RPD may be selected if bone support and residual ridge contour are optimal, or if the partial denture is to be considered transitional to facilitate patient adaptation to a removable prosthesis.

The mesial and distal guide plates must not "lock" onto the abutments during functional movements of the denture bases. Physiologic relief of the guide plates at the framework try-in is essential.

Retentive arm options are the same as those discussed for case 10.3.

Case 10.23

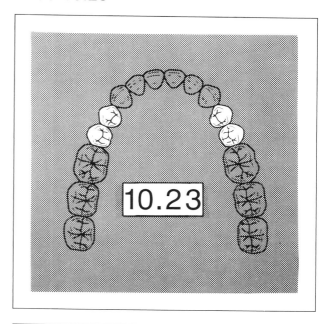

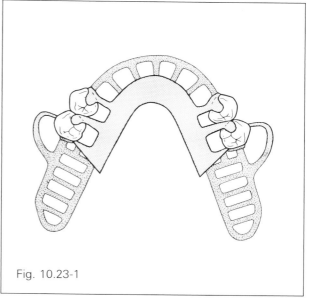

Fig. 10.23-1

The design for case 10.23 is related to that of case 10.1. However, without the canines present, the RPD can be considered as having both anterior and posterior extension areas.

The potential for tissueward movement of *both* the posterior *and* the anterior segments creates significant clasping problems, because no type of retentive arm will release with both types of movement. Thus, retentive arms should be tapered and flexible. Whenever possible, muscular control by the patient is preferred over mechanical retention. The prosthesis is then regarded as a "complete denture," where the four remaining teeth provide horizontal stabilization. Cast buccal arms located *above the height of contour* can be used to facilitate this bracing action.

Case 10.24

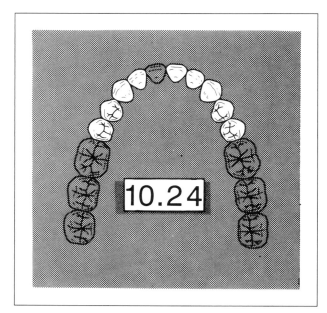

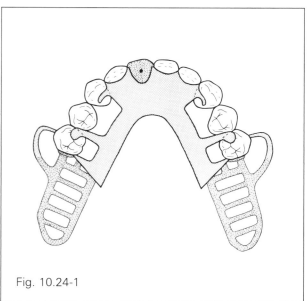

Fig. 10.24-1

The design for case 10.24 is essentially the same as that for case 10.1 with a single-tooth anterior modification space. Changes necessitated by the modification space are considered below. Refer to case 10.1 for discussion of other aspects of the design.

Rests

Because it is often difficult to prepare adequate rest seats on the incisors, vertical stops for the anterior segment are usually placed on the canines. If the teeth next to the modification space exhibit exceptionally good bone support and prominent cinguli, rest seats and rests may be placed on the incisors rather than the canines, and linguoplating of the anterior segment can be eliminated.

The anterior rests are very effective indirect retainers; therefore, mesial rests on the first premolars are usually omitted.

Guide plates

Anterior guide plates must be located on linguoproximal surfaces so that they will not be visible from the labial aspect or interfere with positioning the replacement teeth.

Major connector

If rest seats and rests are placed on incisors rather than canines, linguoplating of the anterior segment can be eliminated.

Retentive arms

The options for clasp assemblies for the second premolars are the same as those for case 10.1. Clasps on the anterior abutments would be unesthetic and lie in front of the axis of rotation; they are rarely, if ever, indicated.

Denture base retentive elements/replacement teeth

With only one tooth in the modification space, a prefabricated facing, a tube tooth, or a custom heat-cured or light-activated resin replacement is almost always used.

Case 10.25

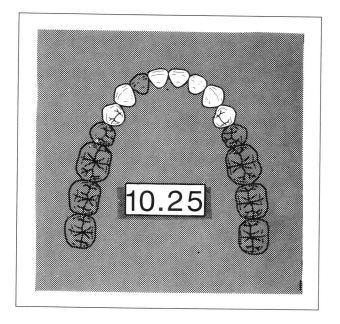

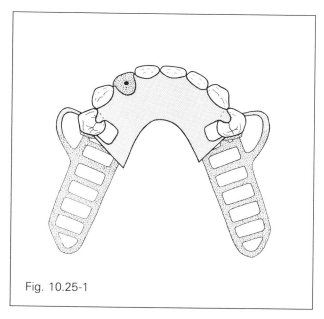

Fig. 10.25-1

The design for case 10.25 is essentially the same as that for case 10.2, with a single-tooth anterior modification space. Changes necessitated by the modification space are considered below. Refer to case 10.2 for discussion of other aspects of the design.

Rests

Rest seats under the linguoplating should be placed on both canines. If the central incisor adjacent to the modification space is periodontally sound and properly shaped, a rest seat and rest may be placed on it and the linguoplating omitted.

Guide plates

Anterior guide plates must be located on linguoproximal surfaces so that they will not be visible from the labial aspect or interfere with positioning the artificial teeth.

Major connector

If an adequate rest seat and rest can be placed on the central incisor, liguoplating of the anterior segment can be omitted.

Retentive arms

The options for clasp assemblies on the first premolars are the same as in case 10.2. Clasps on anterior teeth would be unesthetic and lie in front of the axis of rotation; they are rarely, if ever, indicated.

Denture base retentive elements/replacement teeth

With only one tooth in the modification space, a prefabricated facing, a tube tooth, or a custom heat-cured or light-activated resin replacement is almost always used.

Case 10.26

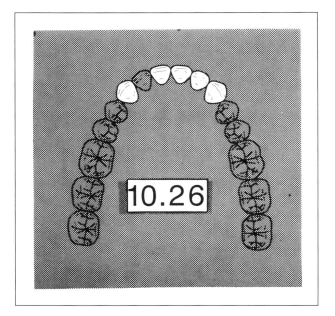

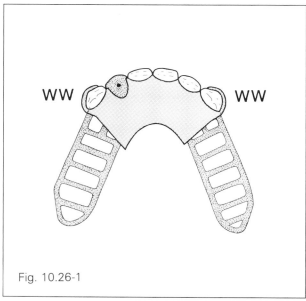

Fig. 10.26-1

Case 10.27

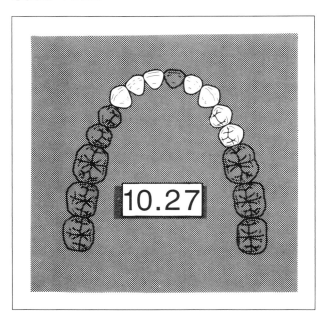

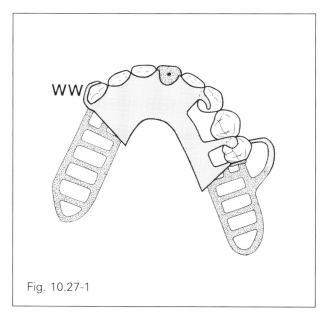

Fig. 10.27-1

The design for case 10.26 is essentially the same as that for case 10.3, with a single-tooth anterior modification space. Changes necessitated by the modification space are similar to those discussed for case 10.25, except that with only five anterior teeth remaining a linguoplate major connector is more commonly selected. Refer to cases 10.3 and 10.25 for further design concepts and variations.

For design concepts and variations, refer to case 10.24 for the anterior segment and case 10.6 for the remainder of the design.

Case 10.28

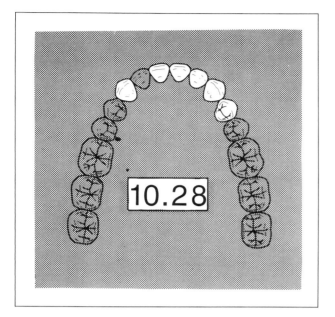

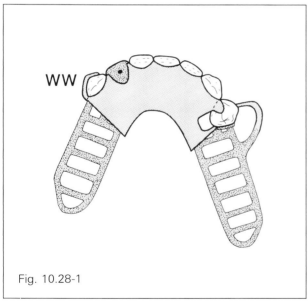

Fig. 10.28-1

For design concepts and variations, refer to case 10.26 for the anterior segment and case 10.7 for the remainder of the design.

Case 10.29

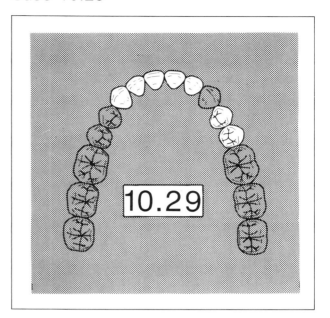

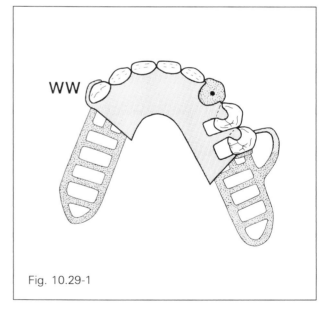

Fig. 10.29-1

The design for case 10.29 is similar to that for case 10.6. Alterations necessitated by the missing canine are discussed below.

Rests

If possible, a rest seat should be placed on the lateral incisor adjacent to the modification space. There is, of course, a rest seat beneath the plating on the remaining canine.

Guide plates

The guide plate on the lateral incisor should be located on the linguoproximal surface so that it will not be visible from the labial aspect or interfere with positioning of the artificial tooth. The labial aspect of the guide plate on the first premolar may also need to be reduced because of esthetic considerations.

Major connector

The missing canine greatly increases the tendency for linguoplating. However, if the lateral incisor exhibits excellent bone support and possesses the lingual contour necessary for placing an adequate cingulum rest, a lingual bar may be selected.

Retentive arms

The clasp assembly options for the posterior abutments are the same as in case 10.6. Clasps on the lateral incisor and first premolar would be unesthetic and lie in front of the axis of rotation; they are rarely, if ever, indicated.

Denture base retentive elements/replacement teeth

With only one tooth in the modification space, a prefabricated facing, a tube tooth, or a custom heat-cured or light-activated resin replacement is almost always selected.

Case 10.30

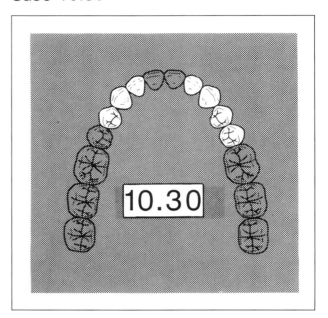

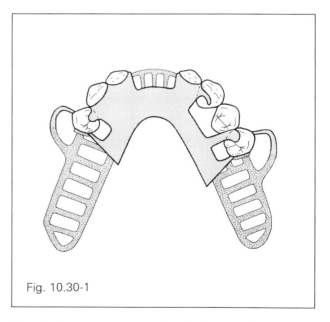

Fig. 10.30-1

For design concepts and variations, refer to case 10.17 for the anterior segment and case 10.5 for the remainder of the design.

Case 10.31

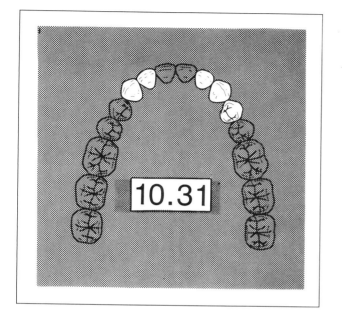

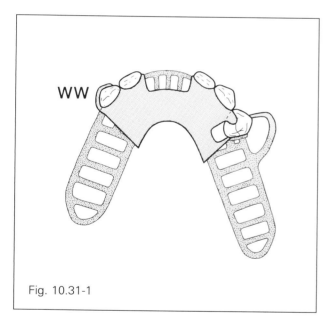

Fig. 10.31-1

Case 10.32

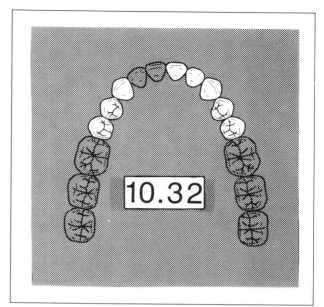

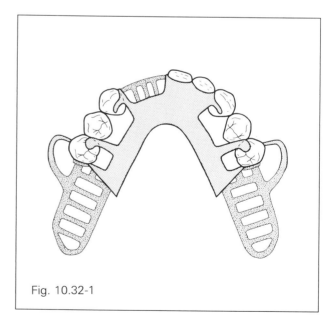

Fig. 10.32-1

For design concepts and variations, refer to case 10.17 for the anterior segment and case 10.7 for the remainder of the design.

The design for case 10.32 is similar to that for case 10.1, with a two-tooth anterior modification space. The changes necessitated by the modification space are discussed below.

Rests

Rest seats should be placed on the incisors if the lingual contours of the teeth are appropriate. Because the rests on the canines and the plating provide indirect retention, mesial rests on the first premolars can be omitted. If the central incisor is periodontally sound and properly shaped, a rest seat and rest may be placed on it and the linguoplating omitted.

Guide plates

Anterior guide plates should be located on linguoproximal surfaces so that they will not be visible from the labial aspect or interfere with positioning the replacement teeth.

Major connector

Although linguoplating would most commonly be used, a lingual bar may be selected if the central incisor is capable of supporting an adequate rest.

Retentive arms

Options for retention on the premolars are the same as in case 10.1. Clasps on anterior teeth would be unesthetic and lie in front of the axis of rotation; they are rarely, if ever, indicated.

Denture base retentive elements/replacement teeth

The central and lateral incisors would most commonly be replaced by denture teeth via retentive network and denture base. However, if the residual ridge is well-healed and exhibits little resorption, and if the width of the space is appropriate for the two missing teeth, acceptable alternatives are facings, tube teeth, or heat-cured or light-activated resin replacements.

Case 10.33

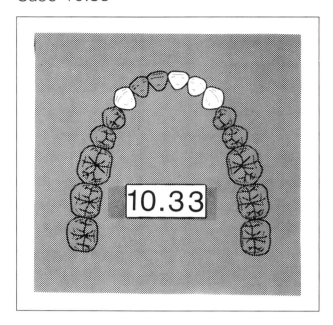

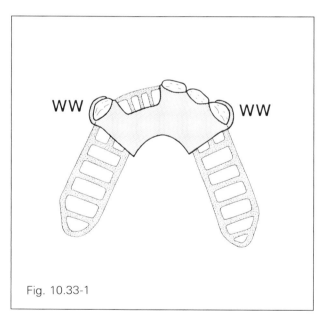

Fig. 10.33-1

For design concepts and variations, refer to case 10.32 for the anterior segment and case 10.3 for the remainder of the design. With only four teeth remaining, linguoplating would almost always be used.

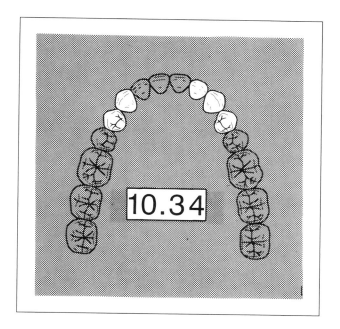

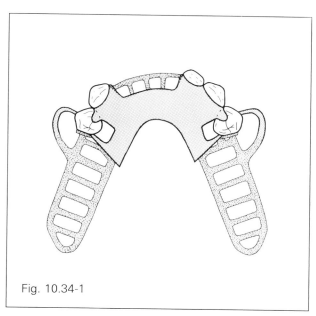

Fig. 10.34-1

The design for case 10.34 is similar to that of case 10.2, with a three-tooth anterior modification space. The changes necessitated by the modification space are discussed below.

Rests

Rest seats must be prepared for the canines and should also be prepared on the lateral incisor if the lingual contour of the tooth permits.

Guide plates

The anterior guide plates should be located on the linguoproximal surfaces so that they will not be visible from the labial aspect or interfere with positioning the replacement teeth.

Major connector

With three teeth in the modification space, linguoplating would almost always be the preferred major connector.

Retentive arms

For clasp assemblies on the premolars, refer to case 10.2. Clasps on the canine and lateral incisor would be unesthetic and lie in front of the axis of rotation; they are rarely, if ever, indicated.

Denture base retentive elements/replacement teeth

With only five teeth remaining and with three teeth in the modification space, denture teeth attached via retentive network and denture base are almost always indicated.

Case 10.35

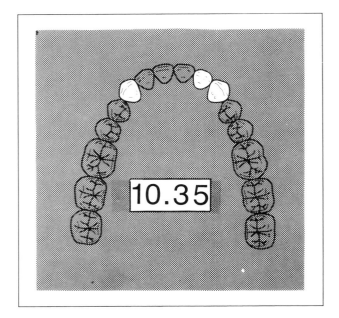

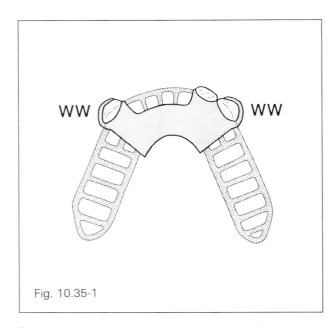

Fig. 10.35-1

Case 10.36

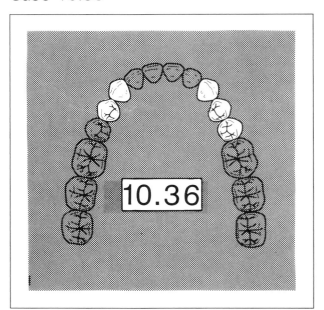

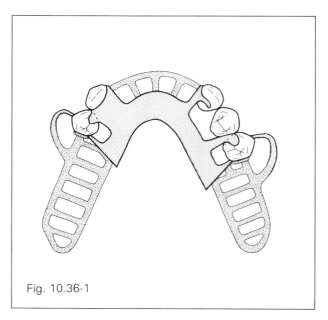

Fig. 10.36-1

For design concepts and variations, refer to case 10.34 for the anterior segment and case 10.3 for the remainder of the design. With only three teeth remaining, linguoplating would always be used.

The design for case 10.36 is similar to that for case 10.5, except for the four-tooth anterior modification space. Changes necessitated by the modification space are discussed below.

Rests

On the right side, the cingulum rest on the canine acts as an indirect retainer. Thus, a rest on the first premolar can be omitted. On the left canine, a rest seat must be placed beneath the plating. If rest seats cannot be placed on the lingual surfaces of the canines, incisal rests must be selected (refer to Fig. 10.20-2).

Guide plates

The anterior guide plates should be located on the linguoproximal surfaces so that they will not be visible from the labial aspect or interfere with positioning the replacement teeth.

Retentive arms

For retentive arms on the premolars, refer to case 10.5. Retentive arms on the canines would compromise esthetics and lie in front of the axis of rotation; they are seldom indicated. If they were used, they would have to be flexible and engage minimal undercuts.

Denture base retentive elements/replacement teeth

Due to the size of the modification space, denture teeth attached via retentive network and denture base are almost always used.

Case 10.37

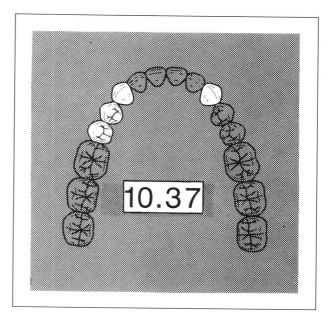

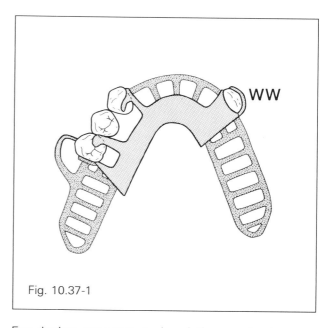

Fig. 10.37-1

For design concepts and variations, refer to case 10.36 for the anterior segment, and the mirror image of case 10.6 for the remainder of the design.

Case 10.38

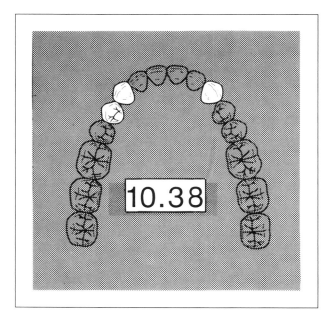

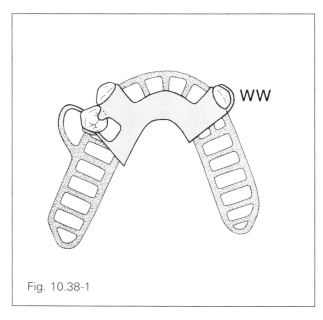

Fig. 10.38-1

Case 10.39

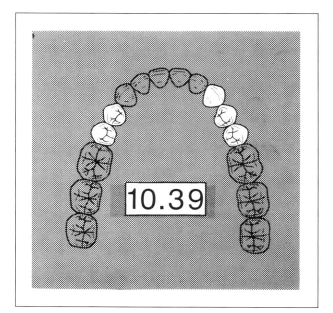

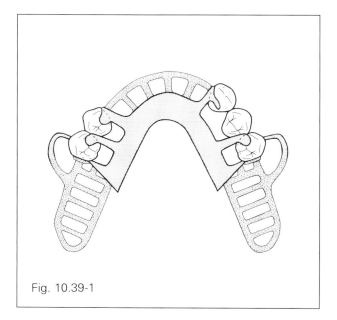

Fig. 10.39-1

For design concepts and variations, refer to case 10.36 for the anterior segment and the mirror image of case 10.7 for the remainder of the design.

The design for case 10.39 is similar to that for case 10.1, except for the very large anterior modification space. The fact that one of the canines is missing creates the tendency to view the RPD as having both anterior and posterior extension areas, particularly if the anterior residual ridge offers less than ideal support.

Rests

If the lingual slope of the canine is inappropriate for a cingulum rest, an incisal rest must be used (refer to Fig. 10.20-2).

Major connector

Additional horizontal stabilization can be achieved by plating the canine and first premolar. Plating of the second premolars should be avoided, if possible, because it will preempt the mesial rests if it extends above the survey line.

Minor connectors

Refer to case 10.1.

Retentive arms

Options for retentive arms on the second premolars are discussed in case 10.1. Retentive arms placed on anterior abutments would tend to engage the teeth during tissueward movement of the distal extension bases; thus, if used, they should be flexible and engage minimal undercuts.

If the anterior abutments are periodontally compromised, and if the support provided by the anterior residual ridge is poor, the RPD should be viewed as possessing both anterior and posterior extension areas. Because the clasps cannot release with both types of movement, all retentive arms should be flexible and engage minimal undercuts. As an alternative, cast (rigid) arms may be placed *above the height of contour* to improve bracing action. The prosthesis is essentially a complete denture with the remaining teeth providing some vertical and horizontal stabilization. Muscular action by the patient must provide the majority of retention for the RPD.

Denture base retentive elements/replacement teeth

Denture teeth attached via retentive network and denture base will almost always be used.

Case 10.40

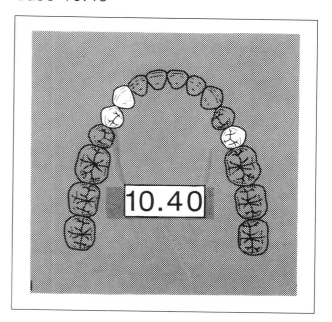

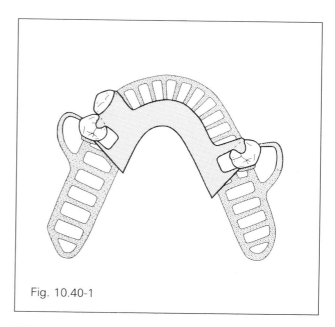

Fig. 10.40-1

The posterior abutments for case 10.40 are the same as those for case 10.5. However, the anterior modification space is so large that the RPD should be viewed as having both anterior and posterior extension areas. Refer to case 10.39 for a discussion of possible variations when both anterior and posterior extension areas are present.

Case 10.41

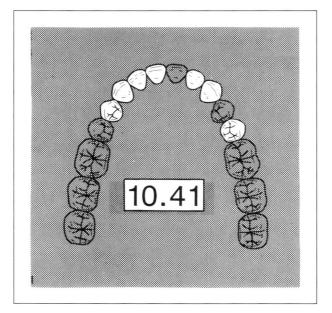

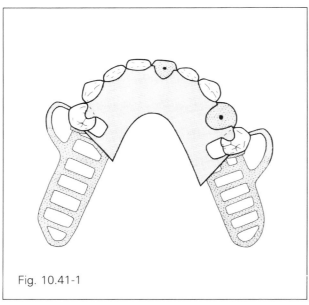

Fig. 10.41-1

Case 10.42

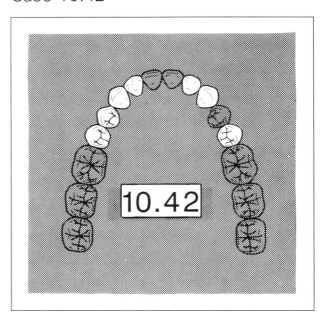

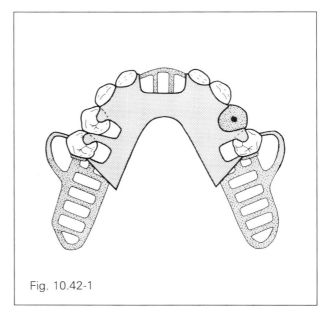

Fig. 10.42-1

For design concepts and variations, refer to case 10.24 for the anterior segment and case 10.14 for the remainder of the design.

For design concepts and variations, refer to case 10.17 for the anterior segment and case 10.14 for the remainder of the design.

Case 10.43

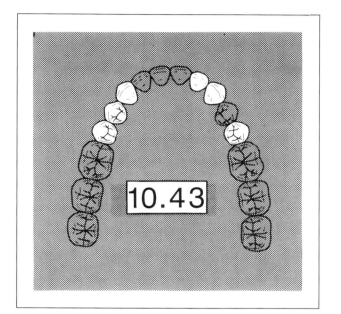

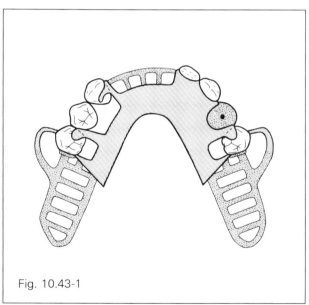

Fig. 10.43-1

Case 10.44

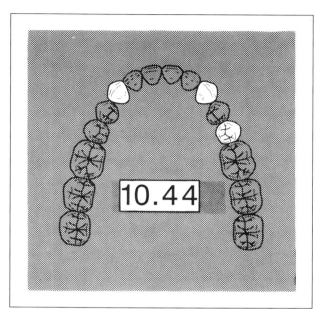

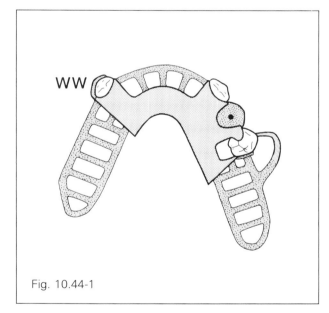

ww

Fig. 10.44-1

For design concepts and variations, refer to case 10.34 for the anterior segment and case 10.14 for the remainder of the design.

For design concepts and variations, refer to case 10.20 for the anterior segment and case 10.16 for the remainder of the design. Because of the number and distribution of the remaining teeth, a complete overdenture should be considered unless the periodontal support is good or the RPD is considered transitional and fabricated to facilitate patient adaptation to a removable prosthesis.

Case 10.45

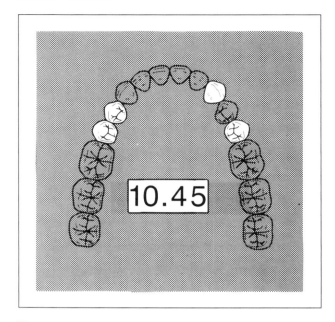

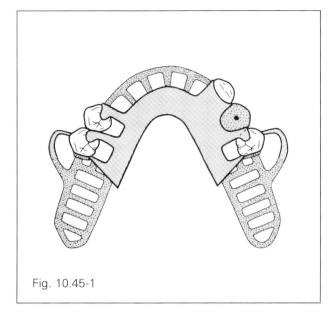

Fig. 10.45-1

The design for case 10.45 is a combination of case 10.14 posteriorly and case 10.39 anteriorly. Because of the number and distribution of the remaining teeth, a complete overdenture should be considered unless the periodontal support is good or the appliance is considered transitional and fabricated to facilitate patient adaptation to a removable prosthesis.

Chapter 11

Mandibular Class II Designs

In our study of 3,000 partially edentulous mandibular arches for which removable partial dentures were fabricated, approximately 25% were Class II. Considering frequency of occurrence, the 43 cases and their variations discussed in chapter 11 cover over 98% of these partially edentulous arches (or their mirror images).

Because a distal extension RPD is seldom fabricated to replace second or third molars, only those situations where at least all the molars are missing will be considered.

Case reference guide	
Without modification space	11.1 to 11.3
With posterior modification space(s) only	
Modification space on extension side only	11.4
Modification space on tooth-supported side only	
Single modification space	
One tooth missing	11.5 to 11.8
Two teeth missing	11.9 to 11.11
Three teeth missing	11.12 to 11.13
Four teeth missing	11.14
Two modification spaces	11.15 to 11.17
Modification spaces on extension and tooth-supported sides	11.18
With anterior modification space(s) only	
Single anterior modification space	
One tooth in space	11.19 to 11.24
Two teeth in space	11.25 to 11.29
Three teeth in space	11.30 to 11.33
Four teeth in space	11.34 to 11.36
Five teeth in space	11.37 to 11.38
Six teeth in space	11.39
Two anterior modification spaces	11.40 to 11.42
With anterior and posterior modifications spaces	11.43

135

Case 11.1

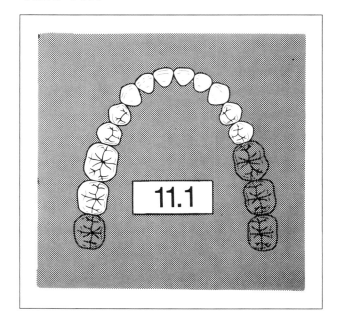

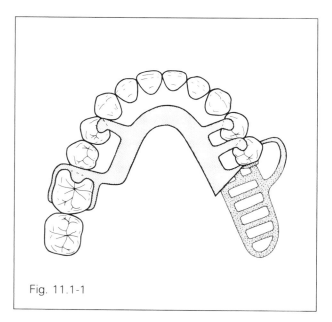

Fig. 11.1-1

Rests

On the extension side, rest location on the terminal (primary) abutment depends on the clasp assembly selected. Refer to case 10.1 for variations.

The rest on the right first premolar is not absolutely essential because the anterior rest on the tooth-supported side will provide adequate indirect retention.

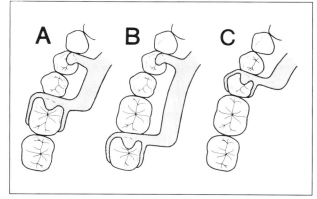

Fig. 11.1-2 On the tooth-supported side, the rest and corresponding embrasure clasp may be placed on the first molar (A), second molar (B), or second premolar (C), depending on the location of an undercut for the clasp tip and on the presence of occlusal interferences. (See also ''Retentive arms,'' below.)

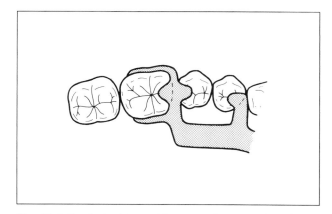

Fig. 11.1-3 A double rest for an embrasure clasp is not usually necessary, but may be selected if there is danger of interproximal food impaction and if the occlusion permits.

Guide plates

Refer to case 10.1 for design concepts. The only guide plate will be located on the distal aspect of the mandibular right second premolar. It will not determine a distinct path of insertion/dislodgement.

Major connector

Refer to case 10.1 for a discussion of options and design concepts.

If the premolars on the tooth-supported side tilt lingually, they may be plated to avoid creation of a space between the superior border of the major connector and the medial aspect of the alveolar ridge. Ordinarily, the terminal abutment on the extension side should not be plated. When it is, the metal must end exactly at the survey line. If the plating ends above the height of contour, it will preempt the planned mesial rest and alter the mechanics of the clasp assembly. If it ends below the height of contour, a space will be created between the major connector and the teeth.

Minor connectors

Refer to case 10.1.

Retentive arms

Case 10.1 discusses clasping options for the extension side. Retention for the tooth-supported side is discussed below.

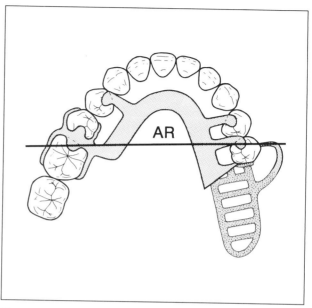

Fig. 11.1-4 On the tooth-supported side, the embrasure clasp may engage a distobuccal or distolingual undercut on the first molar, second molar, or second premolar (see Fig. 11.1-2). The anterior retentive arm *(AR)* would be in front of the axis of rotation and must therefore be flexible (wrought wire). However, because there is seldom sufficient space for a wrought wire clasp, the anterior component of the embrasure clasp is usually omitted. Cast anterior arms may be used, but because of their rigidity they should be placed above the height of contour and should function for bracing only.

Denture base retentive elements/replacement teeth

Refer to case 10.1.

Case 11.2

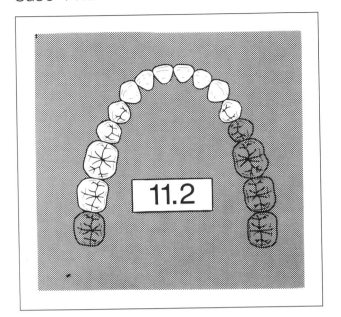

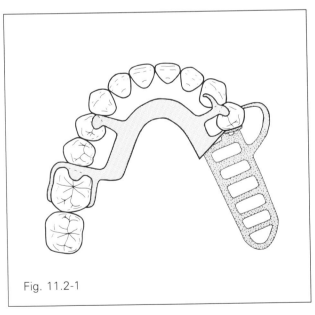

Fig. 11.2-1

For design concepts and variations, refer to case 10.2 for the extension side and case 11.1 for the tooth-supported side.

Case 11.3

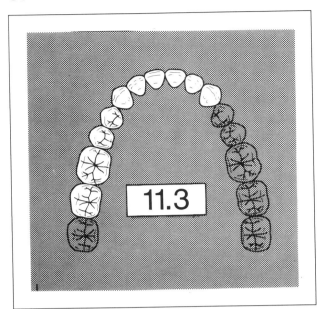

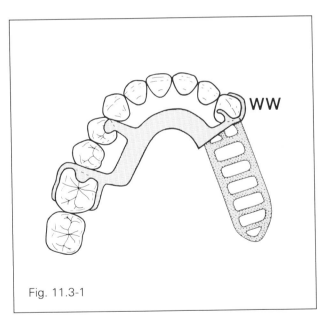

Fig. 11.3-1

For design concepts and variations, refer to case 10.3 for the extension side and case 11.1 for the tooth-supported side.

Case 11.4

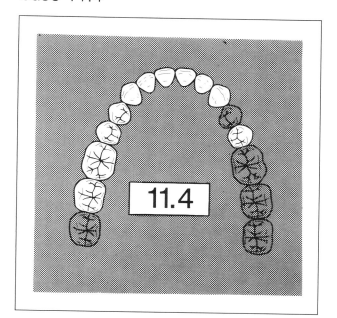

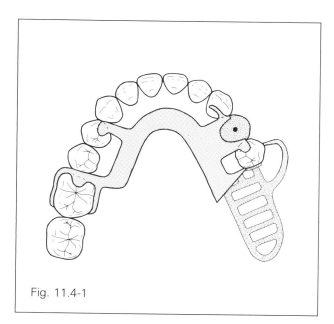

Fig. 11.4-1

For design concepts and variations, refer to case 10.13 for the extension side and case 11.1 for the tooth-supported side.

Case 11.5

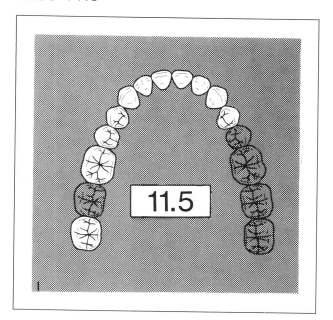

If the extension side varies from that shown, refer to cases 11.1 to 11.4 for the correct configuration.

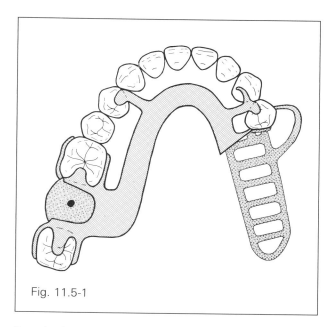

Fig. 11.5-1

For design concepts on the extension side, refer to cases 11.1 to 11.4. Options related to the tooth-supported side are discussed below.

Rests

Because of the long span from the left first molar to the right canine, a rest would usually be placed in the mesial fossa of the left first premolar. This rest would also function as an indirect retainer; therefore, the rest on the right canine could be omitted. The distal rest on the first molar could also be deleted if occlusion interfered with its placement. The rests on the third molar and first premolar would still provide vertical stops for the tooth-supported segment.

Guide plates

Theoretically, the multiple guide surface–guide plate contacts determine a distinct path of insertion/dislodgement, and the I-bar on the extension side could be placed at the greatest mesiodistal curvature of the facial surface. However, placement of the retentive tip slightly in front of the greatest curvature is still recommended, because it provides protection against excessive blockout or excessive reduction of the guide plates during finishing procedures.

Major connector

Refer to case 11.1.

Minor connectors

Refer to case 11.1.

Retentive arms

Because the clasp tip on the first molar is located in front of the axis of rotation, it should be made of wrought wire to increase flexibility. Cast arms may be selected if they are placed above the height of contour and used only for bracing.

If the most posterior abutment has an accessible distobuccal or distolingual undercut, a circumferential clasp assembly is preferred. However, mesiolingual drifting is common, and options utilizing mesiolingual undercuts must be considered.

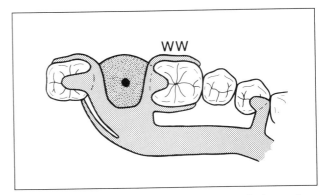

Fig. 11.5-2 If the only available undercut is located on the mesiolingual surface, an I-bar emanating from the inferior border of the major connector is the retentive arm of choice. It is very important that the I-bar be placed near the mesiolingual line angle so that the originating portion of the arm will not stand out medially in the floor of the mouth. A buccal bracing arm may be used with the lingual I-bar.

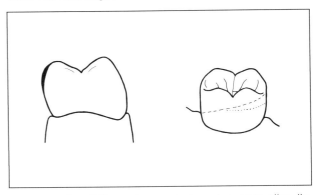

Fig. 11.5-3a When the posterior abutment tilts lingually, retentive arm position can be improved by recontouring—removing the shaded area. The height of contour can be lowered from the dashed line to the dotted line.

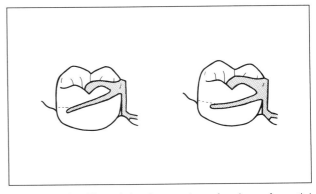

Fig. 11.5-3b The originating portion of a circumferential clasp can be moved gingivally.

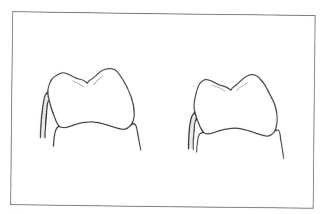

Fig. 11.5-3c The tip of a mesiolingual I-bar can be relocated so that the body of the arm will be closer to the approximating soft tissues.

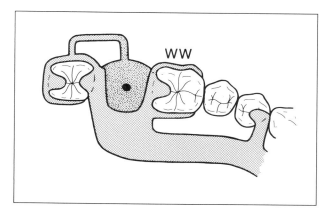

Fig. 11.5-4 A ring clasp may be selected if the only available undercut is located on the mesiolingual surface and a large tissue undercut precludes the use of an I-bar. This clasp should have an auxiliary distal rest and a buccal reinforcing strut. This retainer should be considered last because of inherent hygiene problems.

Denture base retentive elements/replacement teeth

The left molar is usually replaced by a tube tooth or cast entirely of metal as part of the framework. The all-metal tooth is particularly useful when the anterior-posterior or vertical space is reduced.

Case 11.6

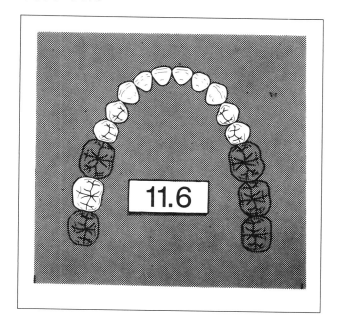

If the extension side varies from that shown, refer to cases 11.2 to 11.4 for the correct configuration.

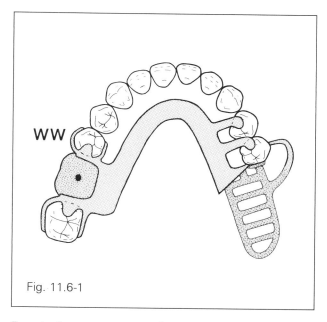

Fig. 11.6-1

For design concepts and variations on the extension side, refer to cases 11.1 to 11.4. Options related to the tooth-supported side are discussed below.

Rests

Although the rest on the left second premolar would function as an indirect retainer, it is very close to a line connecting the retentive tips on the left molar and right premolar, and thus would not be particularly effective. It is probably best to achieve additional indirect retention with a mesial rest on the right first premolar.

If occlusion interferes with placement of the distal rest on the left second premolar, it can be moved forward to the mesial or distal fossa of the first premolar. If it is moved to the first premolar, its effectiveness as an indirect retainer improves, and the indirect retainer on the right first premolar can be deleted.

Guide plates

Refer to cases 11.5 and 11.1.

Major connector

Refer to case 11.1.

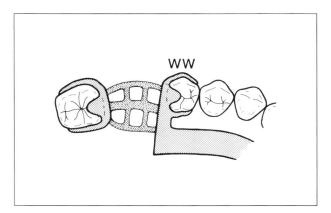

Fig. 11.6-2 As shown in Fig. 11.6-1, the major connector should almost always extend to the posterior abutment on the tooth-supported side. If the prognosis of the tooth is highly questionable, however, a finish line may be placed at the anterior end of the tooth-supported space. Although the design is not considered as hygienic, it does allow for subsequent conversion to a distal extension area.

Retentive arms

Clasping options for the second molar are essentially the same as those for the third molar in case 11.5.

Because the second premolar lies in front of the axis of rotation, a retentive arm, if used, should either be flexible or function for bracing only.

Figs. 11.6-3a to c Retentive arm options for the premolar on the tooth-supported side.

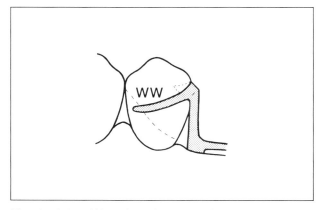

Fig. 11.6-3a Wrought wire circumferential clasp into mesiofacial undercut.

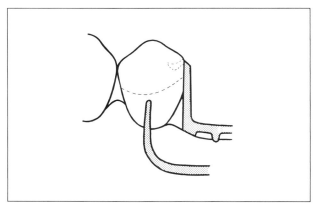

Fig. 11.6-3b I-bar into mesiofacial or midfacial undercut.

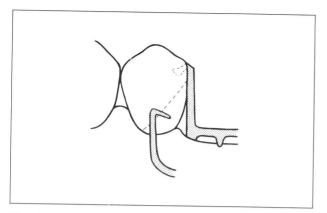

Fig. 11.6-3c   Modified T-bar into distofacial undercut. If a bar clasp is selected, it should be long, tapered, and flexible, or engage a minimal undercut.

Denture base retentive elements/replacement teeth

The first molar can be replaced with either a tube tooth or an all-metal tooth. Restricted vertical space or anterior-posterior space would tend to favor an all-metal replacement.

Case 11.7

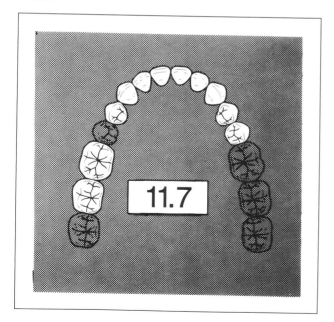

If the extension side varies from that shown, refer to cases 11.2 to 11.4 for the correct configuration.

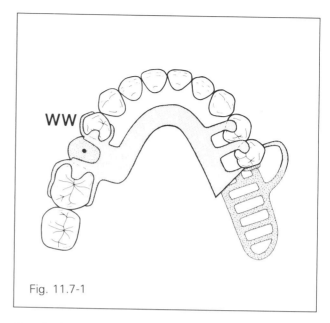

Fig. 11.7-1

For design concepts and variations on the extension side, refer to cases 11.1 to 11.4. Options related to the tooth-supported side are discussed below.

Rests

If occlusal interferences exist, the rest on the left first premolar could be moved to the mesial fossa or to the canine. If it is moved anteriorly, the indirect retainer on the right first premolar could probably be deleted.

Guide plates

Refer to cases 11.5 and 11.1.

Major connector

Refer to cases 11.6 and 11.1.

Minor connectors

Refer to case 11.1.

Retentive arms

Clasping options for the first molar of case 11.7 are essentially the same as those for the third molar of case 11.5. Clasping options for the first premolar of case 11.7 are the same as those for the second premolar in case 11.6.

Denture base retentive elements/replacement teeth

Because of esthetic considerations, the second premolar is usually replaced by a tube tooth or a heat-cured or light-activated facing.

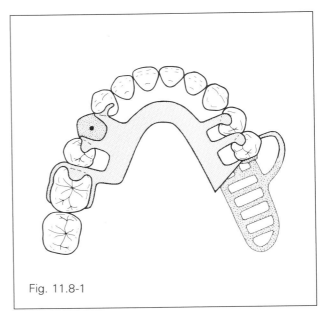

Fig. 11.8-1

For design concepts and variations on the extension side, refer to cases 11.1 to 11.4. Options related to the tooth-supported side are discussed below.

Case 11.8

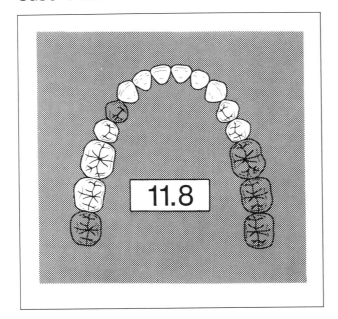

If the extension side varies from that shown, refer to cases 11.2 to 11.4 for the correct configuration.

Rests

The rest on the mesio-occlusal aspect of the left second premolar could be omitted if occlusal interferences exist. Rests on the molar and canine would provide vertical stops for the tooth-supported segment. Variations in rest seats and rests for the canine are discussed in case 10.3. The rest on the right first premolar could be deleted because the rest on the left canine would act as an adequate indirect retainer.

A circumferential clasp assembly may be placed on the left second premolar instead of on the first molar. Some decrease in stability may occur with this design. When the clasp assembly is moved forward, the rest on the canine is a less effective indirect retainer, and the indirect retainer on the right first premolar should probably be included.

Guide plates

Refer to cases 11.5 and 11.1.

Major connector

Refer to cases 11.6 and 11.1.

Minor connectors

Refer to case 11.1.

Retentive arms

The clasping options for the left first molar are the same as those described for case 11.1. A wrought wire circumferential clasp placed into a mesiofacial undercut could be used on the canine. Because the first premolar is missing, there is adequate space for passage of the arm from the lingual to the buccal surface. However, with only one tooth missing, clasping the canine is probably neither necessary nor desirable, particularly since this could sacrifice esthetics.

A circumferential clasp assembly with the retentive arm into either a distofacial or distolingual undercut may be used on the second premolar and the clasp assembly deleted from the first molar. Some stability may be lost with this design.

Denture base retentive elements/replacement teeth

Because of esthetic considerations, the first premolar is almost always replaced by a tube tooth or a heat-cured or light-activated resin facing.

Case 11.9

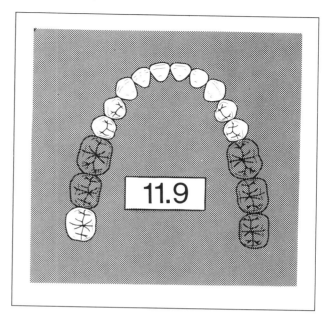

If the extension side varies from that shown, refer to cases 11.2 to 11.4 for the correct configuration.

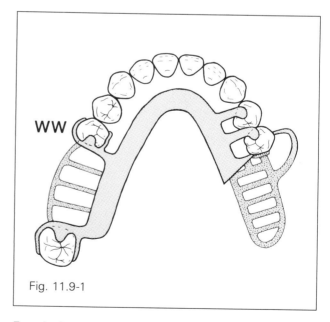

Fig. 11.9-1

For design concepts and variations on the extension side, refer to cases 11.1 to 11.4. Options related to the tooth-supported side are discussed below.

Rests

The rest on the right first premolar can be eliminated since the rest on the left second premolar would provide adequate indirect retention.

Guide plates

Refer to cases 11.5 and 11.1.

Major connector

Refer to cases 11.6 and 11.1.

Minor connectors

Refer to case 11.1.

Retentive arms

Clasping considerations for the left third molar are the same as those described in case 11.5. Clasping considerations for the left second premolar are the same as those described in case 11.6.

Denture base retentive elements/replacement teeth

Artificial teeth attached by retentive network and denture base are almost always used. A metal base may be considered if the vertical space is limited. However, since relining is almost impossible, the residual ridge must be well-healed.

Case 11.10

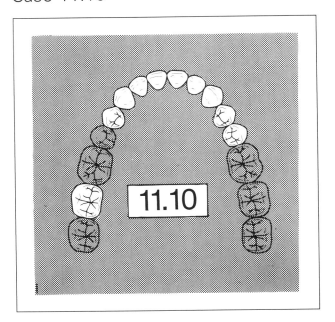

If the extension side varies from that shown, refer to cases 11.2 to 11.4 for the correct configuration.

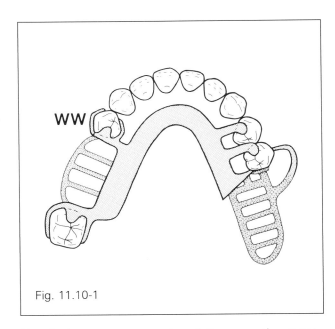

Fig. 11.10-1

For design concepts and variations on the extension side, refer to cases 11.1 to 11.4. Options related to the tooth-supported side are discussed below.

Rests

The rest on the left first premolar could be moved to the mesial fossa if the opposing occlusion prevents placement in the distal fossa.

The rest on the right first premolar could be omitted because the rest on the left first premolar would provide adequate indirect retention.

Guide plates

Refer to cases 11.5 and 11.1.

Major connector

Refer to cases 11.6 and 11.1.

Minor connectors

Refer to case 11.1.

Retentive arms

Clasping considerations for the left second molar are the same as those in case 11.5. Clasping considerations for the left first premolar are the same as those for the second premolar in case 11.6.

Denture base retentive elements/replacement teeth

Refer to case 11.9.

Case 11.11

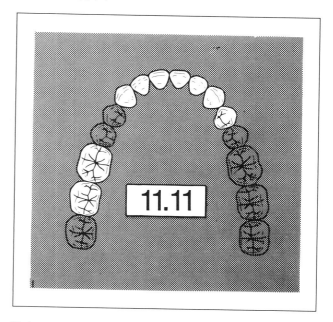

If the extension side varies from that shown, refer to cases 11.1 to 11.4 for the correct configuration.

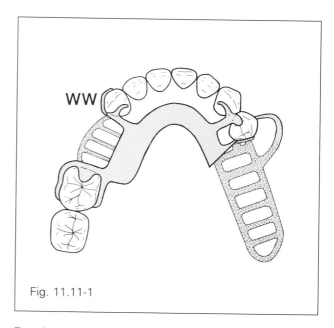

Fig. 11.11-1

For design concepts and variations on the extension side, refer to cases 11.1 to 11.4. Options related to the tooth-supported side are discussed below.

Rests

The indirect retainer on the right side is not absolutely essential, because the rest on the left canine will provide adequate indirect retention.

Refer to case 11.8 for discussion of the canine rest seat and rest.

Guide plates

Refer to cases 11.5 and 11.1.

Major connector

Refer to case 11.1.

Minor connectors

Refer to case 11.1.

Retentive arms

Clasping considerations for the left first molar are the same as those for the third molar in case 11.5.

With a two-tooth edentulous space, a clasp would usually be placed on the canine unless contraindicated by esthetic considerations. A wrought wire arm into a mesiofacial undercut would be most common. However, long, tapered, flexible bar clasps may be used to engage midfacial (I-bar) or distofacial (modified T-bar) undercuts. Refer to case 10.3 for illustrations and further discussion of clasping variations for the canine.

Denture base retentive elements/replacement teeth

Refer to case 11.9.

Case 11.12

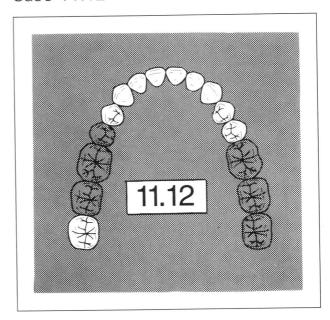

If the extension side varies from that shown, refer to cases 11.2 to 11.4 for the correct configuration.

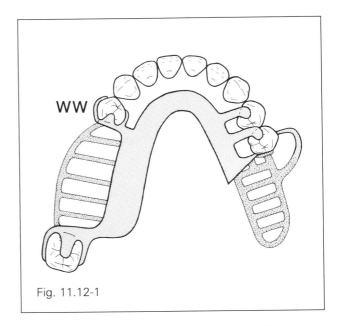

Fig. 11.12-1

For design concepts and variations on the extension side, refer to cases 11.1 to 11.4. Options related to the tooth-supported side are described below.

Rests

The rest on the left first premolar may be moved to the mesial fossa if the opposing occlusion prevents placement in the distal fossa. The rest on the right first premolar is not essential, because the rest on the left first premolar will act as an adequate indirect retainer.

Guide plates

Refer to cases 11.5 and 11.1.

Major connector

Refer to cases 11.6 and 11.1.

Minor connectors

Refer to case 11.1.

Retentive arms

Clasping considerations for the molar are the same as those for case 11.5. Clasping considerations for the first premolar are the same as those for the second premolar in case 11.6.

Denture base retentive elements/replacement teeth

Refer to case 11.9.

Case 11.13

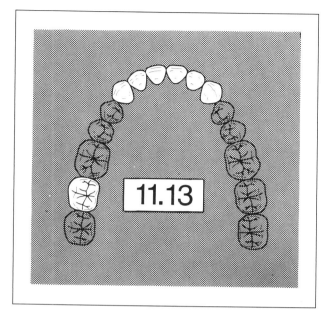

If the extension side varies from that shown, refer to cases 11.1 to 11.4 for the correct configuration.

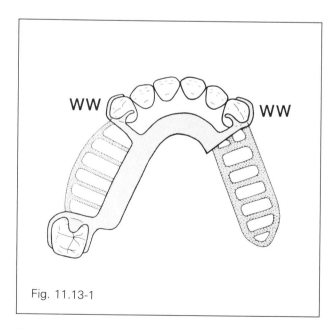

Fig. 11.13-1

For design concepts and variations on the extension side, refer to cases 11.1 to 11.4. Options related to the tooth-supported side are described below.

149

Rests

For variations in the canine rests refer to case 10.3.

Guide plates

Refer to cases 11.5 and 11.1.

Major connector

Refer to cases 11.6 and 11.1.

Minor connectors

Refer to case 11.1.

Retentive arms

Clasping considerations for the second molar are the same as those for the third molar in case 11.5. With the size of the edentulous tooth-supported space, a retentive arm would almost always be used on the canine. Refer to case 11.11 for options.

Denture base retentive elements/replacement teeth

Refer to case 11.9.

Case 11.14

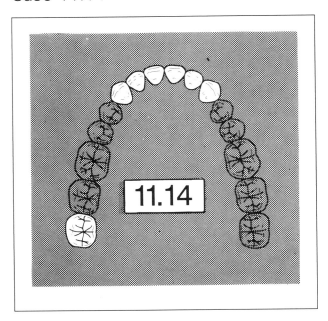

If the extension side varies from that shown, refer to cases 11.1 to 11.4 for the correct configuration.

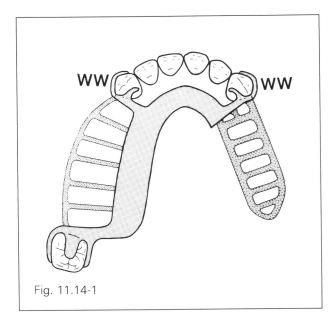

Fig. 11.14-1

For design concepts and variations on the extension side, refer to cases 11.1 to 11.4. Options for the tooth-supported side are essentially the same as those for case 11.13.

Case 11.15

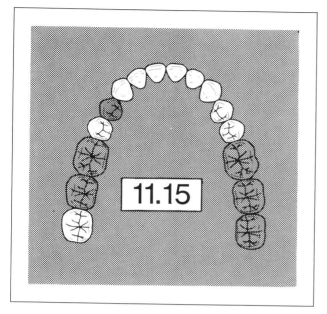

If the extension side varies from that shown, refer to cases 11.2 to 11.4 for the correct configuration.

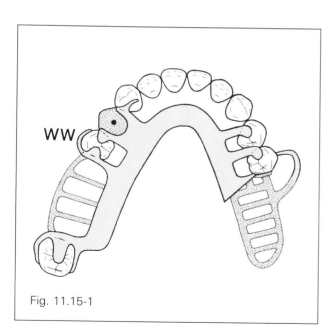

Fig. 11.15-1

For design concepts and variations on the extension side, refer to cases 11.1 to 11.4. Options for the tooth-supported side are discussed below.

Rests

One of the rests on the left second premolar could be deleted if occlusal interferences exist. The rest on the right first premolar could be deleted because the canine rest on the left provides adequate indirect retention. For variations in the canine rest refer to case 11.8.

Guide plates

Refer to cases 11.5 and 11.1.

Major connector

Refer to cases 11.6 and 11.1. The left second premolar should be plated if the mesiodistal width of the opening is less than 4 mm or if the tooth exhibits linguoversion.

Minor connectors

Refer to case 11.1.

Retentive arms

Clasping considerations for the molar are the same as those for case 11.5. Clasping considerations for the premolar are the same as those for case 11.6. A retentive arm may be placed on the canine rather than the first premolar. If this option is selected, refer to case 11.11.

Denture base retentive elements/replacement teeth

Refer to case 11.9.

Case 11.16

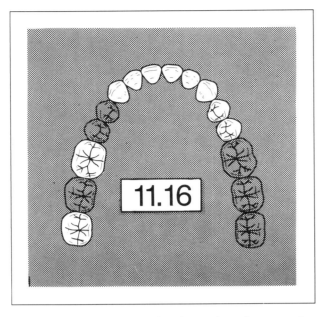

If the extension side varies from that shown, refer to cases 11.2 to 11.4 for the correct configuration.

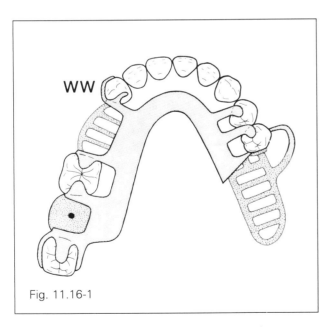

Fig. 11.16-1

For design concepts and variations on the extension side, refer to cases 11.1 to 11.4. Options for the tooth-supported side are discussed below.

Rests

One of the rests on the left first molar can be deleted if occlusal interferences exist. For variations in the canine rest refer to case 11.8. The rest on the right first premolar is not absolutely essential, because the rest on the left canine functions as an adequate indirect retainer.

Guide plates

Refer to cases 11.5 and 11.1.

Major connector

Refer to case 11.1.

Minor connectors

Refer to case 11.1.

Retentive arms

For variations in clasping for the third molar refer to case 11.5. Clasping of the canine (refer to case 11.11) is advisable unless contraindicated by esthetic demands; in this case a wrought wire clasp should be placed on the first molar. It would usually originate from the distal aspect and engage a mesiofacial undercut, but may originate from the mesial aspect and engage a distofacial undercut.

Denture base retentive elements/replacement teeth

Refer to case 11.5 for the posterior and case 11.11 for the anterior tooth-supported spaces.

Case 11.17

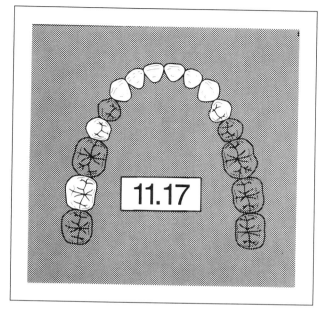

If the extension side varies from that shown, refer to cases 11.1 to 11.4 for the correct configuration.

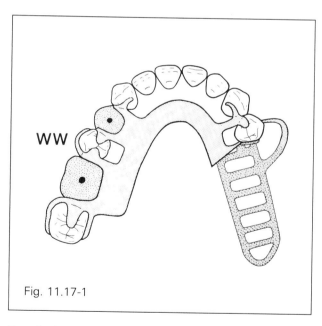

Fig. 11.17-1

For design concepts and variations on the extension side, refer to cases 11.1 to 11.4. Options for the tooth-supported side are discussed below.

Rests

One of the rests on the left second premolar could be deleted if occlusal interferences exist. For variations in the canine rest, refer to case 11.8. The rest on the right canine is not absolutely necessary, because the rest on the left canine is an adequate indirect retainer.

Guide plates

Refer to cases 11.5 and 11.1.

Major connector

Refer to cases 11.6 and 11.1.

Minor connectors

Refer to case 11.1.

Retentive arms

For clasping variations on the molar refer to case 11.5. For clasping variations on the premolar refer to case 11.6. A retentive arm can be placed on the canine instead of the premolar if esthetic demands allow. For clasping variations on the canine refer to case 11.11.

Denture base retentive elements/replacement teeth

With two single-tooth modification spaces, tube teeth would usually be selected. An all-metal tooth could be used to replace the molar and would be particularly indicated if vertical or anterior-posterior space is limited.

Case 11.18

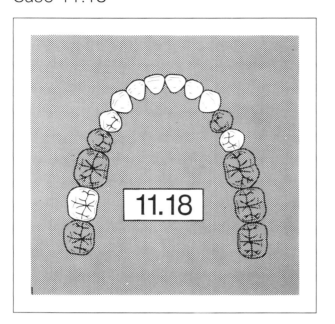

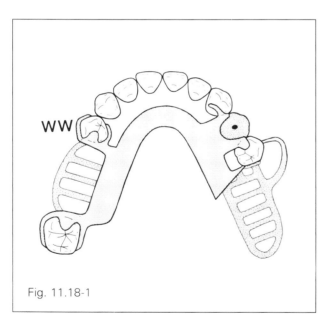

Fig. 11.18-1

For design concepts and variations, refer to case 11.4 for the extension side and case 11.10 for the tooth-supported side.

Case 11.19

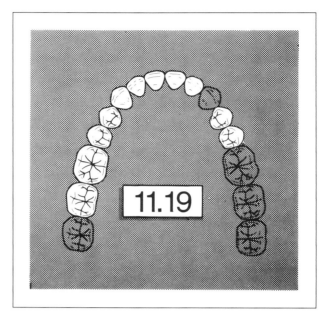

If the first premolar is the only posterior tooth present on the extension side, refer to case 11.2.

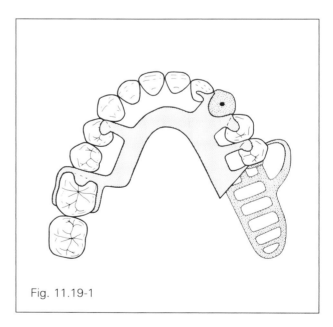

Fig. 11.19-1

The design for case 11.19 is essentially the same as that for case 11.1 with a single-tooth anterior modification space. Changes associated with the modification space are considered below. Refer to

case 11.1 for discussion of other aspects of the design.

Rests

A rest may be placed on the lateral incisor if it possesses good bone support and a prominent cingulum. If these attributes are not present, linguoplating should be used. A rest should be placed at least on the left canine and the rest on the left premolar can be omitted. If possible, a rest seat should be prepared on the lateral incisor.

Guide plates

Refer to case 11.1. The guide plate on the lateral incisor must be located on the linguoproximal surface so that it will not be visible from the labial aspect or interfere with positioning of the replacement tooth.

Major connector

A linguoplate should be selected if the incisors are periodontally weakened and in danger of being lost in the near future.

Retentive arms

The options for clasp assemblies are the same as those for case 11.1. Clasps on the lateral incisor and first premolar would be unesthetic and lie in front of the axis of rotation; they are rarely, if ever, indicated.

Denture base retentive elements/replacement teeth

With only one tooth in the modification space, a prefabricated facing, tube tooth, or a custom heat-cured or light-activated resin replacement is almost always used.

Case 11.20

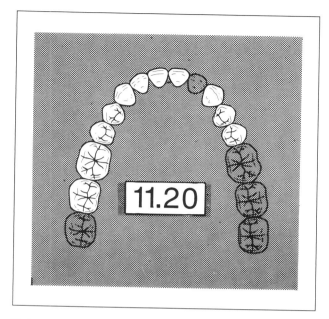

If the extension side varies from that shown, refer to cases 11.2 to 11.4 for the correct configuration.

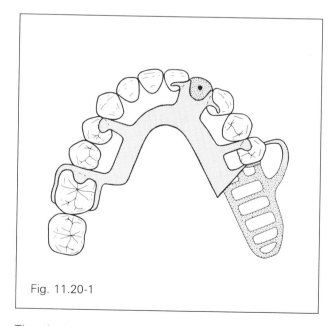

Fig. 11.20-1

The design for case 11.20 is essentially the same as that for case 11.1 with a single-tooth anterior modification space. Changes associated with the modification space are considered below. Refer to

case 11.1 for discussion of other aspects of the design.

Rests

A rest may be placed on the central incisor if it possesses good bone support and a prominent cingulum. If these attributes are not present, linguoplating should be used. Rests should be placed at least on the canines; the rests on the premolar can be omitted. If possible, a rest seat should be prepared on the central incisor.

Guide plates

The anterior guide plates must be located on the linguoproximal surfaces so that they will not be visible from the labial aspect or interfere with positioning of the replacement tooth.

Major connector

A linguoplate should be selected if the incisors are periodontally weakened and in danger of being lost in the near future.

Retentive arms

The options for clasp assemblies are the same as those for case 11.1. Clasps on the anterior teeth would be unesthetic and lie in front of the axis of rotation, and so are rarely, if ever, indicated.

Denture base retentive elements/replacement teeth

Refer to case 11.19.

Case 11.21

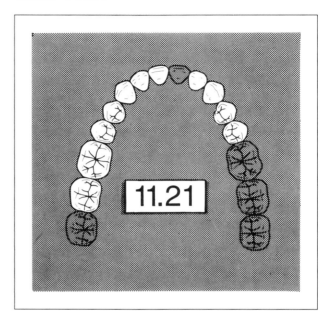

If the extension side varies from that shown, refer to cases 11.2 to 11.4 for the correct configuration.

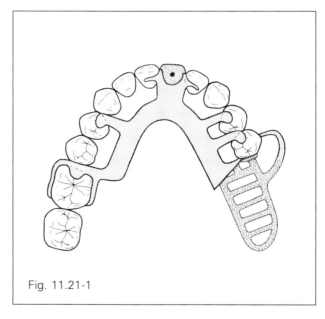

Fig. 11.21-1

The design for case 11.21 is essentially the same as that for case 11.1 with a single-tooth anterior modification space. Changes associated with the modification space are considered below. Refer to

case 11.1 for discussion of other aspects of the design.

Rests

Rest seats and rests may be placed on the incisors adjacent to the modification space if the teeth are periodontally sound and exhibit prominent cinguli. The rests on the first premolars are not absolutely necessary, because the anterior rests will provide adequate indirect retention. If the remaining incisors exhibit significant bone loss, linguoplating should be used. Rest seats and rests should be placed at least on the canines. Then, rests on the first premolar would be unnecessary unless adequate rest seats could not be prepared on the canines.

Guide plates

Refer to case 11.20.

Major connector

A linguoplate should be selected if the remaining incisors are periodontally weakened and in danger of being lost in the near future.

Retentive arms

Refer to case 11.20.

Denture base retentive elements/replacement teeth

Refer to case 11.19.

Case 11.22

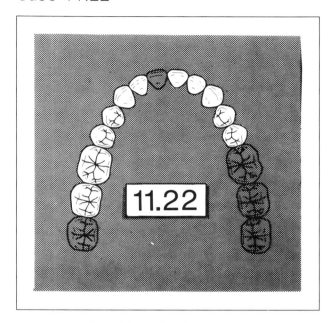

If the extension side varies from that shown, refer to cases 11.2 to 11.4 for the correct configuration.

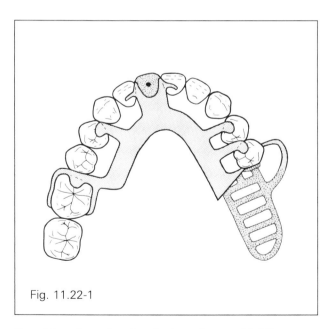

Fig. 11.22-1

Considerations for the design of case 11.22 are essentially the same as those for case 11.21.

Case 11.23

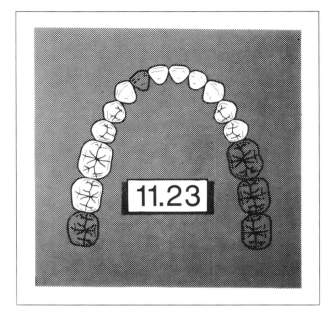

If the extension side varies from that shown, refer to cases 11.2 to 11.4 for the correct configuration.

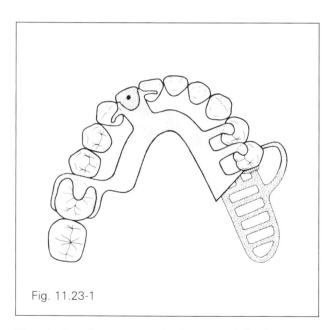

Fig. 11.23-1

The design for case 11.23 is essentially the same as that for case 11.1 with a single-tooth anterior modification space. Changes associated with the modification space are considered below. Refer to

case 11.1 for discussion of the other aspects of the design.

Rests

A rest seat and rest may be placed on the central incisor if it has good bone support and a prominent cingulum. The rest on the right first premolar is not absolutely necessary, because the anterior rests will provide adequate indirect retention. If the remaining incisors exhibit significant bone loss, linguoplating should be used. Rest seats and rests should be placed at least on the canines. Then, rests on the first premolars would be unnecessary unless adequate rest seats could not be prepared on the canines.

Guide plates

The anterior guide plates must be located on the linguoproximal surfaces so that they will not be visible from the labial aspect or interfere with positioning of the replacement tooth.

Major connector

A linguoplate should be selected if the incisors are periodontally weakened and in danger of being lost in the near future.

Retentive arms

Refer to case 11.20.

Denture base retentive elements/replacement teeth

Refer to case 11.19.

Case 11.24

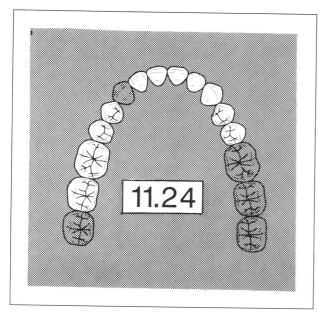

If the extension side varies from that shown, refer to cases 11.2 to 11.4 for the correct configuration.

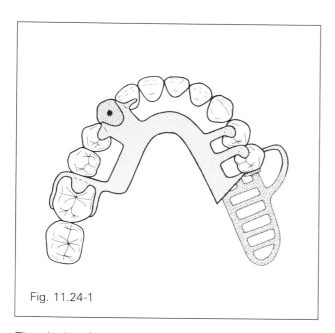

Fig. 11.24-1

The design for case 11.24 is essentially the same as that for case 11.1 with a single-tooth anterior modification space. Changes associated with the modification space are considered below. Refer to case 11.1 for discussion of other aspects of the design.

Rests

A rest seat and rest may be placed on the lateral incisor if it possesses good bone support and a prominent cingulum. The rest on the right first premolar is not absolutely essential, because the anterior rests will provide adequate indirect retention. If the incisors exhibit significant bone loss, linguoplating should be used. A rest seat and rest should be placed at least on the right canine. A rest on the right first premolar would be unnecessary unless an adequate rest seat could not be prepared on the canine.

Guide plates

Refer to case 11.19.

Major connector

A linguoplate should be selected if the incisors are periodontally weakened and in danger of being lost in the near future.

Retentive arms

Refer to case 11.19.

Denture base retentive elements/replacement teeth

Refer to case 11.19.

Case 11.25

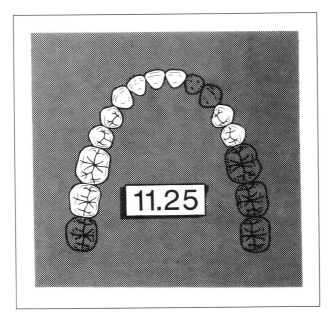

If only the first premolar is present on the extension side, refer to case 11.2.

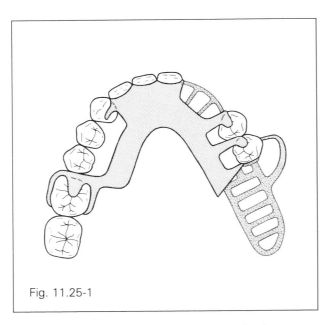

Fig. 11.25-1

The design for case 11.25 is essentially the same as that for case 11.1 with a two-tooth anterior modification space. Changes associated with the modification space are considered below. Refer to case 11.1 for a discussion of the other aspects of the design.

Rests

With two anterior teeth in the modification space (and particularly with the canine missing), linguoplating would almost always be used. A rest seat should be prepared at least on the central incisor. In the rare instance when the central incisor has exceptionally good bone support and a prominent cingulum, a rest seat and rest may be placed on it and linguoplating avoided.

Guide plates

The guide plate on the central incisor must be located on the linguoproximal surface so that it will not be visible from the labial aspect or interfere with positioning of the replacement teeth.

Major connector

Linguoplating of the remaining anterior teeth would almost always be used.

Retentive arms

The options for clasp assemblies are the same as those for case 11.1. Clasps on the central incisor and first premolar would be unesthetic and lie in front of the axis of rotation; they are rarely, if ever, indicated.

Denture base retentive elements/replacement teeth

The two missing teeth are most commonly replaced by denture teeth via retentive network and denture base. However, if the residual ridge is well-healed and exhibits little resorption, and if the width of the space is appropriate for the missing teeth, acceptable alternatives are facings, tube teeth, or heat-cured or light-activated resin replacements.

Case 11.26

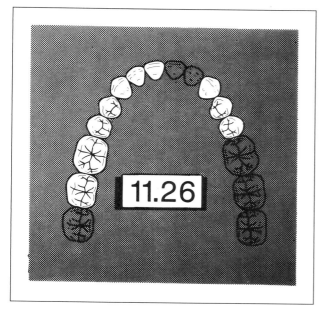

If the extension side varies from that shown, refer to cases 11.2 to 11.4 for the correct configuration.

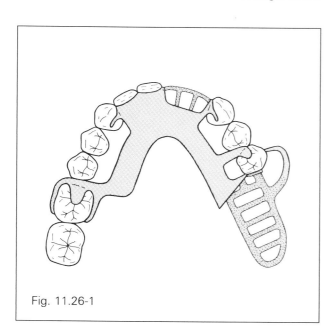

Fig. 11.26-1

The design for case 11.26 is essentially the same as that for case 11.1 with a two-tooth anterior modification space. Changes associated with the modification space are considered below. Refer to

case 11.1 for a discussion of other aspects of the design.

Rests

With two teeth in the modification space, linguoplating of the remaining incisors would almost always be used. If possible, a rest seat should be placed on the central incisor. Rests on the first premolars can be omitted unless it is impossible to place adequate rest seats on the canines.

Guide plates

The anterior guide plates must be located on the linguoproximal surfaces so that they will not be visible from the labial aspect or interfere with positioning of the replacement teeth.

Major connector

Linguoplating of the remaining incisors would almost always be used.

Retentive arms

The options for clasp assemblies are the same as those for case 11.1. Clasps on the anterior teeth would be unesthetic and lie in front of the axis of rotation; they are rarely, if ever, indicated.

Denture base retentive elements/replacement teeth

Refer to case 11.25.

Case 11.27

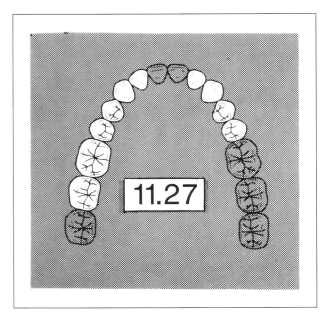

If the extension side varies from that shown, refer to cases 11.2 to 11.4 for the correct configuration.

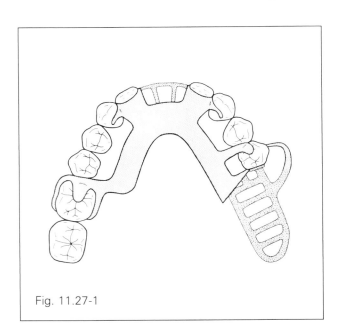

Fig. 11.27-1

Considerations for the design of case 11.27 are essentially the same as those for case 11.26.

Case 11.28

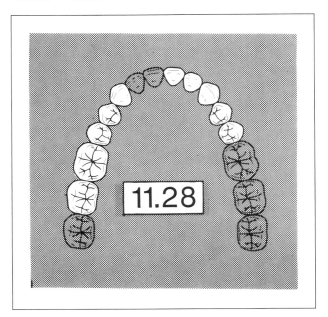

If the extension side varies from that shown, refer to cases 11.2 to 11.4 for the correct configuration.

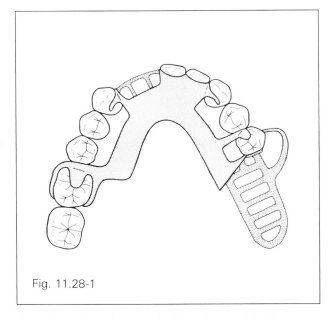

Fig. 11.28-1

Considerations for the design of case 11.28 are essentially the same as those for case 11.26.

Case 11.29

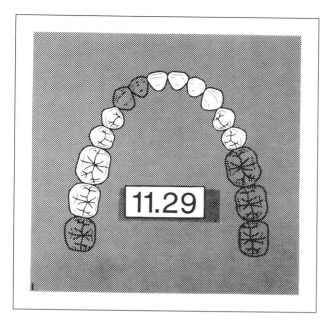

If the extension side varies from that shown, refer to cases 11.2 to 11.4 for the correct configuration.

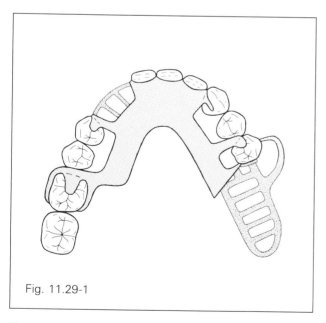

Fig. 11.29-1

Considerations for the design of case 11.29 are essentially the same as those for case 11.25.

Case 11.30

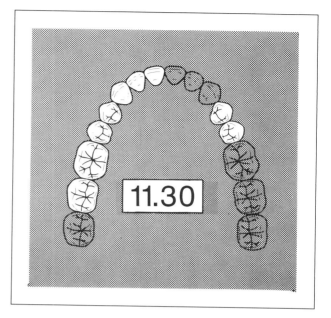

If the second premolar on the extension side is not present, refer to case 11.2 for the correct configuration.

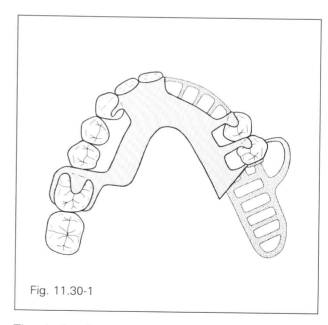

Fig. 11.30-1

The design for case 11.30 is essentially the same as that for case 11.1 with a three-tooth anterior modification space. Changes associated with the modification space are considered below. Refer to case 11.1 for other aspects of the design.

Rests

With a three-tooth modification space, the remaining incisors should almost always be plated. If possible, a rest seat should be prepared at least on the central incisor. If an adequate rest seat cannot be prepared on the canine, it should also be plated and a rest placed on the first premolar.

Guide plates

The guide plate on the central incisor must be located on the linguoproximal surface so that it will not be visible from the labial aspect or interfere with positioning of the replacement teeth.

Major connector

Linguoplating would almost always be used on the remaining incisors.

Retentive arms

The options for clasp assemblies are the same as those for case 11.1. A clasp on the central incisor would be unesthetic and lie in front of the axis of rotation; it is rarely, if ever, indicated.

Denture base retentive elements/replacement teeth

The three missing teeth are almost always replaced by denture teeth via retentive network and denture base. In the rare instance when the residual ridge is well-healed and exhibits very little resorption, and the width of the space is appropriate for the missing teeth, acceptable alternatives are facings, tube teeth, or heat-cured or light-activated resin replacements.

Case 11.31

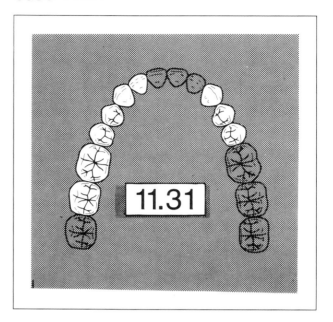

If the extension side varies from that shown, refer to cases 11.2 to 11.4 for the correct configuration.

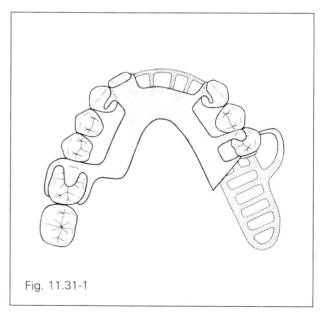

Fig. 11.31-1

The design for case 11.31 is essentially the same as that for case 11.1 with a three-tooth anterior modification space. Changes associated with the modifications space are considered below. Refer to case 11.1 for a discussion of other aspects of the design.

Rests

With a three-tooth modification space, the remaining lateral incisor should be plated. When possible, a rest seat should be prepared on the lateral incisor. If adequate cingulum rest seats cannot be prepared on the canines, they should also be plated, and mesial rests placed on the first premolars.

Guide plates

The guide plates on the anterior teeth must be restricted to the linguoproximal surfaces so that they will not be visible from the labial aspect or interfere with positioning the replacement teeth.

Major connector

Linguoplating should be used on the lateral incisor and may be used on the canines.

Retentive arms

The options for clasp assemblies for case 11.31 are the same as those for case 11.1. Clasps on the canine and lateral incisor would be unesthetic and lie in front of the axis of rotation; they are rarely, if ever, indicated.

Denture base retentive elements/replacement teeth

Refer to case 11.30.

Case 11.32

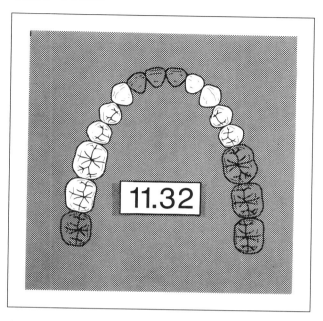

If the extension side varies from that shown, refer to cases 11.2 to 11.4 for the correct configuration.

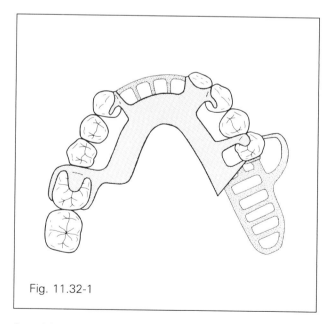

Fig. 11.32-1

Considerations for the design of case 11.32 are essentially the same as those for case 11.31.

Case 11.33

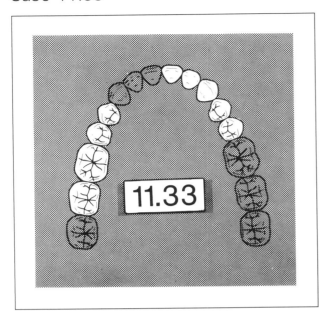

If the extension side varies from that shown, refer to cases 11.2 to 11.4 for the correct configuration.

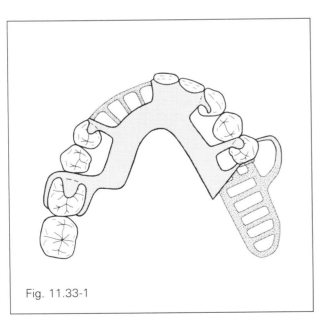

Fig. 11.33-1

Considerations for the design of case 11.33 are essentially the same as those for case 11.30.

Case 11.34

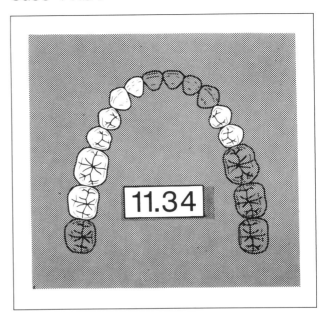

If only the first premolar is present on the extension side, refer to case 11.2.

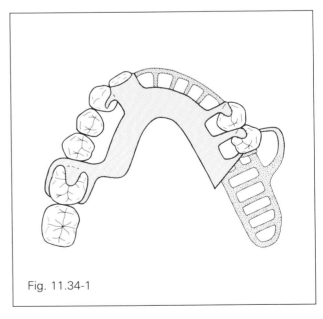

Fig. 11.34-1

The design for case 11.34 is essentially the same as that for case 11.1 with a four-tooth anterior modification space. Changes associated with the modification space are considered below. Refer to case 11.1 for a discussion of other aspects of the design.

Rests

If an adequate cingulum rest seat cannot be prepared on the left canine (and if an incisal rest is esthetically unacceptable), it should also be plated and a mesial rest placed on the first premolar.

Guide plates

The guide plate on the mesial surface of the lateral incisor should be located on the linguoproximal surface so that it will not be visible from the labial aspect or interfere with positioning of the replacement teeth.

Major connector

Linguoplating would always be used on the lateral incisor and may be used on the canine.

Retentive arms

Clasping options are the same as for case 11.1. Retentive arms on the lateral incisor and first premolar would be unesthetic and lie in front of the axis of rotation; they are usually omitted.

Denture base retentive elements/replacement teeth

The four missing teeth are almost always replaced by denture teeth via retentive network and denture base.

Case 11.35

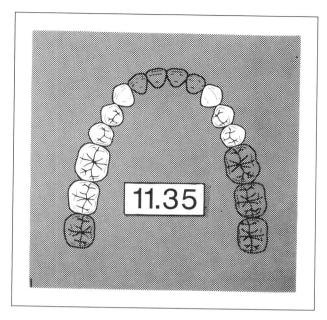

If the extension side varies from that shown, refer to cases 11.2 to 11.4 for the correct configuration.

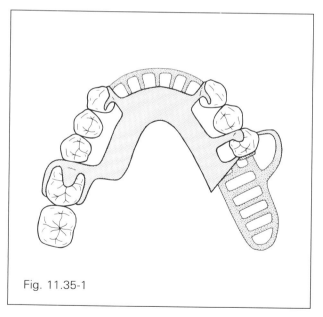

Fig. 11.35-1

The design for case 11.35 is essentially the same as that for case 11.1 with a four-tooth anterior modification space. Changes associated with the modification space are considered below. Refer to case 11.1 for a discussion of other aspects of the design.

Rests

If adequate cingulum rest seats cannot be prepared on the canines (and if incisal rests are esthetically unacceptable), they should be plated and mesial rests placed on the first premolars.

Guide plates

The guide plates on the canines must be located on the linguoproximal surfaces so that they will not be visible from the labial aspect or interfere with positioning of the replacement teeth.

Major connector

Linguoplating may be used on the canines.

Retentive arms

Retentive arms on the canines would be unesthetic and lie in front of the axis of rotation; they are usually omitted.

Denture base retentive elements/replacement teeth

Refer to case 11.34.

Case 11.36

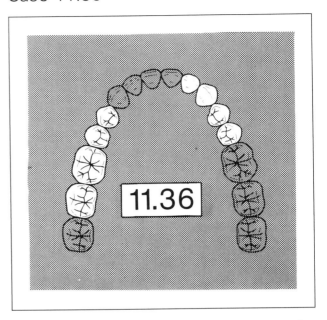

If the extension side varies from that shown, refer to cases 11.2 to 11.4 for the correct configuration.

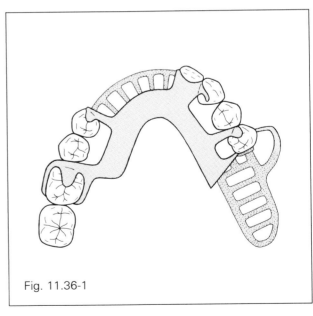

Fig. 11.36-1

Considerations for the design of case 11.36 are essentially the same as those for case 11.34.

Case 11.37

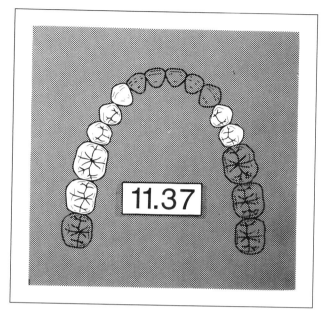

If the extension side varies from that shown, refer to cases 11.3 to 11.4 for the correct configuration.

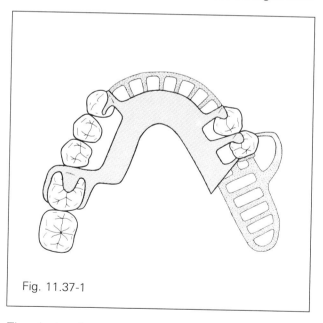

Fig. 11.37-1

The design for case 11.37 is essentially the same as that for case 11.1 with a five-tooth anterior modification space. Changes associated with the modification space are considered below. Refer to case 11.1 for discussion of other aspects of the design.

Rests

If an adequate cingulum rest seat cannot be prepared on the left canine, an incisal rest may be used. If esthetic considerations preclude the use of an incisal rest, the canine should be plated and a mesial rest placed on the first premolar.

Guide plates

The mesial guide plate on the canine must be located on the linguoproximal surface so that it will not be visible from the labial aspect or interfere with positioning of the replacement teeth.

Major connector

Linguoplating may be used on the left canine.

Retentive arms

Retentive arms on the left canine and right first premolar are not usually necessary. If retainers are desired, they should be long, tapered, and flexible bar clasps emanating from the modification space. Wrought wire circumferential clasps would originate high on the mesial surfaces of the abutments; they would be esthetically objectionable.

Denture base retentive elements/replacement teeth

Denture teeth attached via retentive network and denture base would almost always be used.

Case 11.38

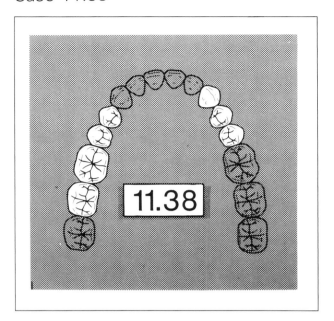

If the extension side varies from that shown, refer to cases 11.2 to 11.4 for the correct configuration.

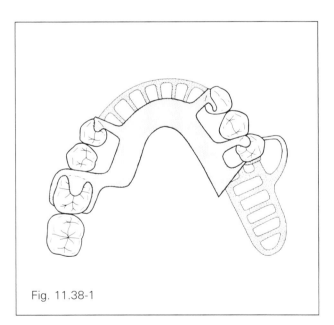

Fig. 11.38-1

Considerations for the design of case 11.38 are essentially the same as those for case 11.37.

Case 11.39

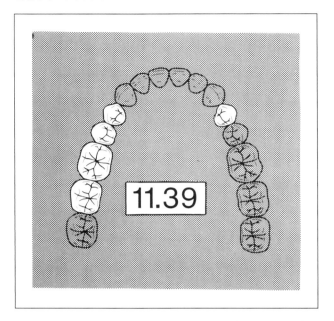

If both premolars are present on the extension side, refer to case 11.1 for the correct configuration.

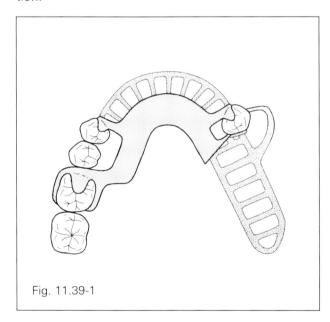

Fig. 11.39-1

The design for case 11.39 is essentially the same as that for case 11.2 with a six-tooth anterior modification space. However, with both canines missing, the modification space could be considered an anterior extension. The dual-extension areas and their effect on the design are the major points of discussion for this case.

Because no clasp can release during tissueward movement of *both* the anterior and posterior extension areas, the I-bar on the right first premolar has the potential for creating torquing forces. As designed in Fig. 11.39-1, the I-bar would engage the tooth when the anterior extension was depressed. If the rest were moved to the distal, the I-bar would engage the tooth when the distal extension was depressed. The same would be true for the left first premolar if a clasp were placed on it. There are essentially three options for decreasing torquing forces. The best would seem to be retaining the root of one of the incisors (preferably a central incisor) for a removable partial overdenture. The root would act as a vertical stop (rest), effectively eliminating the anterior extension, and allowing for normal clasping of the premolars. If a root cannot be retained, the clasp arms utilized on the premolar(s) should be long, tapered, and flexible. Or, rigid circumferential arms may be placed above the height of contour so that they provide for lateral stabilization only (bracing).

Case 11.40

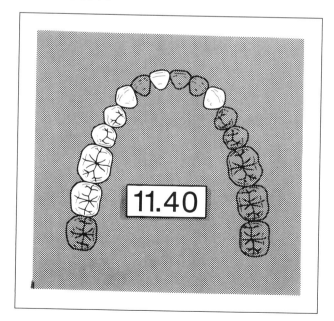

If the extension side varies from that shown, refer to cases 11.2 to 11.4 for the correct configuration.

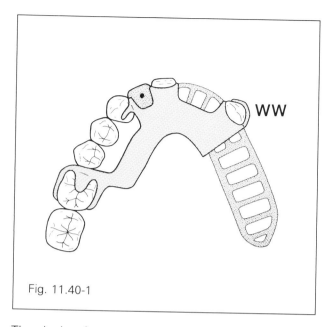

Fig. 11.40-1

The design for case 11.40 is essentially the same as that for case 11.3 with two modification spaces. Refer to case 11.3 for rest and clasping options on the extension side.

The major complicating factor in the design is the lone-standing central incisor. Quite frequently its shape precludes preparation of an adequate rest seat and the plating contacts an inclined plane. In addition, the presence of the central incisor complicates esthetics (both shade matching and tooth placement) for the entire anterior segment. In the great majority of cases it would seem advantageous to provide endodontic therapy and utilize the root of the tooth as an abutment for a removable partial overdenture. The presence of the root would provide an excellent vertical stop (rest) and the absence of the crown would facilitate arrangement of the replacement teeth. The design would then represent a variation of case 11.35.

Case 11.41

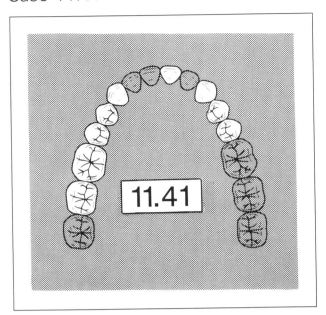

If the extension side varies from that shown, refer to cases 11.2 to 11.4 for the correct configuration.

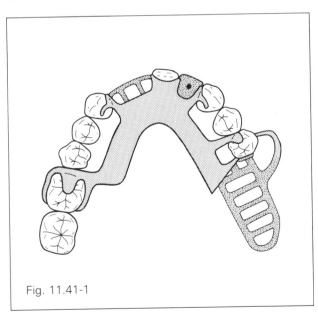

Fig. 11.41-1

Considerations for the design of case 11.41 are essentially the same as those for case 11.40. If the central incisor is used as an abutment for a removable partial overdenture, the design becomes the same as for case 11.35.

Case 11.42

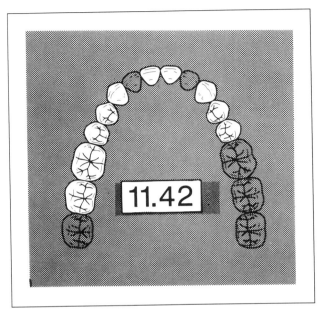

If the extension side varies from that shown, refer to cases 11.2 to 11.4 for the correct configuration.

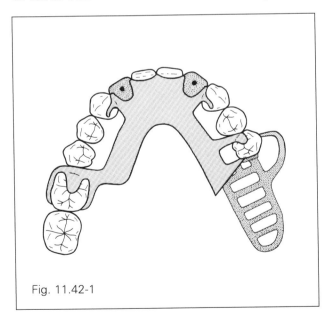

Fig. 11.42-1

The design for case 11.42 is essentially the same as that of case 11.1 with two single-tooth anterior modification spaces. Changes associated with the modification spaces are considered below. Refer to case 11.1 for discussion of other aspects of the design.

Rests

If possible, rest seats should be prepared (beneath the plating) on the central incisors. If adequate rest seats cannot be prepared on the canines, they should be plated and mesial rests placed on the first premolars. If the central incisors exhibit significant loss of bone support, consider utilizing one or both as abutments for a removable partial overdenture. The design would then be the same as that for case 11.35.

Guide plates

The anterior guide plates must be restricted to the linguoproximal surfaces so that they will not be visible from the labial aspect or interfere with positioning of the replacement teeth.

Major connector

Linguoplating should be used on the central incisors and may be used on the canines.

Retentive arms

Retentive arms on the central incisors and canines would be unesthetic and lie in front of the axis of rotation; they are rarely, if ever, indicated.

Replacement teeth

The lateral incisors would usually be replaced by tube teeth or by custom heat-cured or light-activated resin facings.

Case 11.43

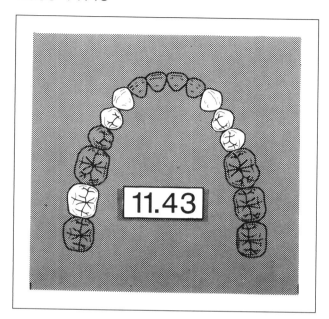

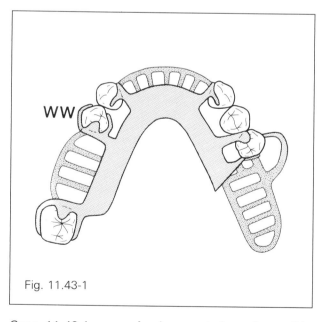

Fig. 11.43-1

Case 11.43 is one of a large number of possible Class II arch forms with both anterior and posterior modification spaces. In order to arrive at the appropriate design, it will be necessary to integrate segments of two or more other designs. The extension area and anterior modification space(s) should usually be considered together, and the posterior modification space should be considered as a separate entity. By consulting the case reference guide at the front of the chapter and examining the partially edentulous arches, it is evident that the design for case 11.43 is a combination of those for cases 11.10 and 11.35. If only one premolar were present on the extension side, the design for case 11.2 would be substituted for case 11.1 in that area.

Chapter 12

Mandibular Class III Designs

In our study of 3,000 partially edentulous mandibular arches for which removable partial dentures were fabricated, slightly less than 25% were Class III. There were 165 different arrangements of missing teeth, and the potential for variations is much greater. Discussion of each possible variation is not practical and, fortunately, not necessary. Because tooth-supported RPDs exhibit no functional motion, the designs are much less complicated and generally follow a fairly straightforward set of guidelines. Consequently, designs for partially edentulous arches not covered can be developed rather easily by extrapolating from or combining the examples presented.

Case reference guide	
Without modification space	
Two teeth in edentulous space	12.1 to 12.3
Three teeth in edentulous space	12.4 to 12.5
Four teeth in edentulous space	12.6
With posterior modification space only	
With posterior space on the same side of the arch	12.7 to 12.10
With posterior space on the opposite side of the arch	
One tooth in the space	12.11 to 12.14
More than one tooth in the space	12.15
With anterior modification space only	
One tooth in space	12.16
Two teeth in space	12.17 to 12.19
Three teeth in space	12.20
Four teeth in space	12.21
Five teeth in space	12.22
Six teeth in space	12.23
With anterior and posterior modification spaces	12.24

Case 12.1

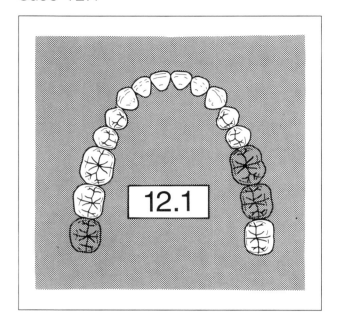

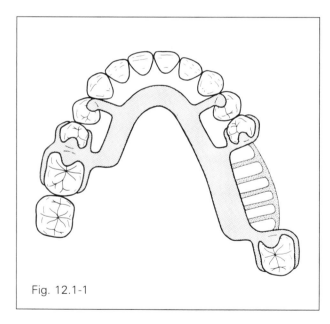

Fig. 12.1-1

Rests

Rests for Class III RPDs are normally located immediately adjacent to the edentulous spaces. However, if occlusal interference or periodontal involvement preclude "normal" placement, rest seats and rests may be relocated as long as the edentulous space lies between the two rest areas. For example, in Fig. 12.1-1, the distal rest on the right second premolar can be omitted if there is a problem with occlusal interference. The mesial rest on the first premolar would provide adequate vertical support at the anterior end of the tooth-supported segment.

There is no axis of rotation in tooth-supported RPDs; thus indirect retainers are not necessary. However, auxiliary rests (those on the premolars in Fig. 12.1-1) may be needed to prevent downward movement of the anterior portion of the major connector—if the arch form is long and narrow or if the slope of the tissues lingual to the anterior teeth is horizontal rather than vertical. The auxiliary rest can be omitted if the lingual tissue slope is vertical and if the arch form is wide and short in an anterior-posterior dimension.

The rest on the right molar may extend to the central fossa. This configuration is especially indicated when the tooth exhibits mesial inclination.

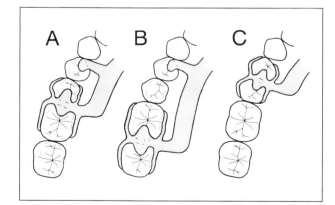

Fig. 12.1-2 The embrasure clasp assembly on the left side may be located at the second premolar/first molar (A), first molar/second molar (B), or first premolar/second premolar (C), depending on occlusion and the location of usable undercuts. The variation has very little effect on the stability of the RPD. If the first premolar/second premolar site is selected, the mesial rest on the first premolar would almost always be omitted.

Guide plates

In Class III RPDs, the path of insertion/dislodgement can be rather strictly defined. The number, length, and parallelism of the guide surface–guide plate contacts all influence the degree of limitation on the path of insertion/dislodgement.

Linguoplating, when used, may extend above the height of contour, even on abutment teeth. The plating will not preempt the rests (as it would for terminal abutments on Class I or II RPDs) because there is no functional movement of the prosthesis.

Major connector

The criteria for selecting a major connector are the same as those discussed for case 10.1.

Because no functional movement occurs in Class III RPDs, linguoplating may extend above the height of contour without affecting the action of retentive arms. However, the use of plating should generally be limited to those areas where (1) the depth of the lingual vestibule is less than 7 to 8 mm, (2) the width of the opening would be less than 4 mm, (3) the premolars or molars are tilted so far lingually that the superior border would stand out in the floor of the mouth, or (4) there is the possibility that future tooth loss would necessitate adding replacement teeth to the RPD.

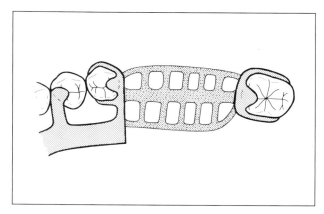

Fig. 12.1-3 The major connector should extend to the terminal abutment unless it is a lone-standing molar with a poor prognosis. In this instance, a finish line is placed distal to the anterior abutment and the clasp assembly on the posterior abutment is connected to the framework via retentive network. The anterior (premolar) clasp assembly should also be modified to be appropriate for the distal extension RPD that would occur if the molar were lost (refer to case 10.1 for clasping options).

Minor connectors

Considerations for minor connectors are the same as those discussed in case 10.1. No special modifications are necessary for Class III RPDs.

Retentive arms

Cast clasps are almost always used for Class III RPDs. The exceptions are when esthetics can be improved by placing wrought wire clasps in undercuts greater than 0.01 in. or when the posterior abutment has a questionable prognosis and the clasp assembly on the anterior abutment must be modified so future conversion to a distal extension RPD is possible. For case 12.1, use of a wrought wire retentive arm on the right second premolar would be recommended.

Circumferential clasps are most commonly selected for tooth-supported RPDs. However, because there is no functional motion or axis of rotation, virtually any type of clasp consistent with the location of the undercut, esthetics, and acceptable hygiene may be selected. Cast bar clasps may be esthetically advantageous on premolars or anterior teeth. Additionally, bar clasps, particularly modified T-bars, may be used on pre-molars when the undercut is located adjacent to the edentulous space. Circumferential clasps are contraindicated because the undercut is located near the point of origin of the arm.

If circumferential clasps are selected, either arm may be retentive. The other should be reciprocating/bracing. Ideally, all retention should be on the buccal or lingual. However, if guide surface–guide plate contacts restrict the path of insertion/dislodgement, a mixture of buccal and lingual retention is acceptable.

Molars posterior to edentulous spaces often exhibit migration and tilting to the degree that the only available undercut is located on the mesiolingual surface. In such cases, mesiolingual I-bars or ring clasps may be indicated (refer to case 11.5 for a discussion of retentive arms for mesiolingual undercuts).

If embrasure clasps are used for areas where there are not modification spaces, both anterior and posterior cast retentive arms are normally used. When the design is modified to make possible future conversion to a Class II RPD, the anterior arms may be omitted or may be removed at the time of the conversion (the anterior arms would lie in front of the axis of rotation in the Class II configuration).

Denture base retentive elements/replacement teeth

With two posterior teeth missing, retentive network, denture teeth, and denture base are most commonly used. Metal teeth and a metal base may be selected if vertical space is limited, if esthetics present no problem, and if the residual ridge is well-healed.

Case 12.2

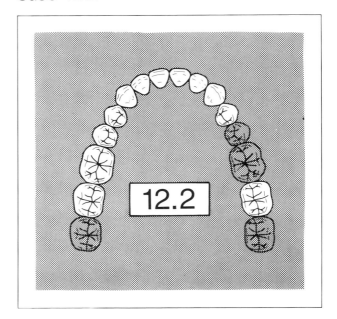

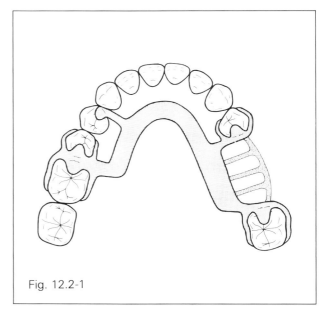

Fig. 12.2-1

Design considerations for case 12.2 are essentially the same as those for case 12.1. The fact that the posterior abutment on the right side is a second molar rather than a third molar does not affect the design.

Case 12.3

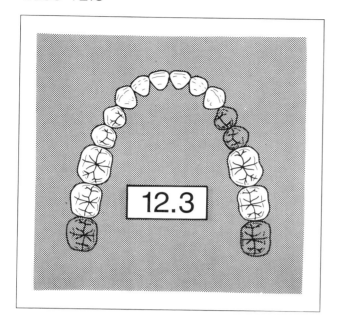

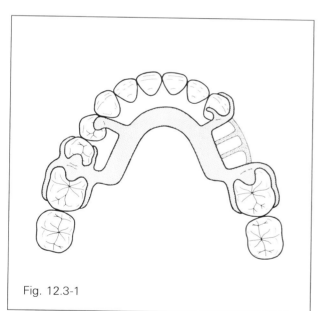

Fig. 12.3-1

Rests

Refer to case 12.1 for options on the left side. Refer to case 10.3 for options on the right canine, and to case 12.1 for options on the right molar.

Guide plates

Refer to case 12.1.

Major connector

Design options for the major connector are essentially the same as those for case 12.1. The major connector should always extend posteriorly to the first molar, unless the second molar is missing.

Minor connectors

Refer to case 12.1.

Rentenive arms

Refer to case 12.1 for clasping options for the left side and the right molar.

A cast circumferential clasp into a mesiofacial undercut is usually selected for the canine. A wrought wire circumferential clasp may be used if esthetics is improved by placing the retentive tip in more than a 0.01-in. undercut. Bar clasps may be used for esthetic reasons if the originating portion of a circumferential clasp would be located near the incisal edge. An I-bar is usually used, but a modified T-bar may be preferred if the undercut is on the distofacial surface, because an I-bar is very short and relatively inflexible. The options are similar to those described for the canines in case 10.3, except that there is no concern for an axis of rotation or functional motion in a tooth-supported RPD.

Denture base retentive elements/replacement teeth

With both premolars missing, retentive network, denture teeth, and denture base are most commonly used. Tube teeth or heat-cured or light-activated resin facings may be selected if the width of the space is appropriate and the residual ridge is well-healed.

Case 12.4

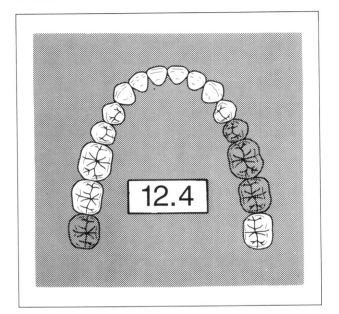

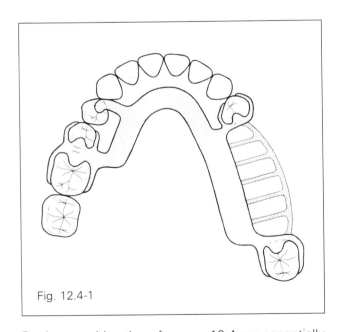

Fig. 12.4-1

Design considerations for case 12.4 are essentially the same as those for case 12.1. The fact that there is a three-tooth edentulous space utilizing the first premolar instead of the second premolar as the anterior abutment does not affect the design.

Case12.5

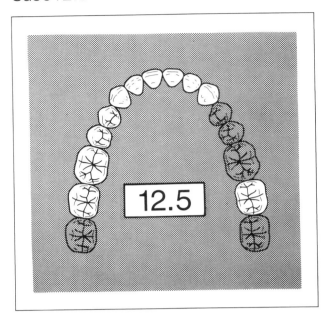

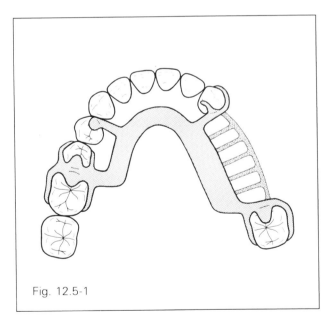

Fig. 12.5-1

Design considerations for case 12.5 are essentially the same as those for case 12.3. The fact that there is a three-tooth edentulous space utilizing the second molar instead of the first molar as the posterior abutment does not affect the design.

Case 12.6

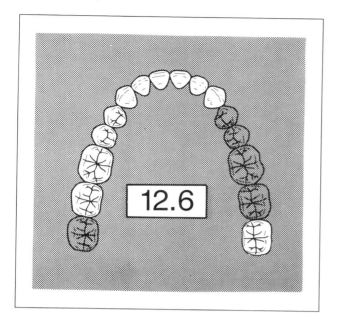

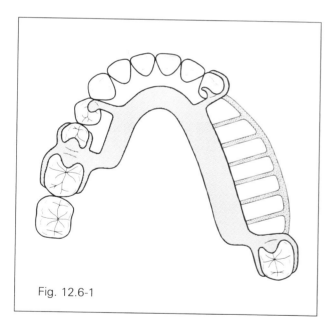

Fig. 12.6-1

The design considerations for case 12.6 are essentially the same as those for case 12.3. The fact that there is a four-tooth edentulous space utilizing the third molar instead of the first molar as the posterior abutment does not appreciably alter the design. However, there would be a greater tendency to end the major connector at the canine, espe-

cially if the long-term prognosis of the third molar were questionable. In addition, with a four-tooth edentulous space, retentive network, denture teeth, and denture base would almost always be used.

Case 12.7

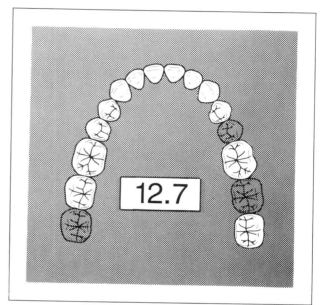

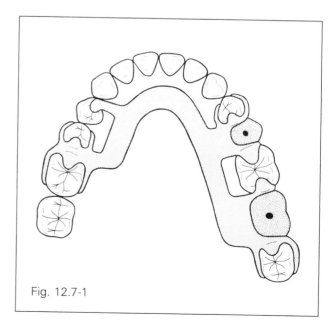

Fig. 12.7-1

Rests

Refer to case 12.1 for the left side. On the right side, one or both rests on the first molar can be omitted if occlusal interferences exist and the orientation and prognosis of the third molar are good. The tooth-supported segment will be adequately supported by the rests on the first premolar and third molar.

Guide plates

If the four guide surface–guide plate contacts are long and parallel, the path of insertion/dislogement will be strictly defined, and the need for mechanical retainers, particularly on the right side, will be minimal.

Major connector

Refer to case 12.1. Because there is no axis of rotation, the right first molar can be plated without affecting the action of the retainers.

Minor connectors

Refer to case 12.1.

Retentive arms

Clasping options for the first premolar and the third molar are the same as those described for case 12.4.

If the retainer on the first premolar is esthetically objectionable, it can be omitted if a circumferential clasp is placed into a mesiobuccal or mesiolingual undercut on the first molar.

Denture base retentive elements/replacement teeth

With single-tooth posterior modification spaces, tube teeth or all-metal pontics are usually used. The all-metal pontic would most often be selected for the molar, and is especially indicated if the anterior-posterior or vertical space is decreased by drifting or extrusion.

Case 12.8

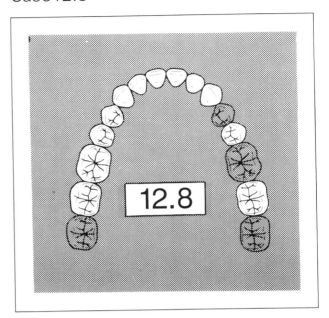

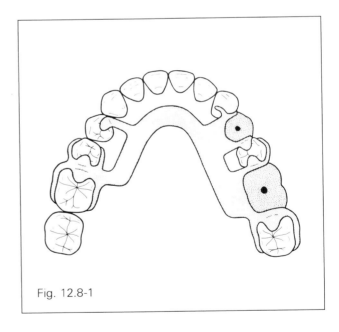

Fig. 12.8-1

Rests

Refer to case 12.1 for the left side. On the right side, one or both rests on the second premolar may be omitted if occlusal interferences exist. Refer to case 10.3 for variations in rests on the canine.

Guide plates

Refer to case 12.7.

Major connector

Refer to case 12.1. Linguoplating should be used on the right second premolar if the width of the opening is less than 4 mm.

Minor connectors

Refer to case 12.1.

Retentive arms

If esthetics is not a problem, a clasp could be placed on the right canine in addition to, or in place of, the retainer on the second premolar. Clasping options for the canine are the same as those discussed for case 10.3. Because there is no axis of rotation in this case, cast clasps would almost always be used.

Denture base retention elements/replacement teeth

Refer to case 12.7.

Case 12.9

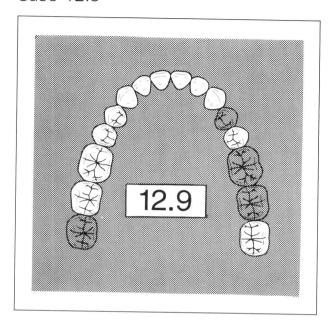

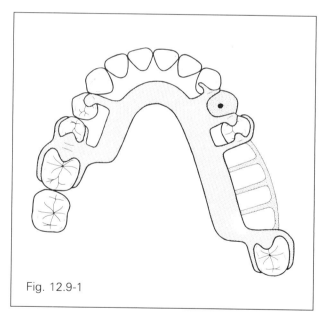

Fig. 12.9-1

Design considerations for case 12.9 are essentially the same as those for case 12.8, except the posterior tooth-supported space is larger. With two molars missing, retentive network, denture teeth, and denture base would usually be used. The major connector may end at the distal aspect of the second premolar if the prognosis of the third molar is questionable. In this instance, the circumferential clasp on the second premolar should be wrought wire.

Case 12.10

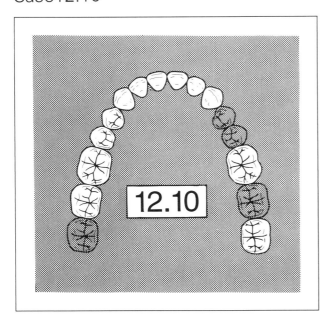

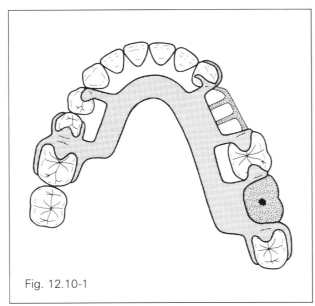

Fig. 12.10-1

The design for case 12.10 is the same as that for case 12.7, except that the anterior edentulous space has two teeth missing instead of one. Refer to case 12.3 for rest and clasp options on the ca-

nine. Although retentive network and denture base would usually be used with a two-tooth space, tube teeth or custom facings may be selected if the width of the space is appropriate and the residual ridge is well-healed.

Case 12.11

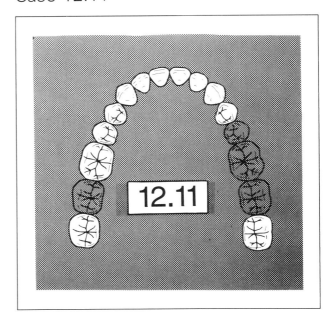

If the right side varies from that shown, refer to cases 12.1 to 12.10 for the correct configuration.

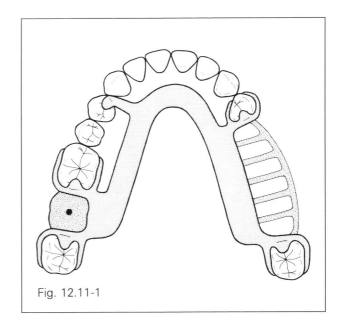

Fig. 12.11-1

For design concepts and variations on the right side, refer to cases 12.1 to 12.10. Options related to the left-side modification space are discussed below.

Rests

An auxiliary rest should be placed on the left first premolar because of the long span of the major connector between the rests on the left first molar and the right first or second premolars.

If occlusal interferences exist, the rest on the left first molar can be omitted, if the rest on the first premolar is present.

Guide plates

Refer to case 12.1.

Major connector

Refer to case 12.1.

Minor connectors

Refer to case 12.1.

Retentive arms

Clasping options for the left third molar of case 12.11 are the same as those for the right third molar of case 12.1.

In the unusual situation where the only usable undercut on the left first molar is on the distofacial surface, a modified T-bar clasp should be used.

Denture base retentive elements/replacement teeth

A tube tooth or all-metal pontic would almost always be used.

Case 12.12

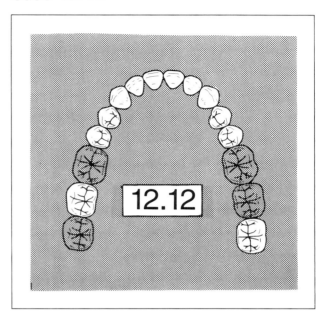

If the right side varies from that shown, refer to cases 12.1 to 12.10 for the correct configuration.

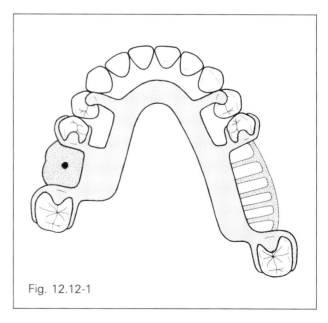

Fig. 12.12-1

For design concepts and variations on the right side, refer to cases 12.1 to 12.10. Options for the left side are essentially the same as those for case 12.11. However, since the span of the major connector is shorter, the auxiliary rests on the first premolars would only be necessary if the arch form is long and tapered.

Case 12.13

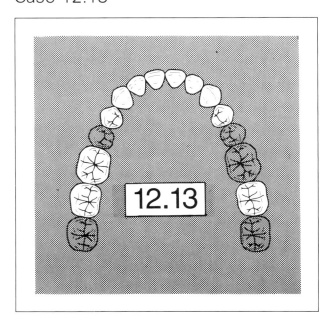

If the right side varies from that shown, refer to cases 12.1 to 12.10 for the correct configuration.

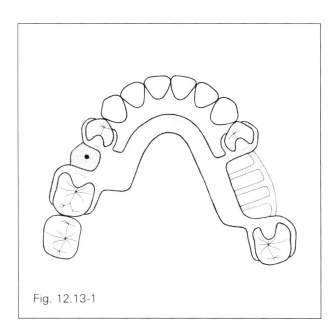

Fig. 12.13-1

For design concepts and variations for the right side, refer to cases 12.1 to 12.10. Options related to the left-side modification space are discussed below.

Rests

The rest on the first premolar may be moved to the mesial if the occlusion interferes with placement on the distal. The first premolar should then be plated if the opening between the minor connectors is less than 4 mm.

Guide plates

Refer to case 12.1.

Major connector

Refer to case 12.1.

Minor connectors

Refer to case 12.1.

Retentive arms

Clasping options for the left first molar are the same as those for the right third molar of case 12.1. Clasping options for the left first premolar are the same as those for the right second premolar of case 12.1.

Denture base retentive elements/replacement teeth

A tube tooth or heat-cured or light-activated resin replacement would usually be used. An all-metal pontic can be selected when esthetics is not important.

Case 12.14

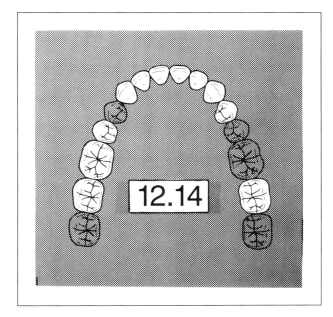

If the right side varies from that shown, refer to cases 12.1 to 12.10 for the correct configuration.

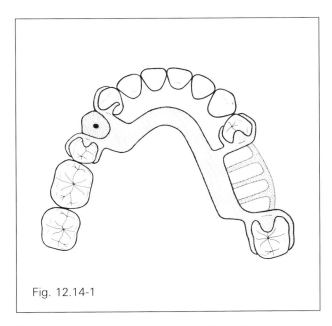

Fig. 12.14-1

For design concepts and variations for the right side, refer to cases 12.1 to 12.10. Options related to the left-side modification space are discussed below.

Rests

Options for the left-canine rest seat and rest are the same as those for the right canine of case 12.3.

Guide plates

Refer to case 12.1.

Major connector

Refer to case 12.1.

Minor connectors

Refer to case 12.1.

Retentive arms

Clasping options for the left canine are the same as those for the right canine of case 12.3. When the major connector is altered to permit later conversion to a Class II RPD in the event that the right posterior abutment is lost, the clasp on the left canine should be wrought wire; after the conversion, it will lie in front of the axis of rotation.

Denture base retentive elements/replacement teeth

A tube tooth, facing, or heat-cured or light-activated resin replacement would almost always be used.

Case 12.15

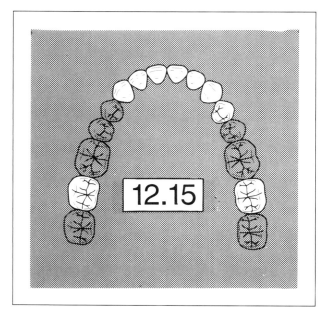

Case 12.15 represents one of a myriad of possible combinations of posterior bilateral tooth-supported spaces. If the arch form varies from that shown, refer to cases 12.1 to 12.10 for right-side configurations and to the mirror images of cases 12.1 to 12.10 for left-side configurations.

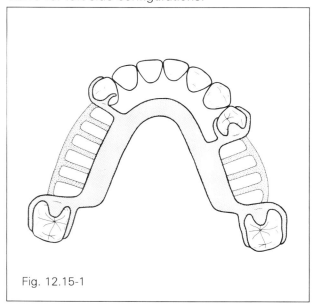

Fig. 12.15-1

Designs for tooth-supported RPDs with bilateral edentulous segments can be created by combining portions of the designs for cases 12.1 to 12.10 (or

their mirror images). The sample design for case 12.15 is a composite of case 12.2 for the right side and the mirror image of case 12.5 for the left side.

Case 12.16

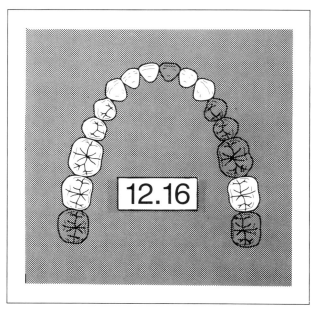

If the right posterior segment varies from that shown, refer to cases 12.1 to 12.10 for the correct configuration. Changes in the location of the anterior modification space have minimal effect on the design.

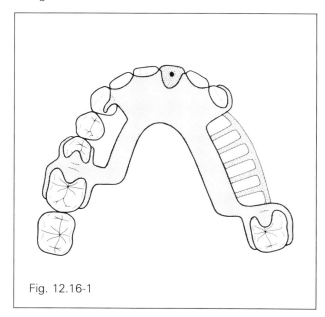

Fig. 12.16-1

Except for the use of linguoplating, the design for case 12.16 is essentially the same as that for case 12.5, with a single-tooth anterior modification space. Options related to the modification space are discussed below. For other aspects of the design, refer to cases 12.1 to 12.10.

Rests

In the design shown, a rest seat should be prepared under the linguoplating *at least on the canine*. If possible, rest seats should also be prepared on the incisors.

Guide plates

Guide plates on the anterior teeth should be located on the linguoproximal surfaces so that they will not be visible from the labial aspect or interfere with positioning of the replacement tooth.

Major connector

With a single tooth in the anterior modification space, linguoplating can often be avoided if the anterior teeth exhibit good bone support and prominent cinguli for rest seats adjacent to the modification space.

Minor connectors

Refer to case 12.1.

Retentive arms

Retentive arms on the anterior teeth would be unesthetic and are rarely, if ever, indicated.

Denture base retentive elements/replacement teeth

With only one tooth in the anterior modification space, a prefabricated facing, tube tooth, or custom heat-cured or light-activated resin replacement is almost always used.

Case 12.17

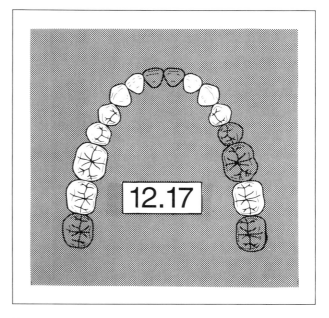

If the right posterior segment varies from that shown, refer to cases 12.1 to 12.10 for the correct configuration.

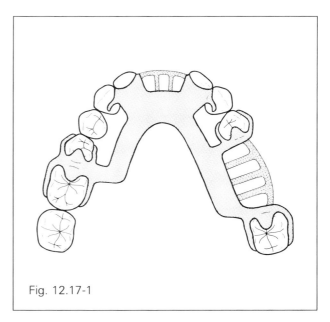

Fig. 12.17-1

The design for case 12.17 is essentially the same as that for case 12.2, with a two-tooth anterior modification space. Options related to the modification space are discussed below. For other aspects of the design, refer to cases 12.1 to 12.10.

Rests

If possible, rest seats should be prepared beneath the plating on the remaining incisors.

Guide plates

Refer to case 12.16.

Major connector

Linguoplating would almost always be used on the remaining incisors.

Minor connectors

Refer to case 12.1.

Retentive arms

Refer to case 12.16.

Denture base retentive elements/replacement teeth

With two or more teeth in the anterior modification space, replacement teeth attached via retentive network and denture base would usually be selected. Commercial facings, tube teeth, or heat-cured or light-activated resin replacements may be used if the residual ridge is well-healed and exhibits minimal resorption.

Case 12.18

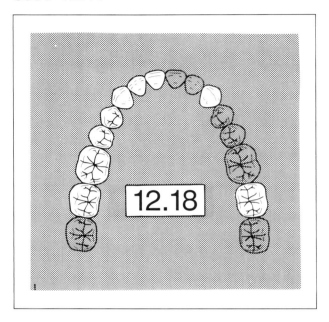

If the right posterior segment varies from that shown, refer to cases 12.1 to 12.10 for the correct configuration.

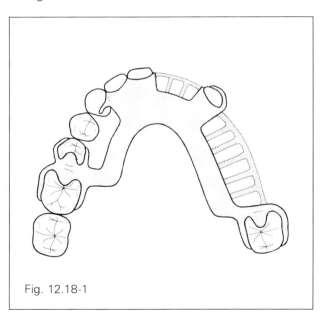

Fig. 12.18-1

The design considerations for case 12.18 are essentially the same as those for case 12.17. A rest seat must be present beneath the plating on the right canine.

Case 12.19

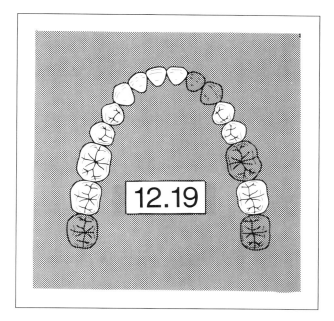

If the right posterior segment varies from that shown, refer to cases 12.1 to 12.10 for the correct configuration.

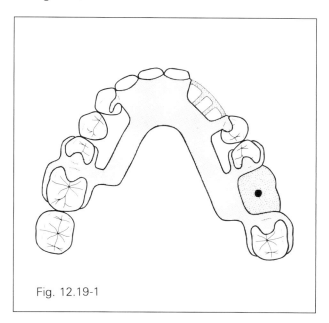

Fig. 12.19-1

For design concepts and variations for the right posterior segment, refer to cases 12.1 to 12.10. Options related to the anterior modification space are discussed below.

Rests

If possible, rest seats should be prepared on the remaining incisors. The distal rest on the right second premolar can be omitted when there are occlusal interferences.

Guide plates

The guide plate on the central incisor should be located on the linguoproximal surface so it will not be visible from the labial aspect or interfere with positioning of the replacement teeth.

Major connector

With a two-tooth anterior modification space, and particularly when the canine is missing, a linguoplate major connector is preferred unless the right central incisor exhibits exceptionally good bone support and a prominent cingulum.

Minor connectors

Refer to case 12.1.

Retentive arms

A retentive arm on the central incisor would be unesthetic; it is rarely, if ever, indicated.

Denture base retentive elements/replacement teeth

Refer to case 12.17 for the anterior segment and to case 12.7 for the posterior segment.

Case 12.20

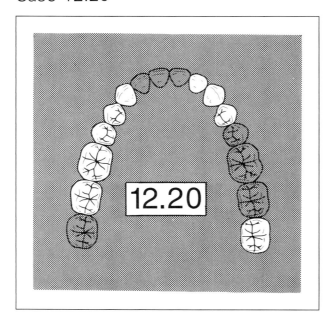

If the right posterior segment varies from that shown, refer to cases 12.1 to 12.10 for the correct configuration.

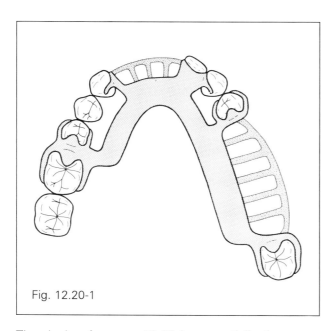

Fig. 12.20-1

The design for case 12.20 is essentially the same as that for case 12.4, with a three-tooth anterior modification space. Design considerations for the

modification space are the same as those for the two-tooth space in case 12.17. Refer to cases 12.1 to 12.10 for other aspects of the design.

Rests

If occlusal interferences exist, the rest on the right first premolar could be moved from the distal to mesial fossa. The canine should then be plated.

Guide plates

Refer to case 12.16.

Major connector

Refer to case 12.1.

Minor connectors

Refer to case 12.1.

Retentive arms

A retentive arm may be placed on the left canine. A bar clasp is usually preferred because it will be less visible. A circumferential clasp engaging a distofacial undercut would often originate near the incisal edge and detract from the esthetic value of the RPD.

Denture base retentive elements/replacement teeth

Refer to case 12.17.

Case 12.21

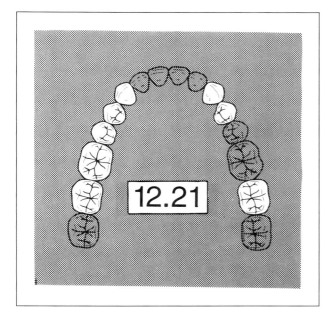

If the right posterior segment varies from that shown, refer to cases 12.1 to 12.10 for the correct configuration.

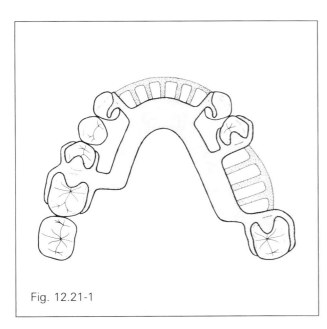

Fig. 12.21-1

The design for case 12.21 is essentially the same as that for case 12.2, with a four-tooth anterior modification space. Design considerations associ-

ated with the anterior modification space are discussed below. Refer to cases 12.1 to 12.10 for other aspects of the design.

Rests

Refer to cases 12.3 and 10.3 for options in canine rests. If adequate cingulum rests cannot be prepared, and if esthetics precludes incisal rests, the canines may be plated and rests placed in the mesial fossae of the first premolars.

Guide plates

Refer to case 12.16.

Major connector

Refer to case 12.1.

Minor connectors

Refer to case 12.1.

Retentive arms

Refer to case 12.20. Rigid metal retention (dual path or rotational path of insertion) should also be considered, especially if esthetics is important.

Denture base retentive elements/replacement teeth

Refer to case 12.17.

Case 12.22

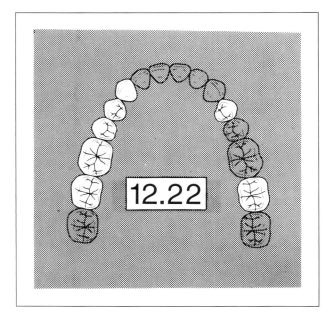

If the right posterior segment varies from that shown, refer to cases 12.1 to 12.10 for the correct configuration.

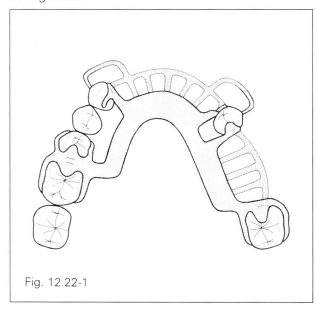

Fig. 12.22-1

With one of the canines missing, the RPD may be considered an anterior extension, particularly if the anterior abutments show loss of bone support, and if the size and contour of the residual ridge is less than ideal.

Rests

If the RPD is considered an anterior extension, it would be best to use a distal rest on the lone-standing premolar. The tip of the I-bar will then release when the anterior extension moves toward the tissue. As designed, the tip of the I-bar on the left canine will not release during functional movements of the anterior segment; the clasp arm should be long, tapered, and flexible. If the canine is periodontally weak, the left anterior rest can be moved to the mesial fossa of the first premolar. Vertical stress will decrease and the I-bar will release during functional movements. If the RPD is considered tooth supported, the anterior rest on the right side could be placed in the mesial fossa of the first premolar, because there is no functional motion or axis of rotation in a Class III RPD.

Guide plates

The guide plate on the canine should be located on the linguoproximal surface so that it will not be visible from the labial aspect or interfere with positioning of the replacement teeth.

Major connector

If the width of the opening lingual to the right first premolar is less than 4 mm, it is best to plate. However, if the RPD is considered an anterior extension, it is best to avoid plating the premolar, because the plating may preempt the planned distal rest during functional movements.

Minor connectors

Refer to case 12.1.

Retentive arms

If the RPD is considered an anterior extension, bar clasps are preferred because of their capacity to release during functional movements. If the RPD is considered tooth supported, cast circumferential clasps could be used—however, the mesial origin of a circumferential clasp on the canine may detract from esthetics.

Denture base retentive elements/replacement teeth

Refer to case 12.17.

Case 12.23

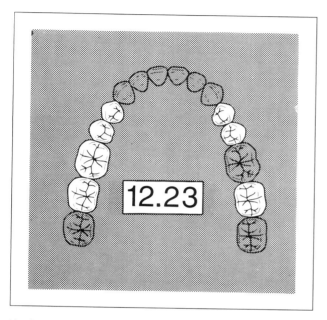

If the right posterior segments vary from that shown, refer to cases 12.1 to 12.10 for the correct configuration.

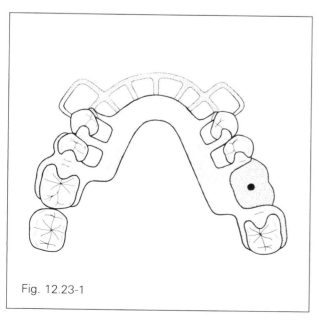

Fig. 12.23-1

With both canines missing, the RPD should be considered an anterior extension.

Rests

Either or both of the distal rests on the second premolars may be omitted if there are occlusal interferences.

Distal rests are preferred for the first premolars because of the anterior extension area. However, mesial rests may be used if alternate clasping is selected (see "Retentive arms," below).

Guide plates

Refer to case 12.22.

Major connector

Refer to case 12.1.

Minor connectors

Refer to case 12.1.

Retentive arms

The retentive arm on the left second premolar is not absolutely necessary as long as a clasp is placed on the first premolar. If esthetic demands preclude clasping the first premolars, clasps should be placed on both second premolars. Rigid metal retention (rotational path or dual path of insertion) may also be considered.

Clasping of the first premolars is designed so the retentive tips will release during functional movements of the anterior extension. If mesial rests must be used due to occlusal interference, bar clasps must be long, tapered and flexible, or wrought wire circumferential clasps should be selected.

Denture base retentive elements/replacement teeth

Refer to case 12.17.

Case 12.24

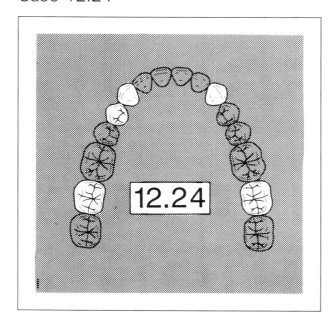

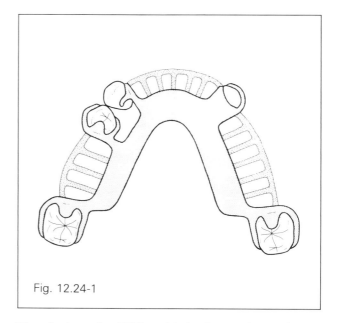

Fig. 12.24-1

Case 12.24 represents one of myriad possible combinations of anterior plus bilateral-posterior tooth-supported spaces. If the arch form varies from that shown, refer to cases 12.1 to 12.10 for the right-posterior configuration to cases 12.16 to 12.23 for the anterior configuration, and to the mirror images of cases 12.1 to 12.10 for the left-posterior configuration.

The designs for RPDs with both anterior and posterior modification spaces can be created by combining portions of cases 12.1 to 12.10 (or their mirror images) for the posterior segments and cases 12.16 to 12.23 for the anterior segments. For example, the design for case 12.24 is a combination of case 12.5 for the right-posterior segment, case 12.21 for the anterior segment, and the mirror image of case 12.2 for the left-posterior segment. Minor alterations will be necessary to arrive at the final composite design.

Mandibular Class IV Designs

According to Applegate's rules for applying the Kennedy Classification, Class IV removable partial dentures cannot have modification spaces. A posterior modification space would take precedence in nomenclature, resulting in a Class III RPD. Thus, the frequency of Class IV RPDs is quite low. In our study of 3,000 partially edentulous mandibular arches for which removable partial dentures were fabricated, less than 2% were truly Class IV. Considering frequency of occurrence, the 12 cases discussed in chapter 13 cover over 95% of these partially edentulous arches (or their mirror images). The partially edentulous arch discussed in case 13.2 comprised almost two thirds of the total.

Case reference guide	
Symmetrical	
Two teeth in space	13.1
Four teeth in space	13.2
Six teeth in space	13.3
Eight teeth in space	13.4
Ten teeth in space	13.5
Asymmetrical	
Three teeth in space	13.6
Four teeth in space	13.7
Five teeth in space	13.8
Six teeth in space	13.9
Seven teeth in space	1310
Eight teeth in space	13.11
Nine teeth in space	13.12

Case 13.1

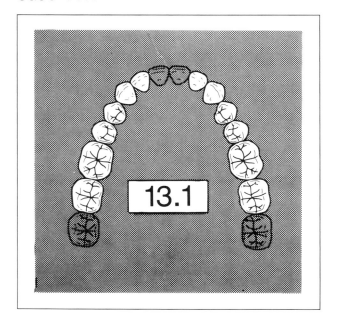

13.1

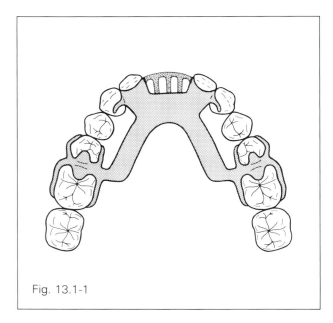

Fig. 13.1-1

Rests

Cingulum rests may be placed on the lateral incisors rather than the canines if the periodontal support is good and the lingual anatomy is appropriate for rest preparations. Incisal rests are seldom used, because with only a two-tooth edentulous segment, minimal cingulum rest preparations suffice. In addition, incisal rests on the lateral incisors would compromise esthetics and could interfere with occlusion.

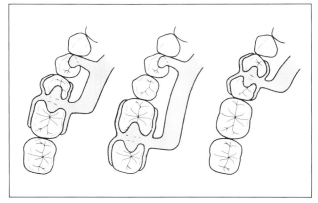

Fig. 13.1-2 The embrasure clasp assemblies may be moved one tooth forward or backward, depending on location of the undercuts and occlusal contacts.

Guide plates

Guide plates on the anterior teeth must be placed on the linguoproximal surfaces so they will not be visible from the labial aspect or interfere with positioning of the replacement teeth.

Major connector

A lingual bar, with or without plating on the lateral incisors, is the preferred major connector. The indications for plating the canines and premolars are the same as those discussed for case 10.1.

Minor connectors

Considerations for minor connectors are the same as those discussed for case 10.1. There are no special considerations for Class IV RPDs.

Retentive arms

Cast clasps are usually used for Class IV RPDs when the edentulous segment is not so large that the prosthesis is considered an anterior extension.

Circumferential (embrasure) clasps are almost always placed to provide posterior retention. Either buccal or lingual undercuts may be used. The portions of the embrasure clasps extending forward may be omitted if there is adequate anterior retention.

If the edentulous space is small (as in case 13.1) anterior retention is usually omitted. When there are proximal undercuts bordering the edentulous space, rigid metal retention may be used (see *dual path* and *rotational path,* p. 70). Bar clasps on the lateral incisors, emanating from the edentulous area, are an acceptable alternative if the arms are hidden by the lower lip. Circumferential clasps would usually originate near the incisal edges and would be esthetically unacceptable.

Denture base retentive elements/replacement teeth

Denture teeth attached via retentive network and denture base, tube teeth, commercial facings, or heat-cured or light-activated resin custom facings are equally acceptable as replacements for the central incisors. Denture teeth are especially indicated if the residual ridge is atrophic or in the process of recontouring, or if the width of the space is inappropriate for the two missing teeth.

Case 13.2

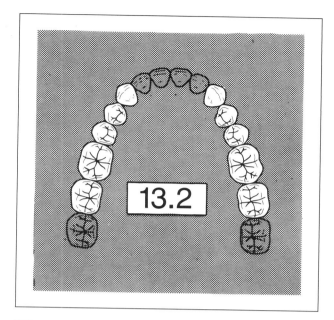

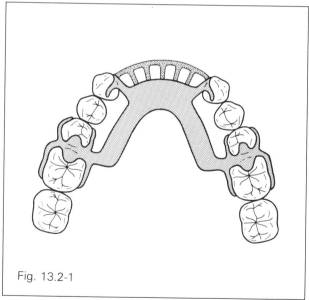

Fig. 13.2-1

Rests

Variations in the location of the embrasure clasp assemblies are essentially the same as those for case 13.1. However, moving the assembly forward onto the premolars tends to decrease the effectiveness of the resistance to biting forces on the anterior segment.

Cingulum rests are selected for the canines if the lingual anatomy is appropriate. When the slope is excessively steep, mesial or distal incisal rests may be preferred. The canines should be plated and mesial rests placed on the first premolars if cingulum rest seats cannot be prepared and if incisal rests are esthetically unacceptable.

Guide plates

Refer to case 13.1.

Major connector

Refer to case 13.1.

Minor connectors

Refer to case 13.1.

Retentive arms

The options for posterior retention are essentially the same as those for case 13.1.

Anteriorly, rigid metal retention (dual path or rotational path) is particularly effective when the four incisors are missing. When the arms are hidden by the lower lip, excellent esthetics and retention can be achieved with bar clasps. I-bars should be used with distofacial or midfacial undercuts, whereas modified T-bars are more appropriate if the undercuts are on the mesiofacial surfaces. Cast circumferential clasps will provide excellent retention but may create severe esthetic problems, particularly if they originate from the mesial guide plates and engage distofacial undercuts. Esthetic problems are decreased if the clasps pass through the embrasures between the first premolars and the canines and engage mesiofacial undercuts. However, this location could interfere with the opposing occlusion. When embrasure clasps are used, the canines should be plated so that the plating will act as an origin for the retentive arms.

Denture base retentive elements/replacement teeth

With four teeth in the edentulous segment, denture teeth would usually be attached via retentive network and denture base. Commercial facings, tube teeth, or heat-cured or light-activated resin replacements may be used if the residual ridge is well-healed and exhibits minimal resorption.

Case 13.3

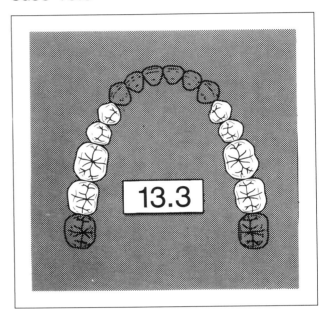

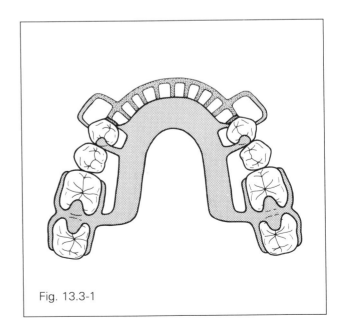

Fig. 13.3-1

When both canines are missing, the RPD should be considered an anterior extension. The axis of rotation will pass through the most anterior rests. Clasp assemblies on the anterior abutments should be designed so that the retentive arms release when the anterior segment moves toward the residual ridge. If this is not possible, the retentive arms should be flexible so that they provide a degree of stress relief to the abutments.

Rests

Distal rests are preferred on the premolars if infrabulge clasps can be used. If occlusion interferes with placement in the distal fossae, the rests may be moved to the mesial fossae. However, the type of retentive arms would usually need to be altered (see "Retentive arms," below).

Guide plates

The principles of guide plate design are the same as those described for the posterior abutments on Class I RPDs (case 10.1), except they are on the mesial surfaces instead of the distal surfaces. Because the guide plates must not bind against the teeth during tissueward movement of the anterior extention, physiologic relief at the framework try-in is essential.

Major connector

A lingual bar is the preferred major connector. If plating is used on the anterior abutments, it must end exactly at the survey line so it will not preempt the distal rests. The indications for plating are the same as those discussed in case 10.1.

Retentive arms

Design principles for the embrasure clasps on the posterior teeth are the same as those discussed for case 13.1, except that the first choice for location is the first molars and second molars, rather than the second premolars and first molars.

Rigid metal retention (see *dual path* and *rotational path*, p. 70) may be used on the premolars if proximal undercuts can be engaged by the guide plates; mesial rests would then be placed.

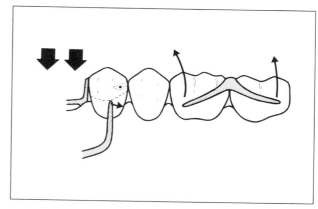

Fig. 13.3-2 Bar clasps on the premolars will release when the anterior segment moves toward the tissues. I-bars are used with midfacial or distofacial undercuts, whereas modified T-bars are preferred if the undercuts are on the mesiofacial surface. Distal rests should be selected with either type of infrabulge clasp. Although retentive arms on the posterior abutments are on the opposite side of the axis of rotation from the extension area, the potential for the development of torquing forces is much less than that for the anterior abutments. Because the posterior retentive tips are farther from the axis of rotation, stresses on the abutments created by tissueward movement of the extension base tend to be vertical rather than torquing. In addition, the posterior teeth are generally stronger and more stable. The potential for the development of excessive stresses can be further reduced by ensuring minimal anterior tooth contact and by periodic relining of the extension base.

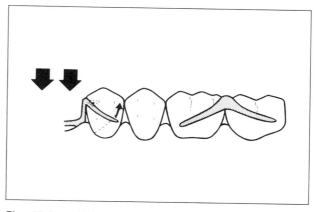

Fig. 13.3-3 If the undercuts are located on the distofacial aspects and infrabulge clasps cannot be used, the rests must be placed on the mesio-occlusal surfaces; wrought wire circumferential clasps originating from the mesial guide plate should be selected. Unfortunately, the mesial origins of the arms will often be near the occlusal surfaces, detracting from esthetics.

Denture base retentive elements/replacement teeth

With six teeth missing, denture teeth would always be attached via retentive network and denture base.

The design for case 13.4 is essentially the same as that for case 13.3. Lingual bracing arms on the first molars are not needed because the combination of mesial and distal minor connectors provides adequate bracing and prevents lingual migration of the teeth.

Case 13.4

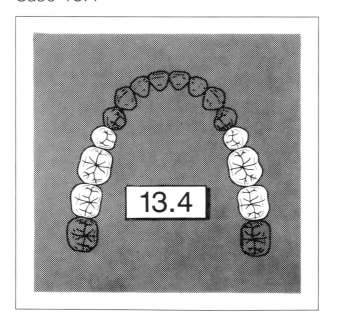

Case 13.5

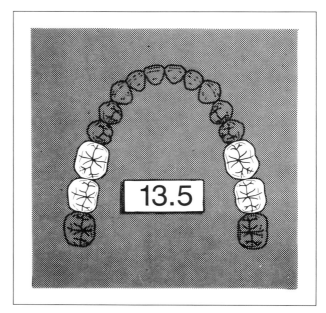

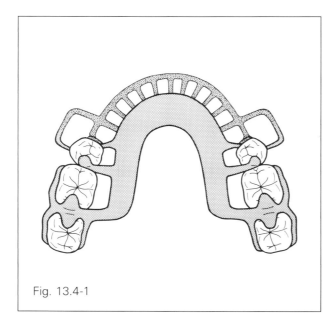

Fig. 13.4-1

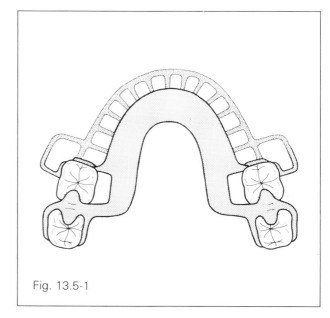

Fig. 13.5-1

The design principles for case 13.5 are essentially the same as those for case 13.3. However, with the very large anterior extension area, special consideration should be given to eliminating torquing forces on the molars. If mesiofacial undercuts are present, modified T-bars are the retentive arms of choice. Although I-bars could be used, the vertical portion of the arm would lie very close to the border of the denture base and complicate finishing and polishing of the plastic. In addition, the small space created would tend to accumulate food and plaque.

If the only undercuts on the first molars are located on the mesiolingual surfaces, cast circumferential clasps emanating from the minor connectors can be selected. Both mesial and distal rests should be used because rigid portions of the clasp arms will be located above the height of contour on inclined surfaces, preempting the distal rests. Because the tips of the retentive arms will lie almost directly under the axis of rotation (which passes through the mesial rests), minimal torquing forces will be applied to the abutments.

Because the extension area is large and the clasp assemblies on the second molars are very close to the axis of rotation, they usually provide bracing only. Both buccal and lingual arms should be rigid and located at or above the survey line. If the abutments are strong and the residual ridge exceptionally good, and if the opposing arch is restored by a complete denture, retention can be on the second molars. Periodic relining of the anterior segment will help reduce undesirable stresses.

Case 13.6

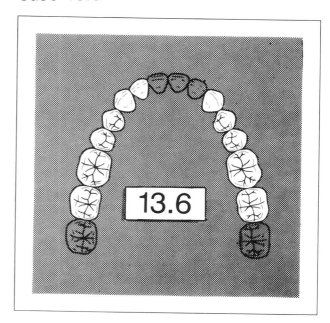

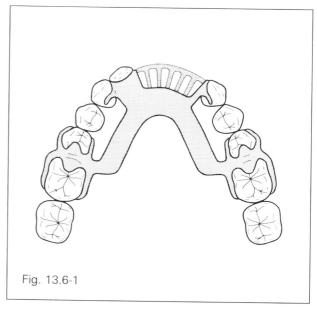

Fig. 13.6-1

For design concepts and variations, refer to case 13.1 for the left side and case 13.2 for the right side.

Case 13.7

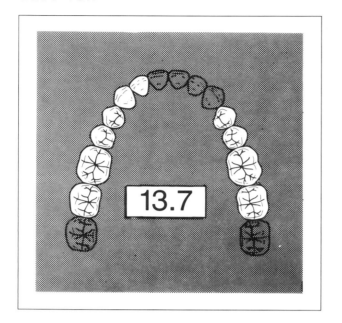

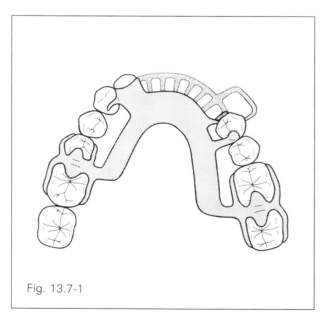

Fig. 13.7-1

Case 13.8

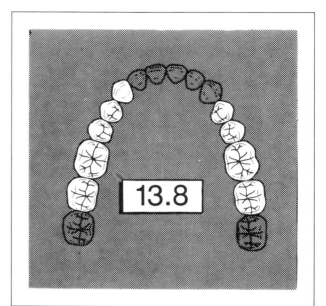

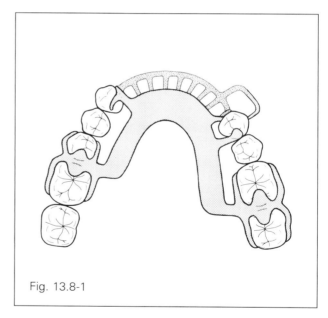

Fig. 13.8-1

For design concepts and variations, refer to case 13.1 for the left side and case 13.3 for the right side.

For design concepts and variations, refer to case 13.2 for the left side and case 13.3 for the right side.

Case 13.9

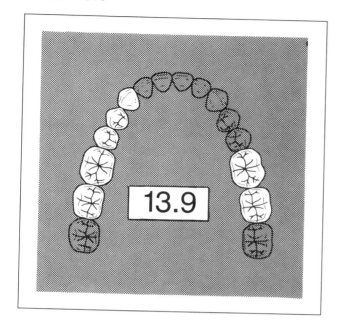

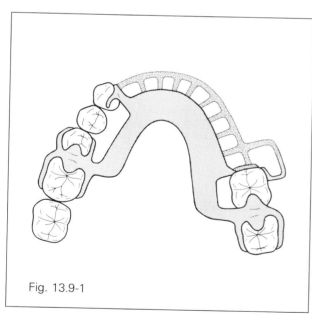

Fig. 13.9-1

For design concepts and variations, refer to case 13.2 for the left side and case 13.5 for the right side.

Case 13.10

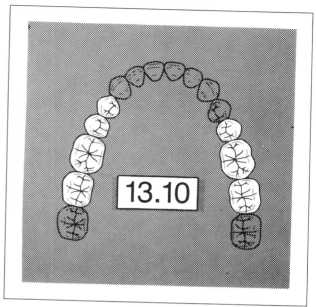

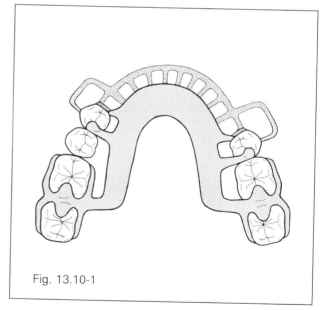

Fig. 13.10-1

For design concepts and variations, refer to case 13.3 for the left side and case 13.4 for the right side.

Case 13.11

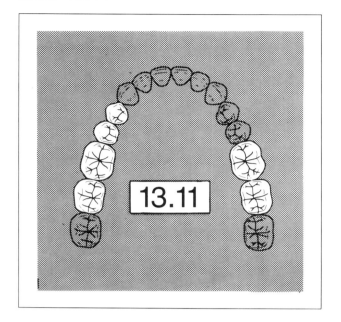

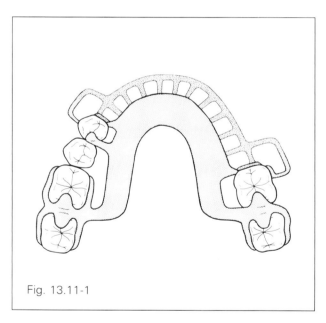

Fig. 13.11-1

For design concepts and variations, refer to case 13.3 for the left side and case 13.5 for the right side.

Case 13.12

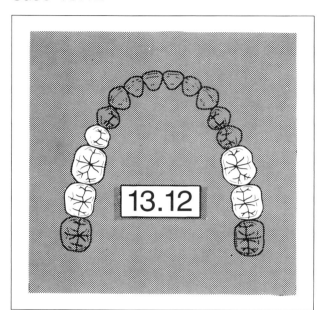

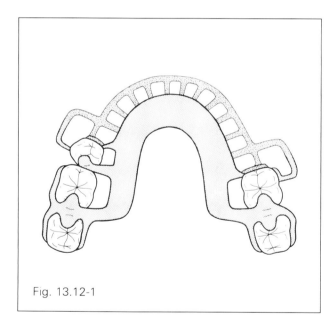

Fig. 13.12-1

For design concepts and variations, refer to case 13.4 for the left side and case 13.5 for the right side.

Maxillary Class I Designs

In our study of almost 2,000 partially edentulous maxillary arches for which removable partial dentures were fabricated, approximately 20% were Class I. Considering frequency of occurrence, the 40 cases discussed in chapter 14 cover over 95% of these partially edentulous arches (or their mirror images).

Because a distal extension RPD is seldom fabricated to replace second or third molars, only those situations where at least all the molars are missing will be considered.

Case reference guide	
Without modification space	
Symmetrical	
All anterior teeth are present	14.1 to 14.3
Canines are missing	14.4
Asymmetrical	
All anterior teeth are present	14.5 to 14.7
Some or all of anterior teeth are missing	14.8 to 14.9
With modification space	
With posterior modification space(s) only	
Symmetrical	14.10
Asymmetrical	14.11 to 14.13
With single anterior modification space only	
Symmetrical	
Two teeth in space	14.14 to 14.16
Four teeth in space	14.17 to 14.19
Asymmetrical	
One tooth in space	14.20 to 14.23
Two teeth in space	14.24 to 14.28
Three teeth in space	14.29 to 14.30
Four teeth in space	14.31 to 14.32
With two anterior modification spaces	14.33 to 14.37
With both anterior and posterior modification spaces	14.38 to 14.40

Case 14.1

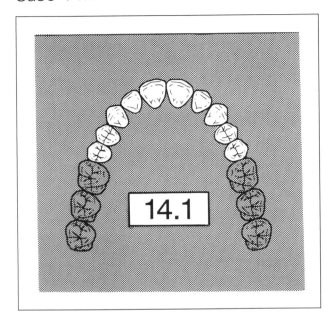

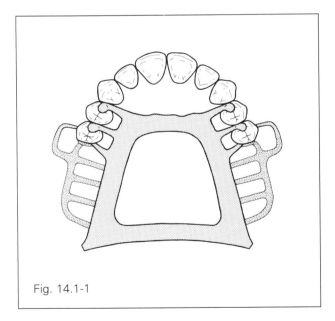

Fig. 14.1-1

Rests

The variations in rest location considered in Figs. 14.1-2 to 14.1-4 apply primarily to the preferred mesial rest, I-bar, and distal guide plate design. However, rest location, particularly that of primary rests, is intimately related to the selection of retentive arms, and is discussed further in that section.

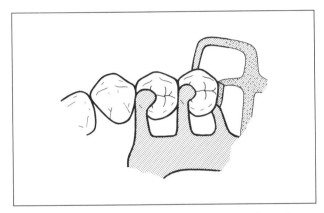

Fig. 14.1-2a On distal extension RPDs, the primary rest is usually placed on the mesio-occlusal aspect of the tooth adjacent to the edentulous space. The indirect retainer would normally be placed in the mesio-occlusal fossa of the first premolar.

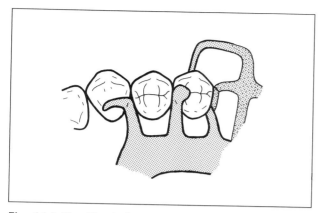

Fig. 14.1-2b   The indirect retainer should be moved to the cingulum of the canine if the mesial fossa of the first premolar is blocked by the opposing occlusion.

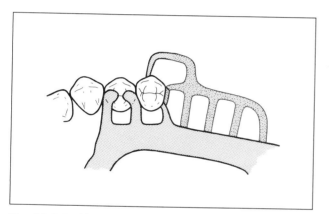

Fig. 14.1-3   If the terminal abutment exhibits significant loss of supporting bone or if the mesio-occlusal fossa is unavailable due to tight interdigitation with an opposing cusp tip, the primary rest may be moved to the disto-occlusal aspect of the next tooth forward. The indirect retainer may remain on the mesio-occlusal aspect of the first premolar or may be placed on the cingulum of the canine.

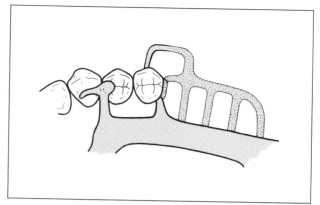

Fig. 14.1-4   If the disto-occlusal fossa of the first premolar is also blocked by the opposing occlusion, the primary rest may be placed in the mesio-occlusal fossa. Although this rest will also function as an indirect retainer, a cingulum rest is usually added on the canine. It will (1) help to offset vertical forces, (2) improve indirect retention (because it lies farther from the retentive tip), and (3) provide bracing when the RPD is fully seated. Because there is now no minor connector between the premolars, the guide surface–guide plate relationship on the distal surface of the second premolar should extend around the distolingual line angle to create reciprocation and/or bracing, and, in combination with the proximal tooth contact, provide 180° encirclement. If necessary, the premolars can be plated. However, the plating must not extend above the height of contour, or it will preempt the planned rest.

Guide plates

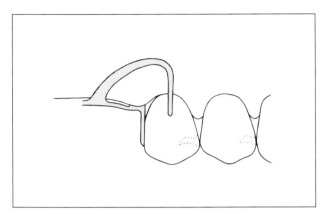

Fig. 14.1-5 Guide surface–guide plate contacts should be parallel to the path of insertion/dislodgement. The occlusogingival dimension of the contact should be one half to two thirds the crown length. If present, a small recess gingival to the guide surface is retained.

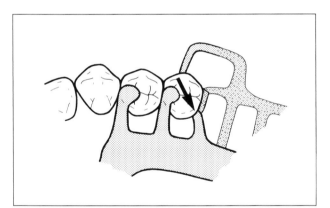

Fig. 14.1-6 The guide plate should curve buccolingually and extend beyond the distolingual line angle *(arrow)* to provide 180° encirclement, bracing, and possibly reciprocation. It should not extend above the height of contour, or it will preempt the planned mesial rest.

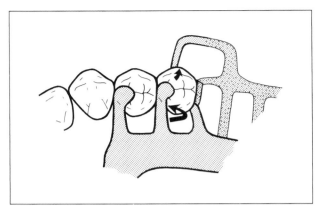

Fig. 14.1-7 In the partially edentulous situation under consideration, the two guide plates do not establish a definite path of insertion/dislodgement. A random dislodging force could cause the RPD to move downward and posteriorly. However, the RPD will resist random dislodging forces and exhibit retention if the retentive tip is placed just in front of the greatest mesiodistal curvature of the facial surface and/or if a small guide surface can be established at the mesiolingual surface of the abutment.

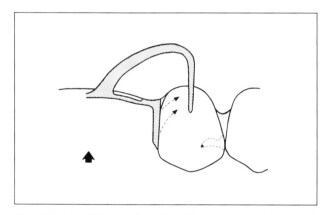

Fig. 14.1-8 When a functional force (toward the residual ridge) is applied to the extension area, the gingival portion of the guide plate may bind against the abutment and must be physiologically relieved at the framework try-in.

Major connector

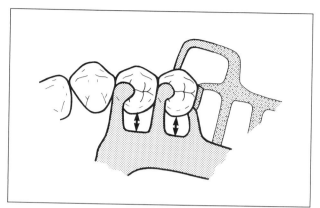

Fig. 14.1-9 For a maxillary RPD, there should be at least 6 mm of space *(arrows)* between the gingival margin and the border of the major connector.

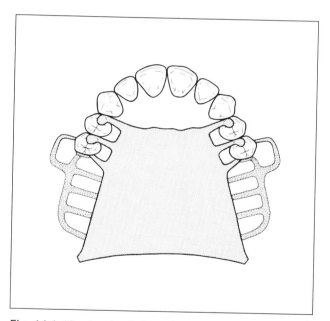

Fig. 14.1-10 A palatal plate should be considered when additional support and denture style retention are needed. Indications include *(1)* atrophic residual ridges, *(2)* periodontally weakened abutments, and *(3)* minimal direct retention from clasps.

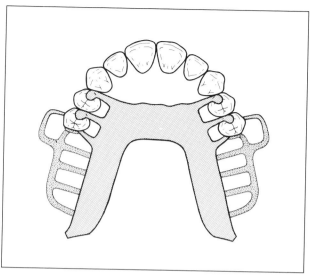

Fig. 14.1-11 A U-shaped major connector may be selected if *(1)* there is an inoperable torus which extends to within 6 to 8 mm of the vibrating line, or *(2)* the patient is unable to tolerate an anterior-posterior palatal strap. The U-shaped connector is the last choice because it often lacks rigidity and covers considerable tissue in an area prone to inflammatory papillary hyperplasia.

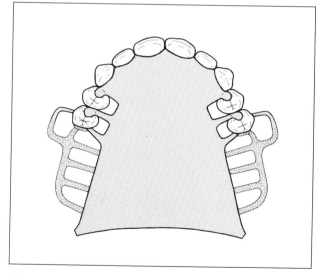

Fig. 14.1-12 Linguoplating may be considered if the long-term prognosis of the anterior teeth is questionable. However, plating should be avoided if possible, because it may interfere with the opposing occlusion and adversely affect speech. If the premolars are also plated, the metal must end exactly at the survey line so that it will not preempt the mesial rests.

Minor connectors

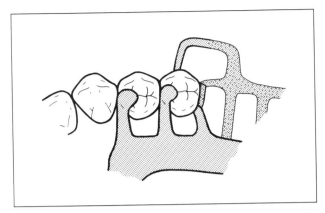

Fig. 14.1-13 Minor connectors that connect rests to major connectors should be positioned in embrasures and form a right angle at the junction with the major connector. Whenever possible, at least 4 mm of space should be present between adjacent vertical minor connectors.

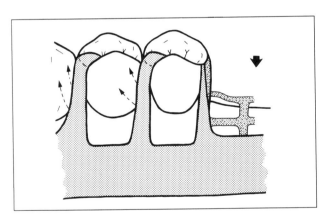

Fig. 14.1-14 When a functional load is placed on the distal extension area, the prosthesis rotates around the primary rests and the minor connectors move occlusally and mesially. The mesial aspects of the minor connectors should be physiologically relieved at the framework try-in.

Retentive arms

Ideally, the tips of retentive arms should release during functional movement of the extension base. If this is not possible, stress-breaking should be achieved with flexible arms (wrought wire or long, tapered bar clasps). When neither of these are possible, consider placing a crown on the abutment, depending on existing or needed restorations and

the compromise in clasping that would be necessary if the crown were not fabricated.

In general, preference for clasp assemblies for terminal abutments on maxillary distal extension RPDs is as follows: *(1)* I-bar with mesial rest, *(2)* T-bar with mesial rest, *(3)* combination clasp with distal rest.

Infrabulge clasps are contraindicated when *(1)* there is a large tissue undercut below the abutment, *(2)* a high frenal attachment or shallow vestibule interferes with the approach arm, *(3)* periodontal considerations preclude crossing the gingival margin with a clasp arm, or *(4)* esthetics is compromised by the visibility of a bar clasp crossing gingival tissue.

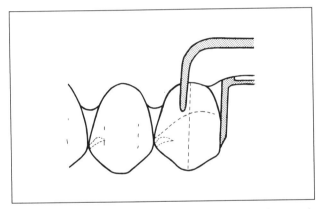

Fig. 14.1-15 When there is an undercut on the mesiofacial surface, the preferred clasp assembly is composed of an I-bar, a mesial rest, and a distal guide plate.

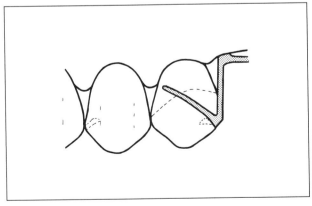

Fig. 14.1-16 When the undercut is located on the mesiofacial surface and a bar clasp is contraindicated, a wrought wire circumferential clasp should be selected. A distal rest is used because the originating portion of

the arm lies above the height of contour and would preempt a mesial rest. Although the clasp will not release during functional movements of the extension base, it will flex and provide some stress relief to the abutment. A distal rest and a wrought wire circumferential clasp are also preferred if the abutment inclines mesially. Here, the entire guide plate lies above the height of contour and will preempt the mesial rest. Relieving the guide plate would result in a space between it and the abutment.

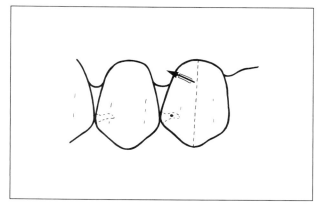

Fig. 14.1-19 If the facial surface exhibits no undercut but is parallel or nearly parallel to the path of insertion/dislodgement, an undercut for an I-bar may be created in the enamel. The retentive groove should be located just ahead of the greatest mesiodistal curvature of the facial surface and should duplicate the path the I-bar will follow *(arrow)* during functional movements of the extension base. When a bar clasp is contraindicated, a mesiofacial undercut may be created and engaged by a wrought wire circumferential clasp. Because the originating portion of the arm will be above the height of contour (and act like a rest), the primary rest should be placed on the distal fossa.

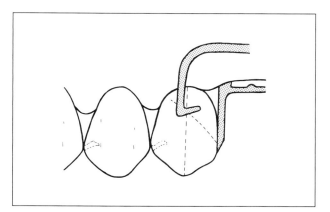

Fig. 14.1-17 When the undercut is located on the distofacial surface, the preferred clasp assembly is composed of a modified T-bar, a mesial rest, and a distal guide plate.

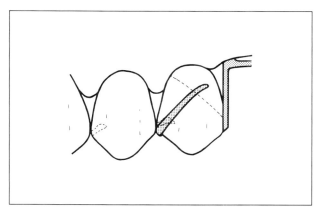

Fig. 14.1-18 When the undercut is located on the distofacial surface and a bar clasp is contraindicated, a circumferential embrasure clasp may be used with a mesial rest. Although the mechanics are not ideal with either a mesial or a distal rest, the mesial is preferred because the tendency for the originating portion of the arm to push the tooth lingually during functional movements of the extension base is resisted by the minor connector and the lingual portion of the distal guide plate. With a distal rest, the retentive tip would move upward and forward, torquing the abutment.

Denture base retentive elements/replacement teeth

Open latticework is the preferred type of denture base retentive element because the attachment of the plastic is stronger. The latticework for a maxillary distal extension RPD should extend approximately two thirds of the distance to the hamular notch.

Mesh should be selected when vertical space is limited. It covers approximately the same area as latticework, but it is generally much thinner. When vertical space is severely restricted, a metal base may be used. However, adjustment is difficult and relining is impossible.

213

Case 14.2

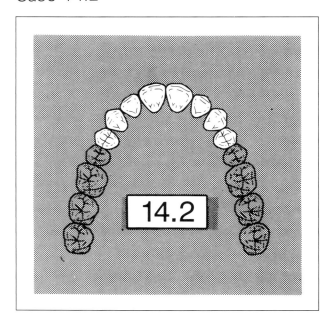

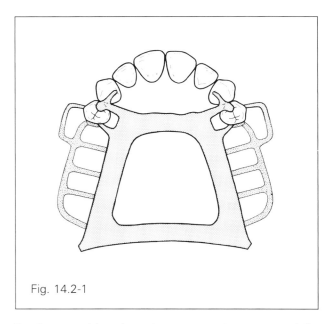

Fig. 14.2-1

Design considerations for case 14.2 are essentially the same as those for case 14.1. Variations in rest location and major connector selection are discussed below.

Rests

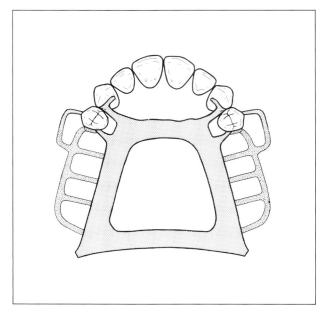

Fig. 14.2-2 If the mesio-occlusal fossa is blocked by the opposing occlusion, the primary rest may be placed on the cingulum of the canine. It would then function as both a primary rest and an indirect retainer.

Major conector

The major connector options are the same as those described for case 14.1. Although the anterior-posterior palatal strap would still be the preferred major connector, the desirability of a palatal plate increases because of the larger extension areas.

Case 14.3

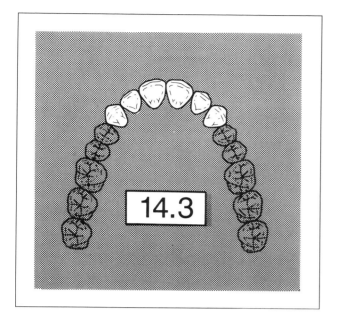

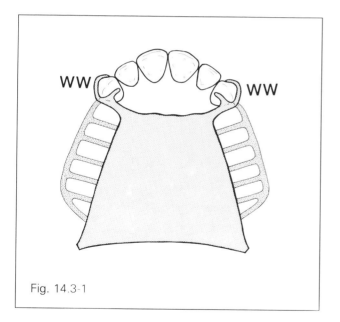

Fig. 14.3-1

Rests

Cingulum rests are almost always used on the canines. Incisal rests would be unesthetic, and they frequently interfere with the occlusion.

Figs. 14.3-2a to c The origins of cingulum rests may vary. It is important to realize, however, that the axis of rotation will pass through the most distal portion of the rests, regardless of their points of origin. Because each functions as a distal rest, the form shown in Fig. 14.3-2a is generally preferred because it is more hygienic.

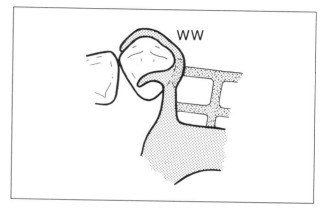

Fig. 14.3-2a Cingulum rest originating from the distal guide plate.

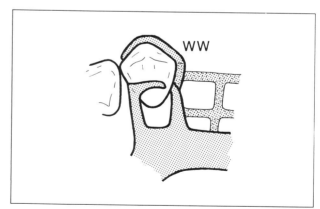

Fig. 14.3-2b Cingulum rest originating from a mesial minor connector.

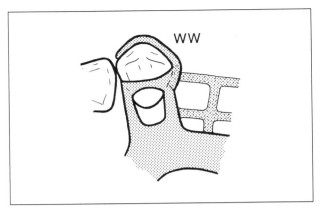

Fig. 14.3-2c   Cingulum rest taking the form of a strap connecting the guide plate and the minor connector.

Guide plates

When only the anterior teeth remain, the contact of guide surfaces and guide plates seldom, if ever, establishes a definite path of insertion/ dislodgement, even if mesial minor connectors or lingual plating are used. Guide surfaces are generally so limited in size that there is insufficient contact with guide plates.

Major connector

With only the six anterior teeth remaining, full palatal coverage (all-metal or part metal and part plastic) would almost always be used to provide additional support and denture style retention.

Denture style retention will help to compensate for the lack of indirect retainers. Although linguo-plating could be selected, it often interferes with the opposing occlusion.

Minor connectors

Refer to case 14.1.

Retentive arms

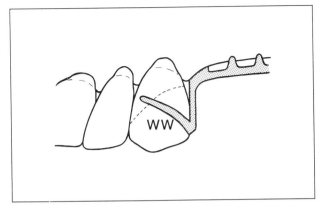

Fig. 14.3-3   Wrought wire circumferential clasps would usually be selected if the gingiva is visible when the patient smiles. Metal on teeth is generally considered more acceptable than metal crossing gingiva.

Figs. 14.3-4a and b   Bar clasps are acceptable if the gingiva is *not* visible when the patient smiles. An I-bar is used when the undercut is located on the mesiofacial surface, and a modified T-bar is used when the undercut is on the distofacial surface. The tip of the I-bar or the approach arm of the modified T-bar should be placed in front of the greatest mesiodistal curvature of the facial surface. Because the retentive area lies in front of the axis of rotation, the bar clasp should be long, tapered, and flexible. Support provided by the full palatal coverage will decrease functional movement and help to reduce the torquing forces applied to the abutments.

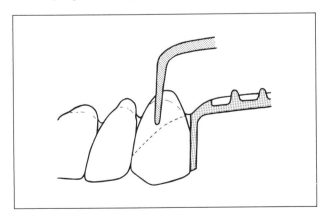

Fig. 14.3-4a   I-bar.

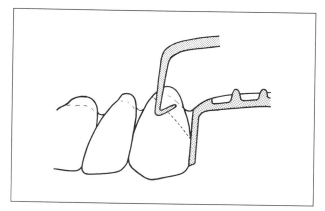

Fig. 14.3-4b Modified T-bar.

Denture base retentive elements/replacement teeth

Refer to case 14.1.

Case 14.4

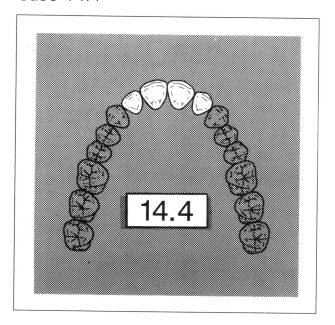

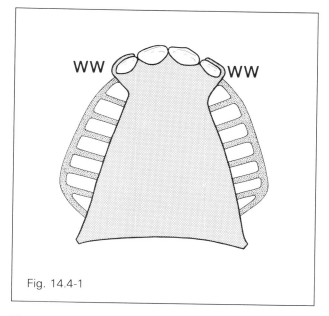

Fig. 14.4-1

The design principles for case 14.4 are essentially the same as those for case 14.3. The incisors should usually be plated and rest seats prepared on all four teeth. The choices for retentive arms are the same as those described for the canines in case 14.3. Unfortunately, all options will present serious compromises in esthetics.

With only four teeth remaining, a complete denture or overdenture should receive serious consideration unless the lateral incisors exhibit exceptionally good bone support and ideal coronal contours.

Case 14.5

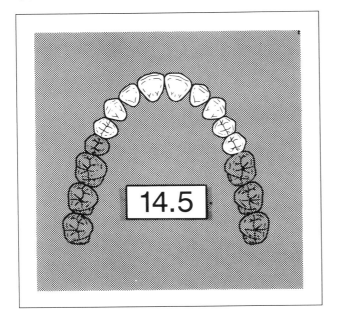

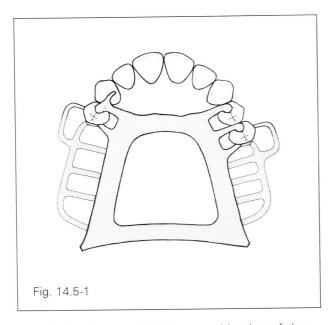

Fig. 14.5-1

The design for case 14.5 is a combination of those for cases 14.1 and 14.2; refer to these cases for design concepts and variations.

Case 14.6

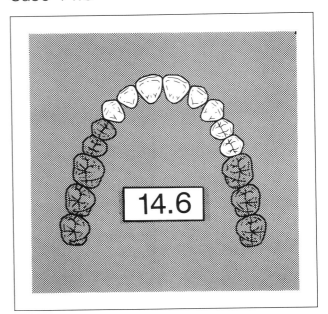

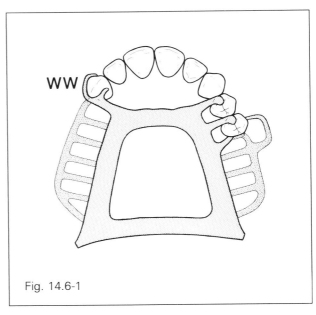

ww

Fig. 14.6-1

The design for case 14.6 is a combination of those for cases 14.1 and 14.3; refer to these cases for design concepts and variations.

Case 14.7

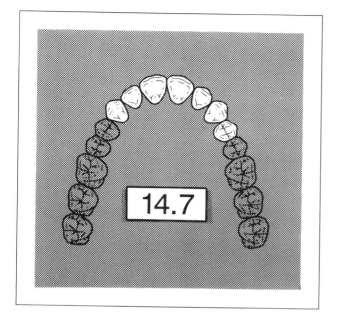

14.7

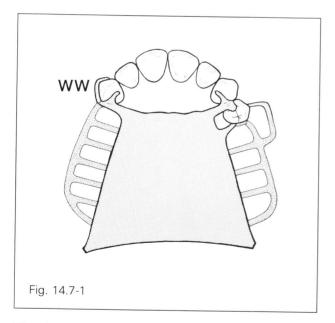

ww

Fig. 14.7-1

Case 14.8

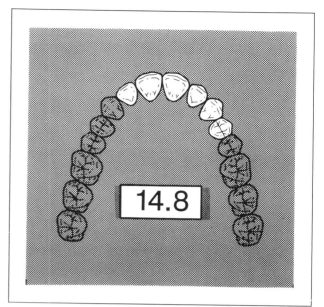

14.8

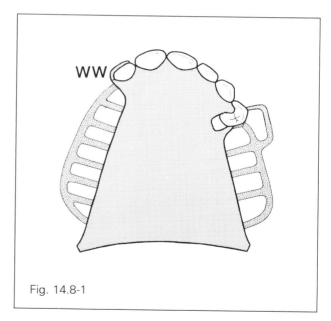

ww

Fig. 14.8-1

The design for case 14.7 is a combination of those for cases 14.2 and 14.3; refer to these cases for design concepts and variations.

The design for case 14.8 is a combination of those for cases 14.2 and 14.4. With a canine missing, linguoplating would usually be selected. Rest seats should be prepared at least on the lateral incisor abutment and the adjacent central incisor. Rest seats on all the remaining anterior teeth are preferred. If the bone support and coronal contours of the lateral incisor abutment are exceptionally favorable, a cingulum rest may be placed on it and the linguoplating omitted. A cingulum rest should then be placed on the remaining canine as an indirect retainer. Refer to cases 14.2 and 14.4 for other design concepts and variations.

Case 14.9

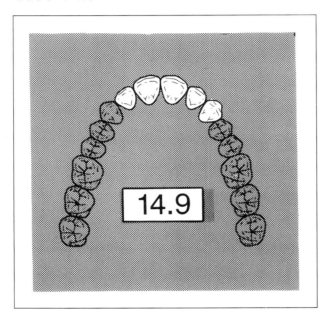

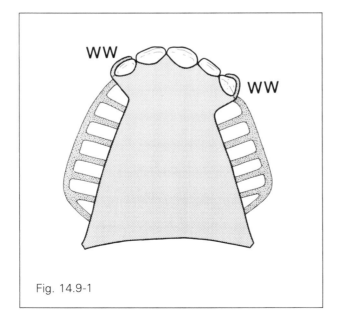

Fig. 14.9-1

The design for case 14.9 is a combination of those for cases 14.3 and 14.4. With a canine missing, linguoplating would usually be selected. Rest seats should be prepared at least on the lateral incisor, the adjacent central incisor, and the remaining canine. Rest seats on all the remaining teeth are preferred. If the bone support and coronal contours of the lateral incisor abutment are exceptionally favorable, a cingulum rest may be placed on it and the linguoplating omitted. If the prognosis for the anterior teeth is questionable, a complete denture or overdenture should be considered. Refer to cases 14.3 and 14.4 for other design concepts and variations.

Case 14.10

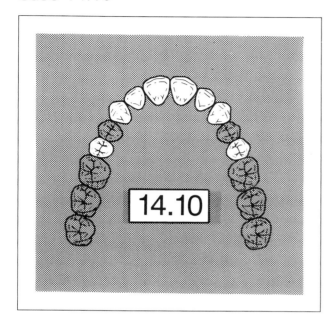

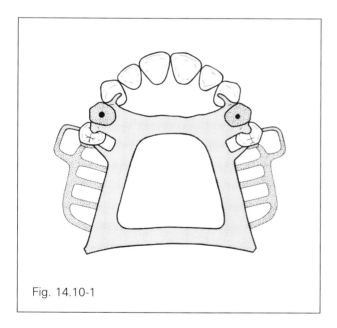

Fig. 14.10-1

Rests

The location of rests on the second premolars depends on the type of retentive arms selected (see case 14.1). Cingulum rests on the canines provide indirect retention.

Guide plates

With the first premolars missing, six guide surface–guide plate contact areas exist and a definite path of insertion/dislodgement can be established. However, "locking" of the lone-standing abutments between the mesial and distal guide plates will transfer torquing forces during functional movements of the extension bases; this should be prevented by physiologically relieving the guide plates at framework try-in.

Major connector

Refer to case 14.1. There might be a slightly greater tendency to use full palatal coverage because of the lone-standing abutments.

Minor connectors

Refer to case 14.1.

Retentive arms

Refer to case 14.1.

Denture base retentive elements/replacement teeth

In addition to the tube teeth shown in Fig. 14.10-1, the first premolars may be replaced by heat-cured or light-activated resin teeth or by denture teeth attached via denture base and retentive network. The last option is more commonly selected when (1) there is an incompletely healed residual ridge, (2) there is a defect in the contour of the residual ridge, or (3) the space is wider than that for a normal premolar.

Case 14.11

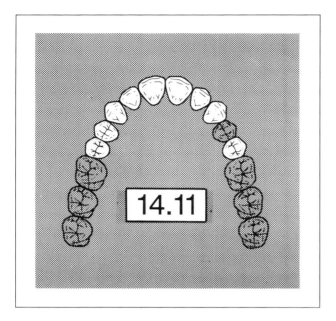

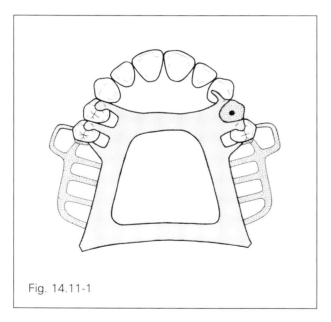

Fig. 14.11-1

The design for case 14.11 is a combination of those for cases 14.1 and 14.10; refer to these cases for design concepts and variations.

Case 14.12

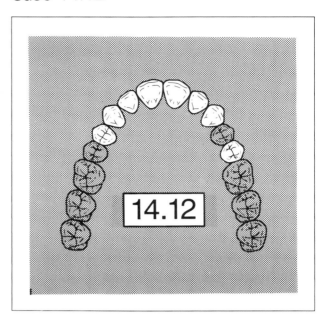

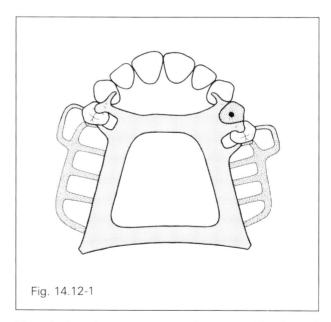

Fig. 14.12-1

The design for case 14.12 is a combination of those for cases 14.2 and 14.10; refer to these cases for design concepts and variations.

Case 14.13

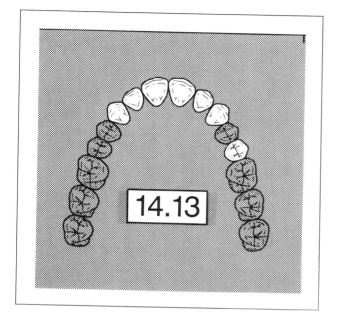

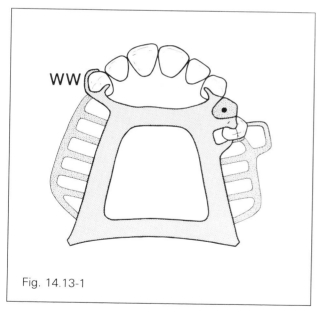

Fig. 14.13-1

The design for case 14.13 is a combination of those for cases 14.3 and 14.10; refer to these cases for design concepts and variations.

Case 14.14

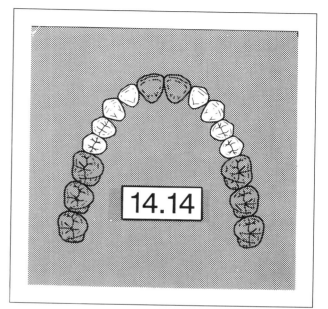

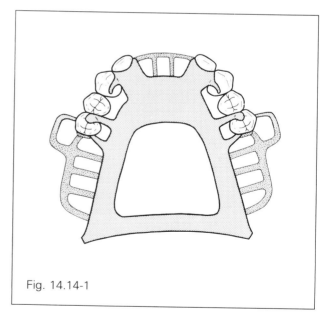

Fig. 14.14-1

The design for case 14.14 is essentially the same as that for case 14.1, with a two-tooth anterior modification space. Only those changes necessitated by the modification space are considered below. Refer to case 14.1 for discussion of other aspects of the design.

Rests

If the lateral incisors have exceptionally good bone support and prominent cinguli, rests may be placed on them instead of the canines. Because the anterior rests (canines or laterals) provide adequate indirect retention, mesial rests on the first premolars can be omitted.

Guide plates

Guide plates on the lateral incisors must be located on the mesiolingual surfaces so that they will not be visible or interfere with placement of the central incisors. For discussion of the guide plates on the premolars, refer to case 14.1.

Retentive arms

The options for clasp assemblies on the second premolars are the same as those for case 14.1. Clasps on the lateral incisors or canines would be unesthetic and lie in front of the axis of rotation; they are seldom, if ever, indicated.

Denture base retentive elements/replacement teeth

The central incisors would most commonly be replaced by denture teeth via retentive network and denture base. However, if the residual ridge is well-healed and exhibits little resorption, and if the width of the space is appropriate for the missing teeth, acceptable alternatives are facings, tube teeth, or heat-cured or light-activated resin replacements.

Case 14.15

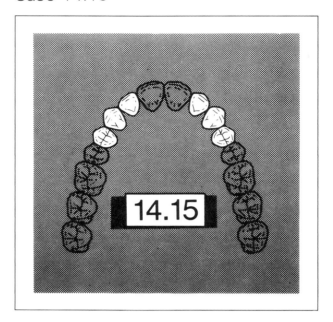

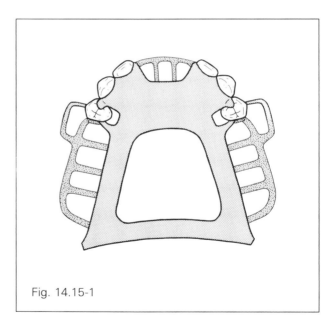

Fig. 14.15-1

The design for 14.15 is a combination of those for cases 14.2 and 14.14; refer to these cases for design concepts and variations.

Case 14.16

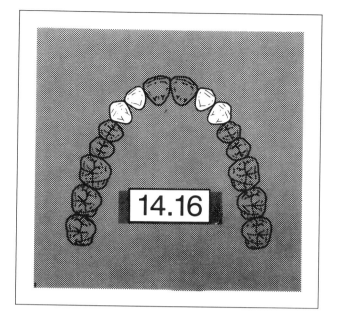

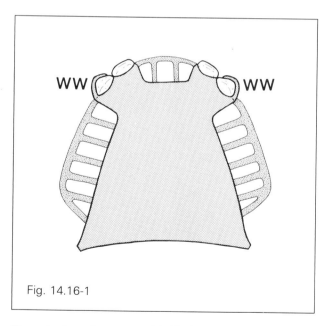

Fig. 14.16-1

The design for case 14.16 is a combination of those for cases 14.3 and 14.14; refer to these cases for design concepts and variations.

Case 14.17

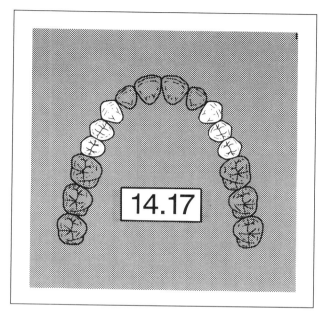

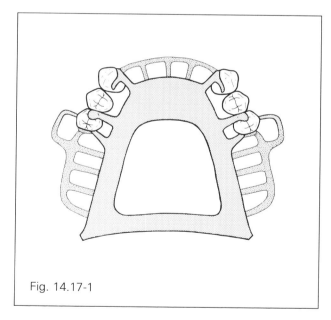

Fig. 14.17-1

The design for case 14.17 is essentially the same as that for case 14.1, with a four-tooth anterior modification space. Only those changes necessitated by the modification space are considered below. Refer to case 14.1 for discussion of other aspects of the design.

Rests

Because the rests on the canines are very effective indirect retainers, rests are not needed on the first premolars.

Guide plates

The anterior guide plates should be located on the linguoproximal surfaces of the canines so that they will not be visible or interfere with placement of the denture teeth.

Retentive arms

The options for clasp assemblies for the second premolars are the same as those described for case 14.1. Clasps on the canines would lie in front of the axis of rotation, may be esthetically displeasing, and are usually unnecessary.

Case 14.18

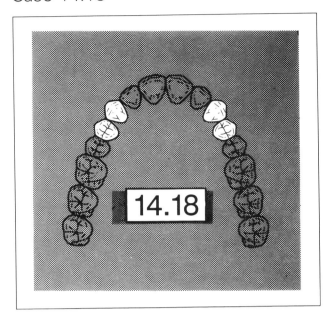

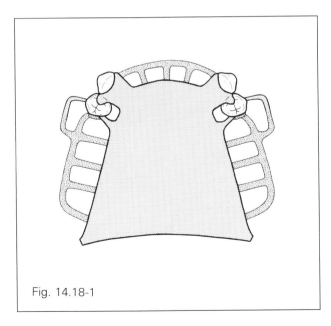

Fig. 14.18-1

The design for case 14.18 is a combination of those for cases 14.2 and 14.17; refer to these cases for design concepts and variations.

Case 14.19

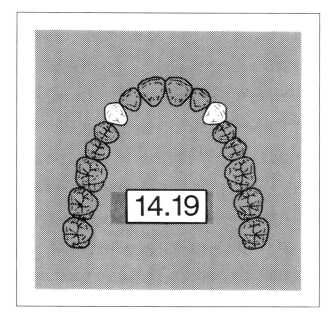

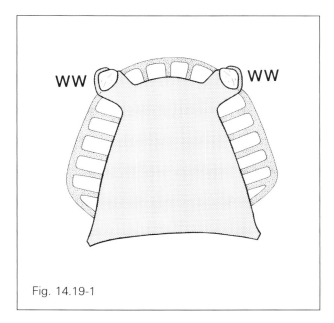

Fig. 14.19-1

Case 14.20

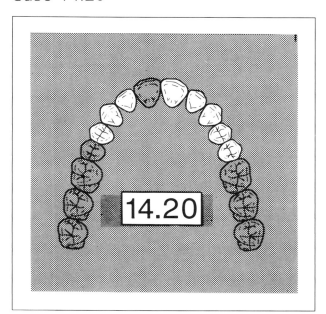

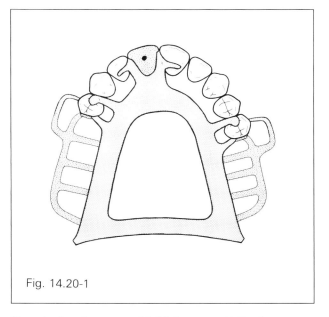

Fig. 14.20-1

The design for case 14.19 is a combination of those for cases 14.3 and 14.17. However, with only the two canines remaining, a conventional denture or overdenture should receive serious consideration unless the teeth have exceptionally good bone support. Refer to cases 14.3 and 14.17 for design concepts and variations.

The design for case 14.20 is essentially the same as that for case 14.5, with a single-tooth anterior modification space. Only those changes necessitated by the modification space are considered below. Refer to case 14.5 for discussion of other aspects of the design.

Rests

Cingulum rests should be placed on both of the anterior abutments if possible. If the lateral incisor has poor bone support or a steeply sloped lingual surface, the rest on it may be omitted as long as a definite rest seat can be prepared on the central incisor.

Because the anterior rests provide excellent indirect retention, rests on the left first premolar and right canine are unnecessary.

Guide plates

The anterior guide plates must be located on the linguoproximal surfaces so that they will not be visible from the labial aspect or interfere with positioning of the replacement tooth.

Denture base retentive elements/replacement teeth

With only one tooth in the modification space, a prefabricated facing, tube tooth, or custom heat-cured or light-activated resin replacement is almost always used.

Case 14.21

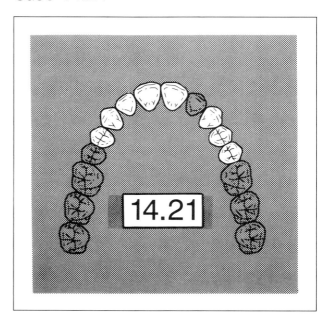

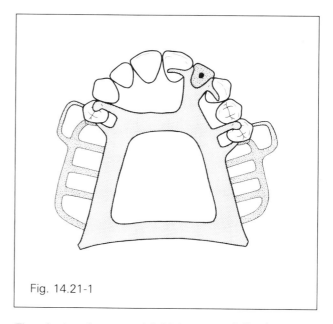

Fig. 14.21-1

The design for case 14.21 is essentially the same as that for case 14.20 (case 14.5 with a single-tooth modification space). Refer to case 14.20 for design concepts and variations.

Case 14.22

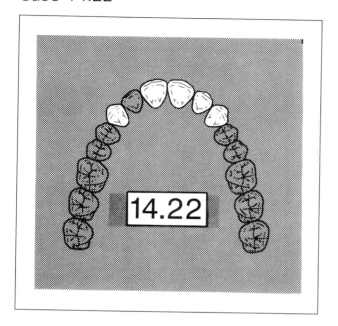

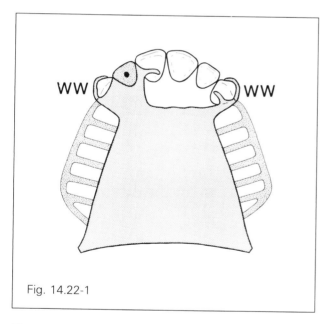

Fig. 14.22-1

The design for case 14.22 is essentially the same as that for case 14.3, with a single-tooth anterior modification space. Only those changes necessitated by the modification space are considered below. Refer to case 14.3 for a discussion of other aspects of the design.

Rests

A rest seat must be prepared beneath the plating on the right canine. The rest on the central incisor will function as an indirect retainer.

Guide plates

The anterior guide plates must be located on the linguoproximal surfaces so that they will not be visible from the labial aspect or interfere with positioning of the replacement tooth.

Denture base retentive elements/replacement teeth

With only one tooth in the modification space, a prefabricated facing, tube tooth, or custom heat-cured or light-activated resin replacement is almost always used.

Case 14.23

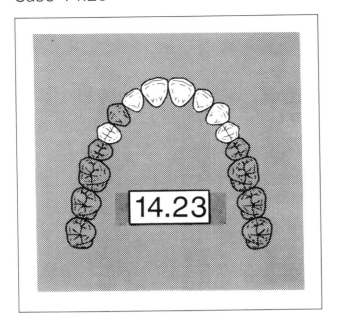

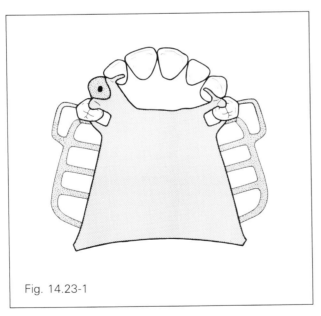

Fig. 14.23-1

The design for case 14.23 is essentially the same as that for case 14.2 with a single-tooth modification space. Only those changes necessitated by the modification space are considered below. Refer to case 14.2 for a discussion of other aspects of the design.

Rests

If the lateral incisor is periodontally compromised, or the lingual slope is too steep to prepare an adequate rest seat, the lateral incisor can be plated and a cingulum rest placed on the central incisor.

Guide plates

The guide plate on the lateral incisor must be located on the distolingual surface so that it will not be visible from the labial aspect or interfere with positioning of the replacement tooth.

Denture base retentive elements/replacement teeth

With only one tooth in the modification space, a prefabricated facing, tube tooth, or custom heat-cured or light-activated resin replacement is almost always used.

Case 14.24

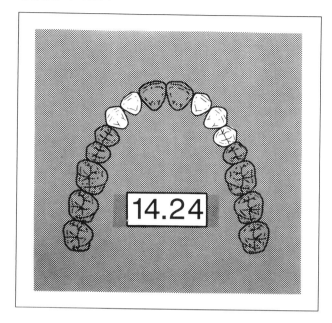

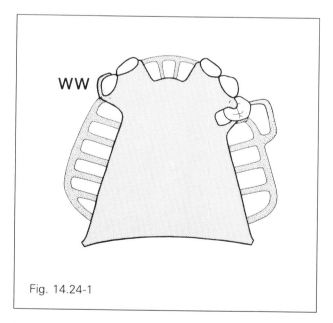

Fig. 14.24-1

The design for case 14.24 is essentially the same as that for case 14.7 with a two-tooth anterior modification space. Only those changes necessitated by the modification space are considered below. Refer to case 14.7 for discussion of other aspects of the design.

Rests

Rest seats should be prepared beneath the plating at least on the canines, and preferably also on the lateral incisors.

Guide plates

The guide plates on the mesial surfaces of the lateral incisors must be located on the linguoproximal surfaces so that they will not be visible from the labial aspect or interfere with positioning of the replacement teeth.

Major connector

Although linguoplating would usually be used, it can be avoided if the lateral incisors are periodontally sound and have lingual surfaces capable of accepting adequate cingulum rest preparations.

Retentive arms

Retentive arms on the lateral incisors would be unesthetic and lie in front of the axis of rotation; they are rarely, if ever, indicated.

Denture base retentive elements/replacement teeth

The incisors would most commonly be replaced by denture teeth via retentive network and denture base. However, if the residual ridge is well-healed and exhibits little resorption, and if the width of the space is appropriate for the two missing teeth, facings, tube teeth, or heat-cured or light-activated resin replacements are acceptable alternatives.

Case 14.25

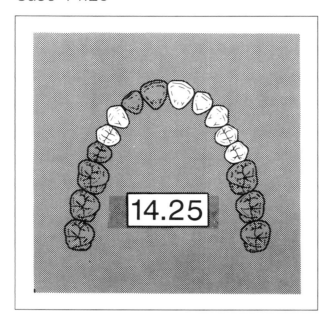

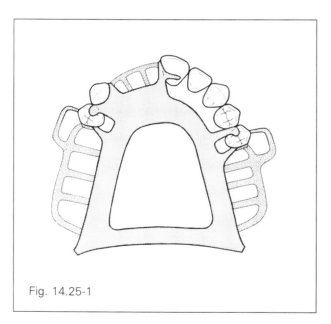

Fig. 14.25-1

The design for case 14.25 is essentially the same as that for case 14.5, with a two-tooth modification space. Only those changes necessitated by the modification space are considered below. Refer to case 14.5 for discussion of other aspects of the design.

Rests

A rest seat should be prepared beneath the plating on the canine.

Guide plates

The guide plates on the canine and central incisor must be located on the linguoproximal surfaces so that they will not be visible from the labial aspect or interfere with positioning of the replacement teeth.

Retentive arms

Retentive arms on the anterior abutments would be unesthetic and lie in front of the axis of rotation; they are rarely, if ever, indicated.

Denture base retentive elements/replacement teeth

Refer to case 14.24.

Case 14.26

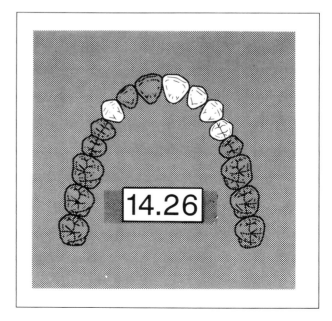

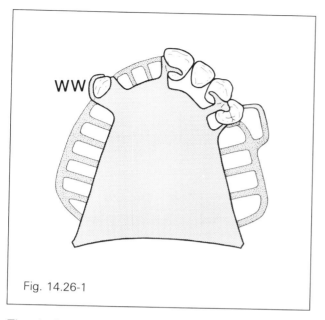

Fig. 14.26-1

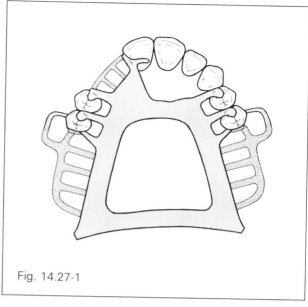

Fig. 14.27-1

The design for case 14.26 is a combination of case 14.7 posteriorly and case 14.25 anteriorly; refer to these cases for design concepts and variations.

The design for case 14.27 is essentially the same as that for case 14.1 with a two-tooth modification space. Only those changes necessitated by the modification space are considered below. Refer to case 14.1 for discussion of other aspects of the design.

Case 14.27

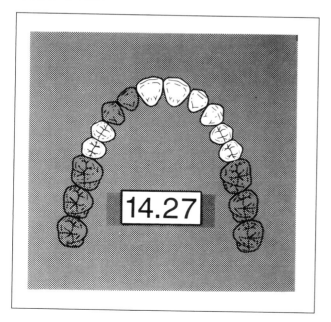

Rests

Because the rests on the central incisor and right first premolar will act as indirect retainers, the rest on the left first premolar may be omitted if desired.

Guide plates

The guide plate on the distal surface of the central incisor must be located on the linguoproximal surface so that it will not be visible from the labial aspect or interfere with positioning of the replacement teeth.

Retentive arms

A retentive arm is rarely, if ever, used on the central incisor. A clasp may be placed on the right first premolar, but since it lies in front of the axis of

233

rotation, it should be flexible (wrought wire or long, tapered bar clasp).

Denture base retentive elements/replacement teeth

Refer to case 14.24.

The design for case 14.28 is a combination of that for case 14.6 posteriorly and the mirror image of case 14.27 anteriorly; refer to these cases for design concepts and variations.

Case 14.28

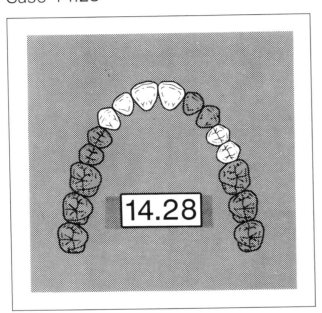

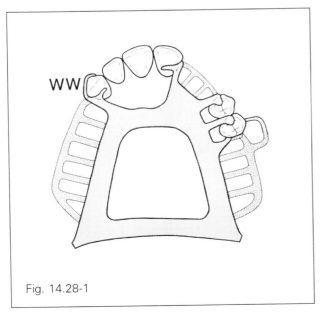

Fig. 14.28-1

Case 14.29

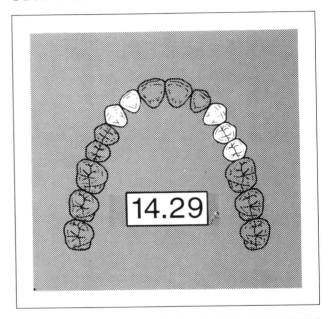

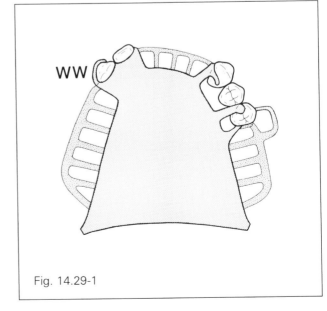

Fig. 14.29-1

The design for case 14.29 is essentially the same as that for case 14.6, with a three-tooth modification space. Only those changes necessitated by the modification space are considered below. Refer to case 14.6 for discussion of other aspects of the design.

Rests

Rest seats should be prepared beneath the plating on the canine and, if possible, on the lateral incisor.

Guide plates

The guide plates on the anterior teeth must be located on the linguoproximal surfaces so that they will not be visible from the labial aspect or interfere with positioning of the replacement teeth.

Retentive arms

Retentive arms on the right lateral incisor and left canine would be unesthetic and lie in front of the axis of rotation; they would rarely, if ever, be indicated.

Denture base retentive elements/replacement teeth

With three teeth in the modification space, denture teeth attached via retentive network and denture base would almost always be used.

Case 14.30

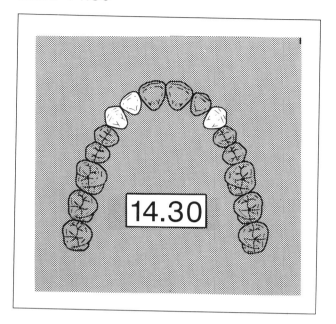

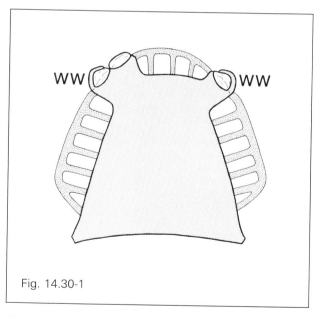

Fig. 14.30-1

The design for case 14.30 is a combination of that for case 14.3 posteriorly and case 14.29 anteriorly; refer to these cases for design concepts and variations.

Case 14.31

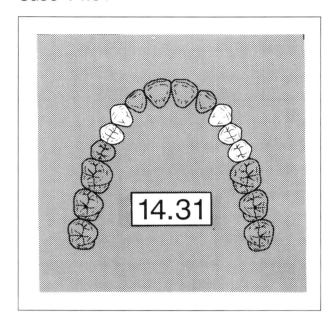

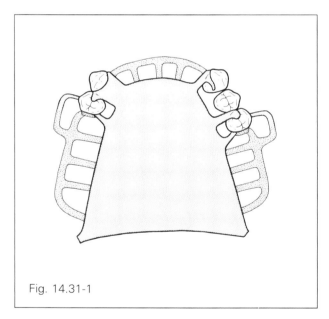

Fig. 14.31-1

The design for case 14.31 is essentially the same as that for case 14.5, with a four-tooth anterior modification space. Only those changes necessitated by the modification space are considered below. Refer to case 14.5 for discussion of other aspects of the design.

Rests

A cingulum rest seat must be placed beneath the plating on the right canine.

Guide plates

The mesial guide plates on the canines must be located on the linguoproximal surfaces so that they will not be visible from the labial aspect or interfere with positioning of the replacement teeth.

Retentive arms

Clasps on the canines lie in front of the axis of rotation, may compromise esthetics, and are usually omitted. If they are used, they should be flexible (wrought wire or long, tapered bar clasps).

Denture base retentive elements/replacement teeth

With four teeth in the modification space, denture teeth attached via retentive network and denture base would almost always be used.

Case 14.32

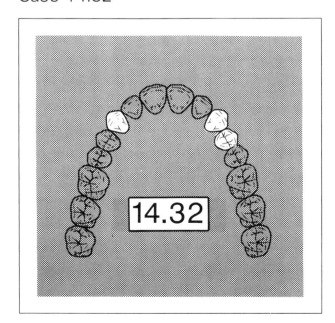

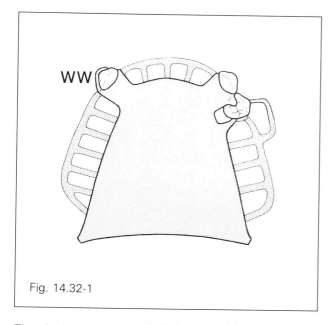

Fig. 14.32-1

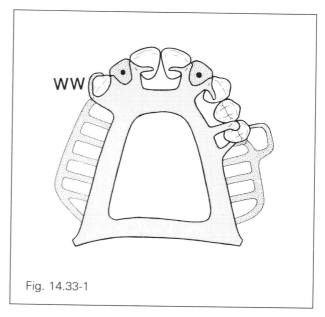

Fig. 14.33-1

The design for case 14.32 is a combination of that for case 14.7 posteriorly and case 14.31 anteriorly; refer to these cases for design concepts and variations.

The design for case 14.33 is essentially the same as that for case 14.6, with two single-tooth anterior modification spaces. Only those changes necessitated by the modification spaces are considered below. Refer to case 14.6 for other aspects of the design.

Case 14.33

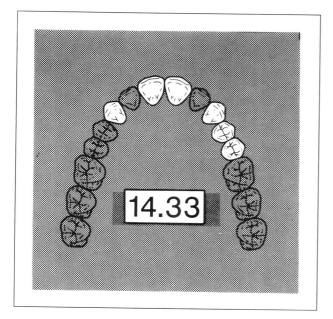

14.33

Guide plates

Anterior guide plates must be located on the linguoproximal surfaces so that they will not be visible from the labial aspect or interfere with positioning of the replacement teeth.

Retentive arms

Retentive arms on teeth other than those shown in Fig. 14.33-1 would be unesthetic and lie in front of the axis of rotation; they are rarely, if ever, indicated.

Denture base retentive elements/replacement teeth

With single-tooth modification spaces, prefabricated facings, tube teeth, or custom heat-cured or light-activated resin replacements are almost always used.

Case 14.34

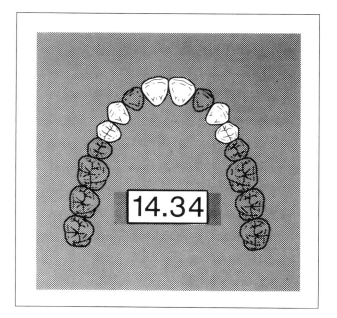

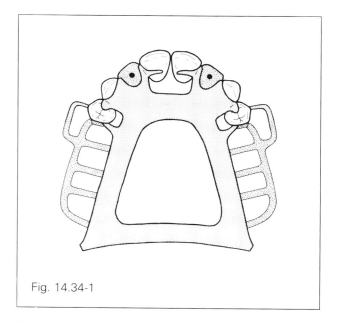

Fig. 14.34-1

Case 14.35

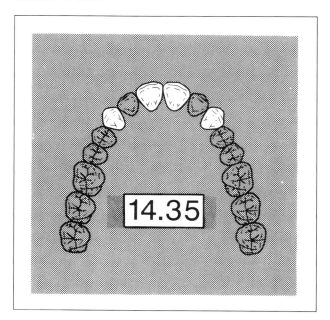

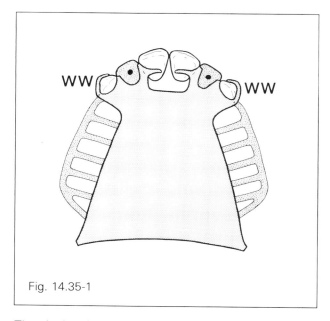

Fig. 14.35-1

The design for case 14.34 is a combination of that for case 14.2 posteriorly and case 14.33 anteriorly; refer to these cases for design concepts and variations.

The design for case 14.35 is a combination of that for case 14.3 posteriorly and case 14.33 anteriorly; refer to these cases for design concepts and variations.

Case 14.36

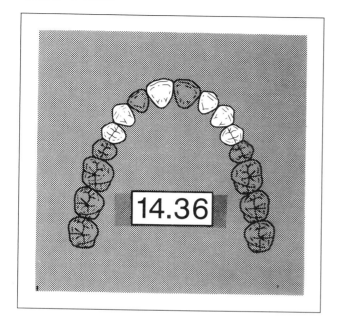

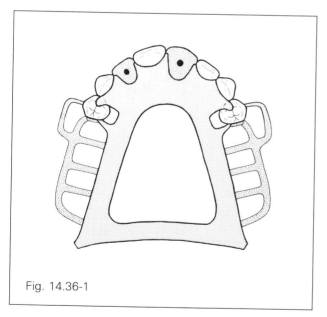

Fig. 14.36-1

The design for case 14.36 is essentially the same as that for case 14.2, with two single-tooth anterior modification spaces. Only those changes necessitated by the modification spaces are considered below. Refer to case 14.2 for other aspects of the design.

Rests

Rest seats must be prepared beneath the plating on the anterior teeth.

Guide plates

Guide plates on the anterior teeth must be located on the linguoproximal surfaces so that they will not be visible from the labial aspect or interfere with positioning of the replacement teeth.

Retentive arms

Retentive arms on teeth other than the first premolars would be unesthetic and lie in front of the axis of rotation; they are rarely, if ever, indicated.

Denture base retentive elements/replacement teeth

Refer to case 14.33.

Case 14.37

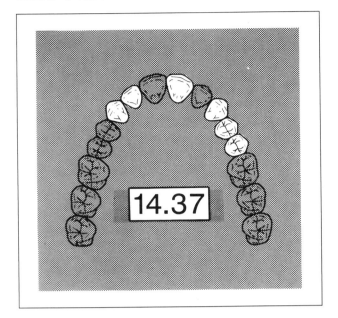

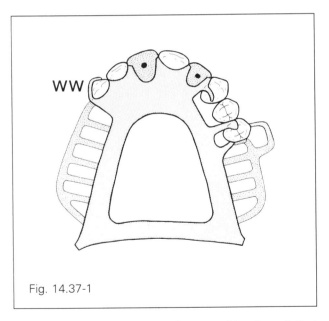

Fig. 14.37-1

The design for case 14.37 is a combination of that for case 14.6 posteriorly and case 14.36 anteriorly; refer to these cases for design concepts and variations.

Case 14.38

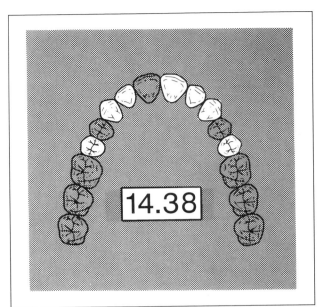

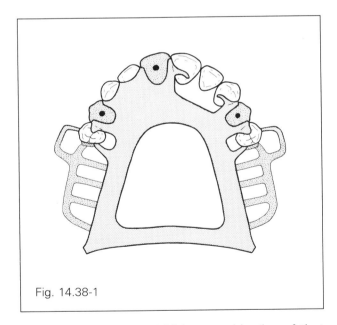

Fig. 14.38-1

The design for case 14.38 is a combination of that for case 14.10 posteriorly and case 14.20 anteriorly; refer to these cases for design concepts and variations.

240

Case 14.39

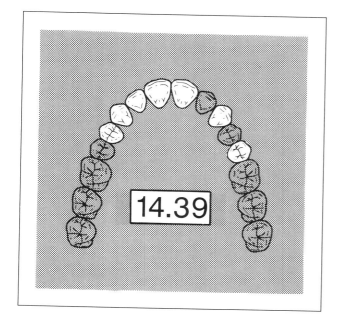

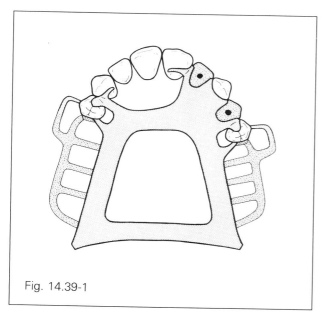

Fig. 14.39-1

The design for case 14.39 is a combination of that for case 14.12 posteriorly and case 14.21 anteriorly; refer to these cases for design concepts and variations.

Case 14.40

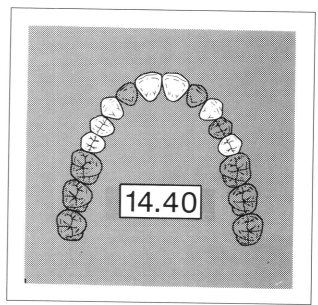

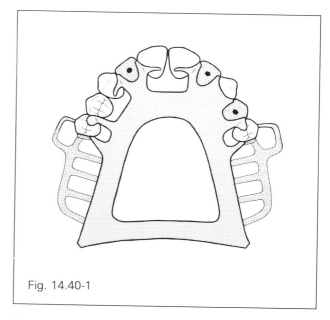

Fig. 14.40-1

The design for case 14.40 is a combination of that for case 14.11 posteriorly and case 14.33 anteriorly; refer to these cases for design concepts and variations.

Maxillary Class II Designs

In our study of almost 2,000 partially edentulous maxillary arches for which removable partial dentures were fabricated, just under 30% were Class II. Considering frequency of occurrence, the 31 cases and their variations discussed in chapter 15 cover almost 98% of these partially edentulous arches (or their mirror images).

Because a distal extension RPD is seldom fabricated to replace second or third molars, only those situations where at least all the molars are missing will be considered.

Case reference guide	
Without modification space	
With posterior modification space(s) only	15.1 to 15.4
Modification space on extension side only	15.5
Modification space on tooth-supported side only	
Single modification space	
One tooth in space	15.6 to 15.8
Two teeth in space	15.9 to 15.11
Three teeth in space	15.12 to 15.13
Four teeth in space	15.14
Two modification spaces	15.15 to 15.16
Modification spaces on both extension and tooth-supported sides	15.17
With anterior modification space(s) only	
Single anterior modification space	
One tooth space	15.18 to 15.20
Two teeth in space	15.21 to 15.23
Three teeth in space	15.24 to 15.25
Four teeth in space	15.26 to 15.28
Two anterior modification spaces	15.29 to 15.30
With anterior and posterior modification spaces	15.31

Case 15.1

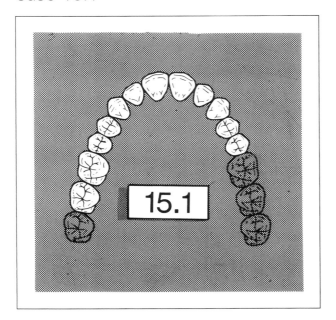

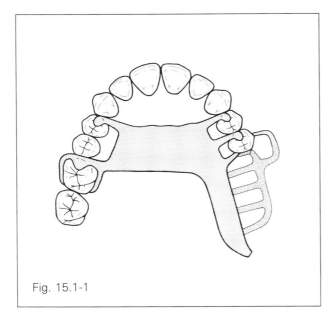

Fig. 15.1-1

Rests

On the extension side, rest location on the terminal (primary) abutment depends on the clasp assembly selected. Refer to case 14.1 for variations.

The rest on the left first premolar is not absolutely essential because the anterior rest on the tooth-supported side will provide adequate indirect retention.

On the tooth-supported side, the rest and corresponding embrasure clasp may be placed on the first molar, second molar, or second premolar, depending on the location of the undercut for the clasp tip and the presence of occlusal interferences.

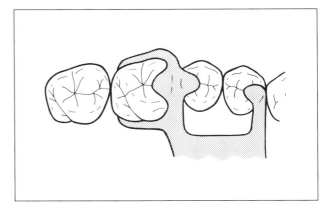

Fig. 15.1-2 A double rest for this type of embrasure clasp is usually not necessary but may be selected if there is danger of interproximal food impaction and if the occlusion permits.

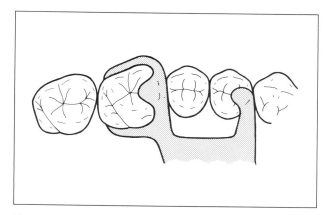

Fig. 15.1-3 Posterior rest placed on first molar.

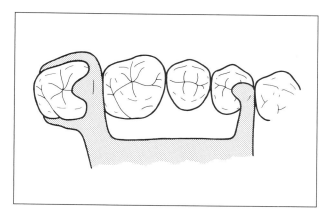

Fig. 15.1-4 Posterior rest placed on second molar.

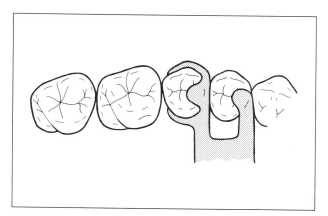

Fig. 15.1-5 Posterior rest placed on second premolar.

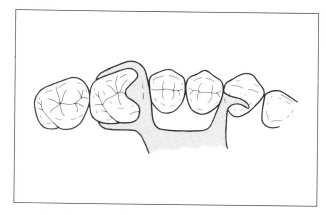

Fig. 15.1-6 The indirect retainer on the tooth-supported side may be moved to the cingulum of the canine if the occlusion does not permit placement in the mesial fossa of the first premolar.

Guide plates

Refer to case 14.1 for design concepts. The only guide plate will be located on the distal aspect of the left second premolar. It will not determine a distinct path of insertion/dislodgement.

Major connector

If there is no modification space on the tooth-supported side or if the modification space is small, a modified palatal plate is almost always the major connector of choice for a Class II RPD.

If the premolars on the tooth-supported side tilt lingually, they may be plated without affecting the mechanics of the RPD during functional movements. However, on the extension side, plating has the potential to act as a rest on an inclined surface, and it should be avoided if at all possible. The plating must not end above the survey line or it will preempt the planned mesial rest.

Refer to case 14.1 for additional design options and concepts.

Minor connectors

Refer to case 14.1.

Retentive arms

Case 14.1 discusses clasping options for the extension side. Retention for the tooth-supported side is considered below.

On the tooth-supported side, an embrasure clasp will almost always engage a distobuccal undercut on the first molar, second molar, or second premolar. If an anterior retentive arm were incorporated in the embrasure clasp assembly, it would lie in front of the axis of rotation and would therefore need to be flexible (wrought wire). However, because there is seldom enough space for a wrought wire clasp to pass through the embrasure, the anterior arm is usually omitted. Cast anterior arms may be used, but because of their rigidity, should be placed above the height of contour and function for bracing only.

Denture base retentive elements/replacement teeth

Refer to case 14.1.

Case 15.2

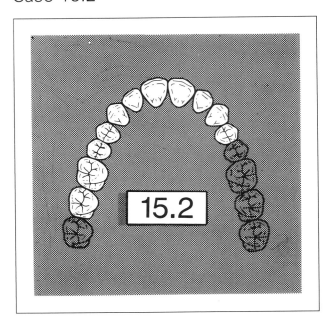

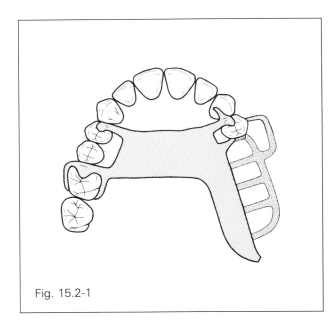

Fig. 15.2-1

For design concepts and variations, refer to case 14.2 for the extension side and case 11.1 for the tooth-supported side.

Case 15.3

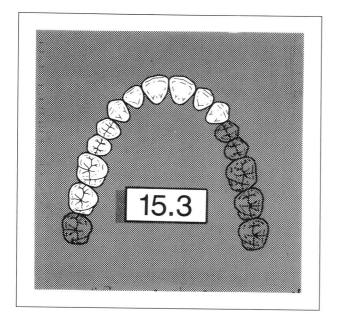

Case 15.4

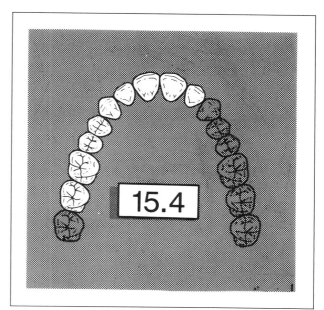

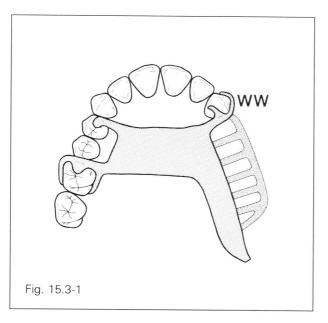

Fig. 15.3-1

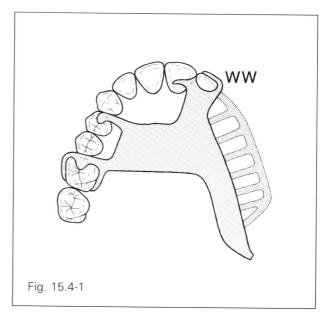

Fig. 15.4-1

For design concepts and variations, refer to case 14.3 for the extension side and case 11.1 for the tooth-supported side.

For design concepts and variations, refer to case 14.4 for the extension side and case 11.1 for the tooth-supported side.

Case 15.5

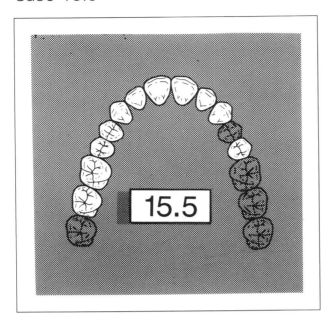

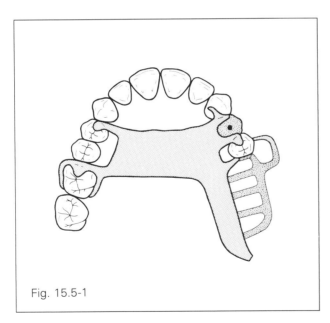

Fig. 15.5-1

For design concepts and variations, refer to case 14.10 for the extension side and case 11.1 for the tooth-supported side.

Case 15.6

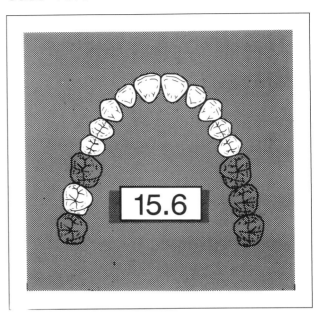

If the extension side varies from that shown, refer to cases 15.1 to 15.5 for the correct configuration.

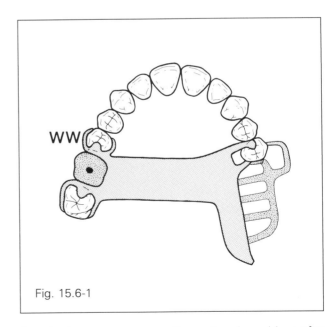

Fig. 15.6-1

For design concepts on the extension side, refer to cases 15.1 to 15.5. Options related to the tooth-supported side are discussed below.

Rests

The anterior rest on the tooth-supported side may be moved forward if occlusion interferes with placement in the distal fossa of the second premolar. If the rest is placed in the mesial fossa of the second premolar or distal fossa of the first premolar, the lingual arm can be omitted because the minor connector will provide reciprocation or bracing and 180° encirclement. If the rest must be moved to the mesial fossa of the first premolar or the cingulum of the canine, the lingual arm should be retained.

Guide plates

Theoretically, the multiple guide surface–guide plate contacts determine a distinct path of insertion/dislodgement and the I-bar on the extension side could be placed at the greatest mesiodistal curvature of the facial surface. However, placement of the retentive tip in front of the greatest curvature is still recommended, as it provides protection against excessive blockout or excessive reduction of the guide plates during finishing procedures.

Major connector

A modified palatal plate major connector is almost always used if the modification space is small. However, if the anterior rest must be moved to the mesial fossa of the first premolar or cingulum of the canine to avoid occlusal interferences, an anterior-posterior palatal strap could be considered.

Retentive arms

Because the anterior retentive tip on the tooth-supported side is in front of the axis of rotation, it should be wrought wire to provide increased flexibility. A cast circumferential arm may be selected if it is placed above the height of contour and used only for bracing.

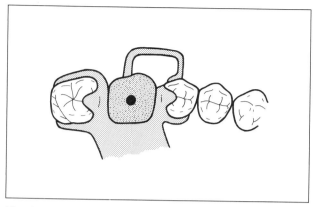

Fig. 15.6-2 If the undercut on the anterior abutment is on the distofacial surface, a long, tapered, and flexible modified T-bar may be used. An alternative would be to omit the retentive arm.

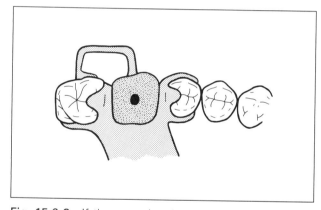

Fig. 15.6-3 If the posterior abutment on the tooth-supported side has a distobuccal undercut, a cast circumferential clasp is preferred. However, if the tooth is mesially inclined, the undercut is usually located on the mesiobuccal surface and a modified T-bar is the retainer of choice.

Denture base retentive elements/replacement teeth

The single tooth in the modification space is usually replaced by a tube tooth or heat-cured or light-activated resin facing. If vertical space is severely limited and esthetics is no problem, an all-metal replacement may be used.

Case 15.7

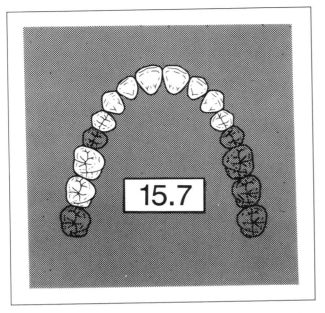

If the extension side varies from that shown, refer to cases 15.1 to 15.5 for the correct configuration.

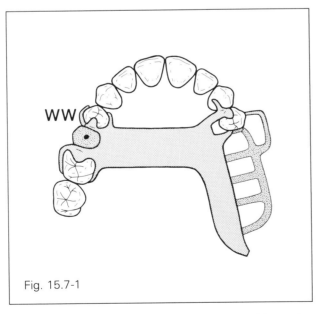

Fig. 15.7-1

For design concepts on the extension side, refer to cases 15.1 to 15.5. Options related to the tooth-supported side are discussed below.

Rests

The rest on the right first premolar could be moved to the mesial fossa or to the canine if occlusal interferences exist.

Because the anterior rest on the tooth-supported side will act as an indirect retainer, the cingulum rest on the left canine could be omitted.

Guide plates

Refer to cases 15.6 and 15.1.

Major connector

Refer to cases 15.6 and 15.1.

Retentive arms

Clasping options for the first molar of case 15.7 are essentially the same as those for the second molar of case 15.6. Clasping options for the first premolar of case 15.7 are the same as those for the second premolar of case 15.6.

Denture base retentive elements/replacement teeth

Because of esthetic considerations, the second premolar is usually replaced by a tube tooth or heat-cured or light-activated facing.

Case 15.8

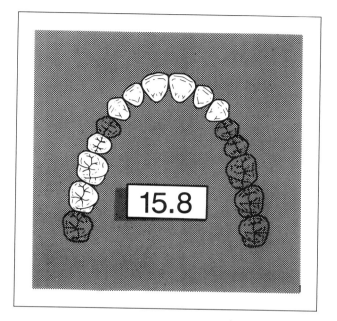

If the extension side varies from that shown, refer to cases 15.1 to 15.5 for the correct configuration.

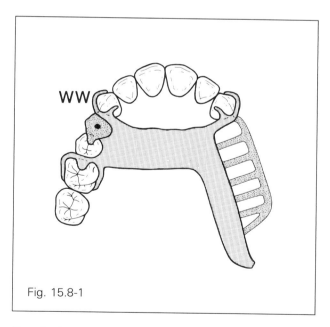

Fig. 15.8-1

For design concepts on the extension side, refer to cases 15.1 to 15.5. Options related to the tooth-supported side are discussed below.

Rests

The rest in the mesial fossa of the right second premolar could be omitted if occlusal interferences exist. Rests on the molar and canine would provide vertical stops for the tooth-supported segment. Variations in rest seats and rests for the canine are discussed in case 15.3.

The posterior circumferential clasp assembly on the tooth-supported side may be moved forward to the second premolar. However, some decrease in stability may occur with this design.

Guide plates

Refer to cases 15.6 and 15.1.

Major connector

Refer to case 15.1.

Retentive arms

The posterior circumferential clasp assembly on the tooth-supported side may be placed on the second premolar rather than the first molar.

A wrought wire circumferential clasp engaging a mesiofacial undercut would often be used on the canine, especially if gingiva were visible when the patient smiled. Because the first premolar is missing, there is adequate space to pass the retentive arm from the lingual to the buccal surfaces.

A long, tapered, and flexible bar clasp may also be used on the canine if the approach arm crossing the gingiva is not visible. An I-bar would usually be selected if the undercut is on the mesiofacial surface and a modified T-bar if the undercut is on the distofacial surface. Occasionally, an I-bar may be hidden by placing the tip into a distofacial undercut. However, such a retentive arm would tend to be very short and rigid and, if selected, should engage a minimal undercut. If esthetics is of paramount importance, a retentive arm on the canine may be omitted altogether.

Denture base retentive elements/replacement teeth

Because of esthetic considerations, the first premolar is almost always replaced by a tube tooth or heat-cured or light-activated resin facing.

Case 15.9

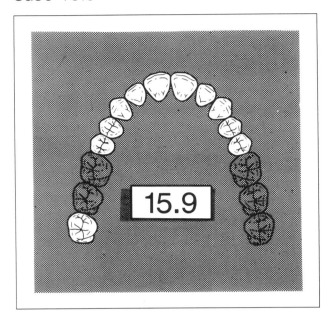

If the extension side varies from that shown, refer to cases 15.1 to 15.5 for the correct configuration.

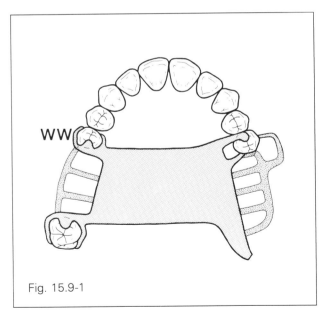

Fig. 15.9-1

For design concepts on the extension side, refer to cases 15.1 to 15.5. Options related to the tooth-supported side are discussed below.

Rests

Because the anterior rest on the tooth-supported side will function as an indirect retainer, no indirect retainer is required on the extension side.

The anterior rest on the tooth-supported side may be moved forward if occlusal contacts interfere with the location shown in Fig. 15.9-1.

Guide plates

Refer to cases 15.6 and 15.1.

Major connector

Although a modified palatal plate major connector would usually be selected, an anterior-posterior palatal strap may be used if the anterior-posterior dimension of the opening is at least 15 mm. This would most likely occur if the anterior rest on the tooth-supported side was moved forward to avoid occlusal interferences.

Retentive arms

Refer to case 15.6.

Denture base retentive elements/replacement teeth

With two teeth in the modification space, retentive network, denture teeth, and denture base would usually be used.

Case 15.10

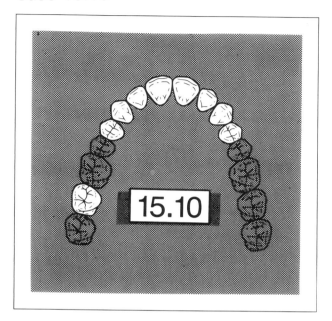

If the extension side varies from that shown, refer to cases 15.1 to 15.5 for the correct configuration.

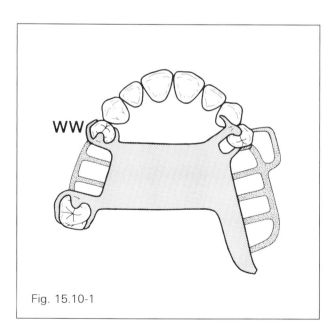

Fig. 15.10-1

For design concepts on the extension side, refer to cases 15.1 to 15.5. Design considerations on the tooth-supported side are essentially the same as those for case 15.9.

Case 15.11

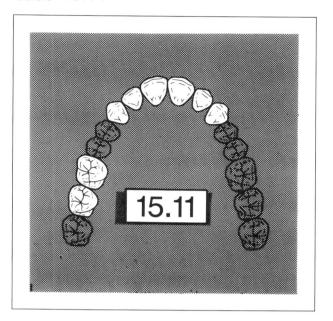

If the extension side varies from that shown, refer to cases 15.1 to 15.5 for the correct configuration

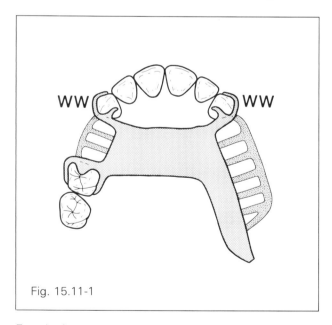

Fig. 15.11-1

For design concepts on the extension side, refer to cases 15.1 to 15.5. Design considerations on the tooth-supported side are similar to those described for case 15.9. Clasping options for the right canine are discussed in case 15.8.

Case 15.12

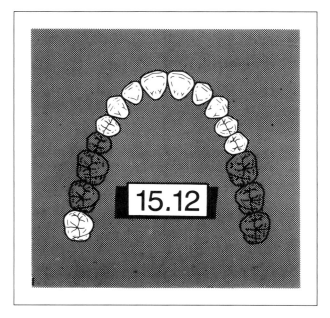

If the extension side varies from that shown, refer to cases 15.1 to 15.5 for the correct configuration.

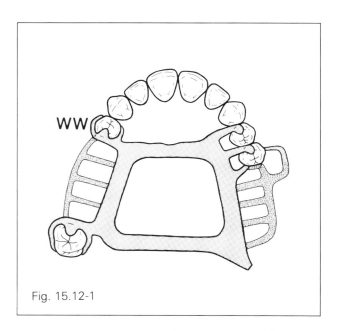

Fig. 15.12-1

For design concepts on the extension side, refer to cases 15.1 to 15.5. Options related to the tooth-supported side are discussed below.

Rests

The rest on the right first premolar may be moved to the mesial fossa or to the canine if the opposing occlusion prevents placement in the distal fossa. The rest on the left first premolar is not absolutely essential because the anterior rest on the opposite side will act as an indirect retainer.

Guide plates

Refer to cases 15.6 and 15.1.

Major connector

With three teeth missing in the modification area, the space is large enough to permit use of an anterior-posterior palatal strap major connector. However, a modified palatal plate may still be indicated if the abutments are weak or the residual ridges are poor and additional palatal support is needed.

Minor connectors

Refer to case 15.1.

Retentive arms

Clasping considerations for the third molar are the same as those for the second molar of case 15.6. Clasping considerations for the first premolar of case 15.12 are the same as those for the second premolar of case 15.6.

Denture base retentive elements/replacement teeth

With three teeth in the modification space, retentive network, denture teeth, and denture base would almost always be used.

Case 15.13

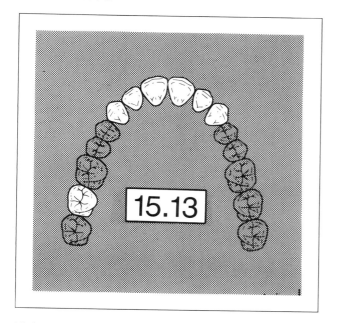

If the extension side varies from that shown, refer to cases 15.1 to 15.5 for the correct configuration.

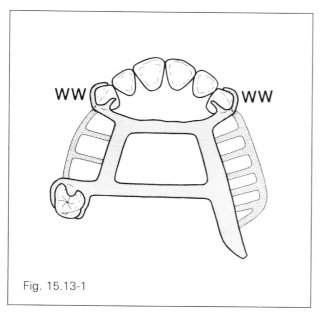

Fig. 15.13-1

For design concepts on the extension side, refer to cases 15.1 to 15.5. Options related to the tooth-supported side are discussed below.

Rests

Rest placement is always as shown in Fig. 15.13-1.

Guide plates

Refer to cases 15.6 and 15.1.

Major connector

Refer to case 15.12.

Retentive arms

Clasping considerations for the second molar are the same as those described for case 15.6. With the size of the modification space, a retentive arm would almost always be used on the right canine. Refer to case 15.8 for options.

Denture base retentive elements/replacement teeth

Refer to case 15.12.

Case 15.14

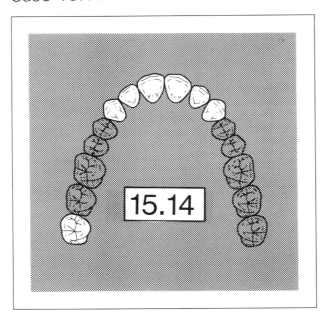

If the extension side varies from that shown, refer to cases 15.1 to 15.5 for the correct configuration.

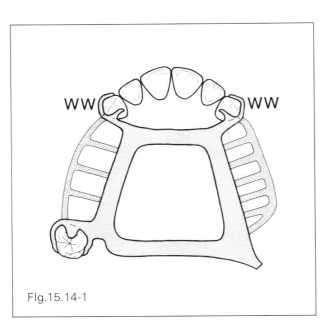

Fig.15.14-1

For design concepts and variations on the extension side, refer to cases 15.1 to 15.5. Options for the tooth-supported side are essentially the same as those for case 15.13.

Case 15.15

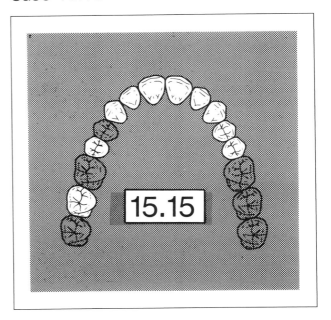

If the extension side varies from that shown, refer to cases 15.1 to 15.5 for the correct configuration.

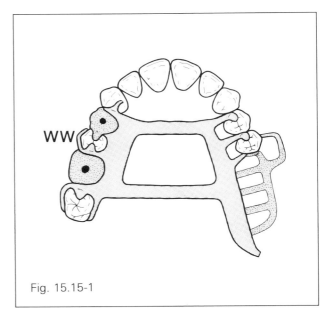

Fig. 15.15-1

For design concepts and variations on the extension side, refer to cases 15.1 to 15.5. Options for the tooth-supported side are discussed below.

Rests

One or both of the rests on the right second premolar could be deleted if occlusal interferences exist. The rest on the left first premolar could be omitted since the rest on the right canine provides excellent indirect retention.

Guide plates

Refer to cases 15.6 and 15.1.

Major connector

Refer to cases 15.12 and 15.1. Plating can be omitted from the right second premolar if the width of the opening is at least 4 mm.

Retentive arms

Clasping considerations for the molar and premolar are the same as those described for case 15.6. If esthetics permits, a retentive arm may be placed on the canine rather than the premolar. If this option is selected, refer to case 15.8.

Denture base retentive elements/replacement teeth

With two single-tooth modification spaces, tube teeth or heat-cured or light-activated resin facings are usually selected.

Case 15.16

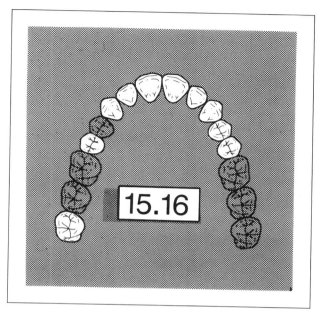

If the extension side varies from that shown, refer to cases 15.1 to 15.5 for the correct configuration.

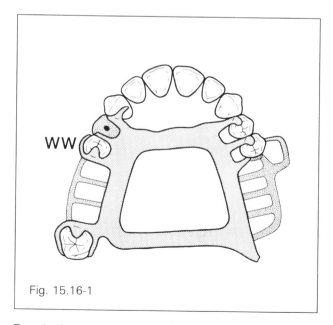

Fig. 15.16-1

For design concepts on the extension side, refer to cases 15.1 to 15.5. Options related to the tooth-supported side are discussed below.

Rests

If occlusion allows, an additional rest may be placed in the mesial fossa of the right second premolar. The rest on the left first premolar may be omitted since the canine rest on the opposite side will act as an excellent indirect retainer.

Guide plates

Refer to cases 15.6 and 15.1.

Major connector

Refer to cases 15.12 and 15.1. Plating can be omitted from the right second premolar if the width of the space is at least 4 mm.

Retentive arms

Clasping considerations for the molar and premolar are the same as those discussed for case 15.6. If esthetics permits, the anterior retentive arm may be placed on the canine rather than the second premolar. If this option is selected, refer to case 15.8.

Denture base retentive elements/replacement teeth

A tube tooth or heat-cured or light-activated resin facing is usually used in the single-tooth anterior modification space. Retentive network and denture teeth would most commonly be selected for the two-tooth posterior modification space.

Case 15.17

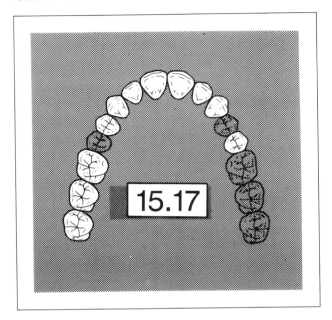

If the tooth-supported side varies from that shown, refer to cases 15.6 to 15.16 for the correct configuration.

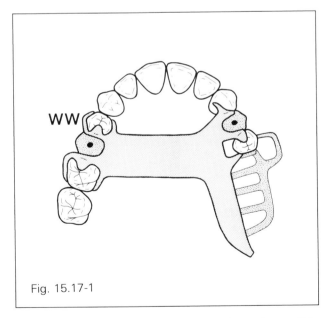

Fig. 15.17-1

Case 15.17 is one of a large number of possible Class II arch forms with posterior modification spaces on both the extension and the tooth-supported sides. Design concepts for the extension side are described under case 15.5. Those for the tooth-supported side are considered under cases 15.6 to 15.16. Consult the "Case reference guide" at the beginning of the chapter in order to find the design for a specific tooth-supported segment. For example, in case 15.17, there is a single tooth in the modification space on the tooth-supported side. In the "Case reference guide," this arrangement corresponds to cases 15.6 to 15.8. After reviewing individual drawings for these partially edentulous arches, it is evident that case 15.7 has exactly the same modification space. Thus, the design for case 15.17 is a combination of those for cases 15.5 and 15.7. Similarly, if the right second premolar and first molar were both missing, the design would be a combination of cases 15.5 and 15.10.

Case 15.18

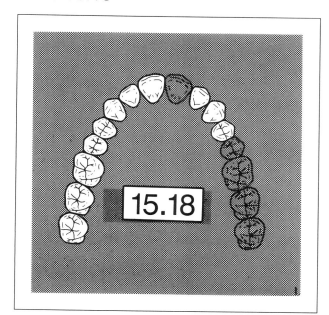

If the extension side varies from that shown, refer to cases 15.1 to 15.5 for the correct configuration.

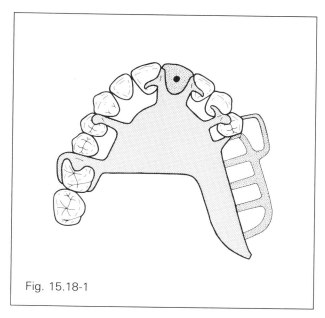

Fig. 15.18-1

The design for case 15.18 is essentially the same as that for case 15.2 with a single-tooth anterior modification space. Changes associated with the modification space are considered below. Refer to case 15.2 for discussion of other aspects of the design.

Rests

Although rests would usually be placed as shown in Fig. 15.18-1, several other combinations are possible, depending on diagnostic information. A rest on the lateral incisor is preferred if the tooth exhibits good bone support and a prominent cingulum. The cingulum rest on the left canine could be omitted since the rests on the anterior teeth and the right first premolar provide excellent indirect retention.

If the lateral incisor does not possess good bone support or lingual anatomy, two possibilities exist. First, the rest could be omitted because adequate vertical stops will be provided by the left premolar and canine and right first premolar. Or, the lateral incisor and canine may be plated if the occlusion permits. If this option is selected, the canine should have a rest seat prepared beneath the plating. If possible, a rest seat should also be placed on the lateral incisor.

Guide plates

The anterior guide plates must be located on the linguoproximal surfaces so that they will not be visible from the labial aspect or interfere with positioning of the replacement tooth.

Major connector

An anterior-posterior palatal strap might be selected if the opening between the straps would be large enough to be of significant benefit.

Minor connectors

Refer to case 15.1.

Retentive arms

The options for clasp assemblies are the same as those for case 15.2. Clasps on the incisors or right first premolar would be unesthetic and lie in front of the axis of rotation; they are rarely, if ever, indicated.

Denture base retentive elements/replacement teeth

With only one tooth in the modification space, a prefabricated facing, tube tooth, or custom heat-cured or light-activated resin replacement is almost always used.

Case 15.19

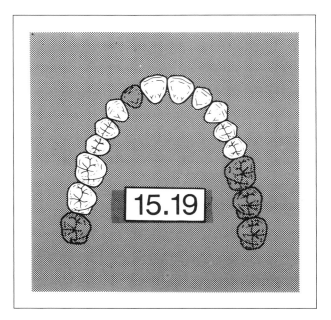

If the extension side varies from that shown, refer to cases 15.1 to 15.5 for the correct configuration.

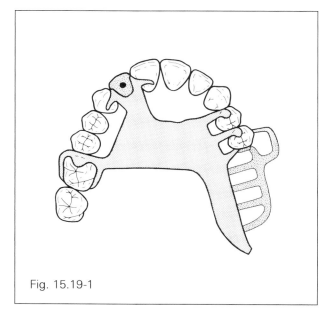

Fig. 15.19-1

The design for case 15.19 is essentially the same as that for case 15.1, with a single-tooth anterior modification space. Changes associated with the modification space are considered below. Refer to

case 15.1 for discussion of other aspects of the design.

Rests

The auxiliary rest on the extension side is not absolutely necessary because the rests adjacent to the modification space will provide excellent indirect retention.

Guide plates

Refer to case 15.18.

Major connector

Refer to case 15.18.

Minor connectors

Refer to case 15.1.

Retentive arms

The options for clasp assemblies are the same as those described for case 15.1. Clasps on the anterior teeth would be unesthetic and lie in front of the axis of rotation; they are rarely, if ever, indicated.

Denture base retentive elements/replacement teeth

Refer to case 15.18.

Case 15.20

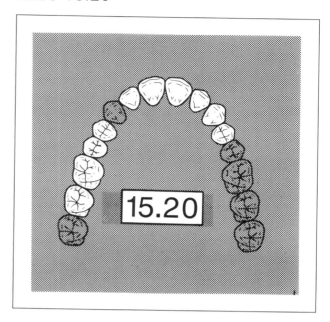

If the extension side varies from that shown, refer to cases 15.1 to 15.5 for the correct configuration.

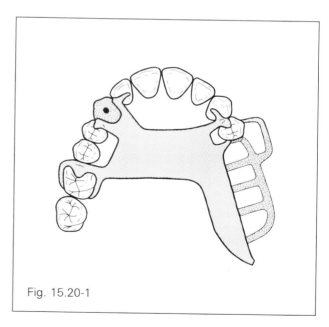

Fig. 15.20-1

The design for case 15.20 is essentially the same as that for case 15.2, with a single-tooth anterior modification space. Changes associated with the modification space are considered below. Refer to

case 15.2 for discussion of other aspects of the design.

Rests

The rest on the left canine is not absolutely essential, since the rests on the right lateral incisor and first premolar will function as indirect retainers.

If the right lateral incisor exhibits poor bone support or lacks the appropriate lingual anatomy for placement of a cingulum rest, two alternatives exist. Either the rest may be omitted from the lateral incisor or the lateral incisor may be plated and a cingulum rest placed on the central incisor.

Guide plates

Refer to case 15.18.

Major connector

Refer to case 15.18.

Minor connectors

Refer to case 15.1.

Retentive arms

The options for clasp assemblies are the same as those described for case 15.2. Retentive arms on the lateral incisor and first premolar would be unesthetic and lie in front of the axis of rotation; they are seldom, if ever, indicated.

Denture base retentive elements/replacement teeth

Refer to case 15.18.

Case 15.21

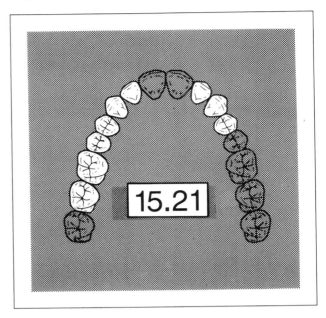

If the extension side varies from that shown, refer to cases 15.1 to 15.5 for the correct configuration.

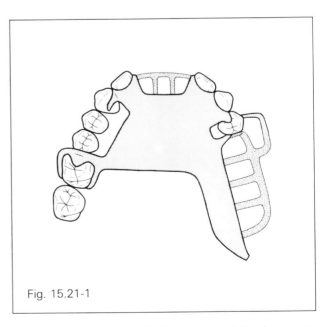

Fig. 15.21-1

The design for case 15.21 is essentially the same as that for case 15.2, with a two-tooth anterior modification space. Changes associated with the modification space are considered below. Refer to

case 15.2 for discussion of other aspects of the design.

Rests

If the lateral incisors exhibit exceptionally good bone support and lingual anatomy, rest seats and rests may be placed on them, and the plating and rests on the canines omitted.

Guide plates

The anterior guide plates should be located on the linguoproximal surfaces so that they will not be visible from the labial aspect or interfere with positioning of the replacement teeth.

Major connector

Refer to case 15.18.

Minor connectors

Refer to case 15.1.

Retentive arms

The options for clasp assemblies are the same as those for case 15.2. Retentive arms on the lateral incisors would be unesthetic and lie in front of the axis of rotation; they are rarely, if ever, indicated.

Denture base retentive elements/replacement teeth

With two teeth in the modification space, retentive network, denture teeth, and denture base are most commonly used. However, if the residual ridge exhibits little resorption, and the space is appropriate for the missing teeth, facings, tube teeth, or heat-cured or light-activated resin replacements may be selected.

Case 15.22

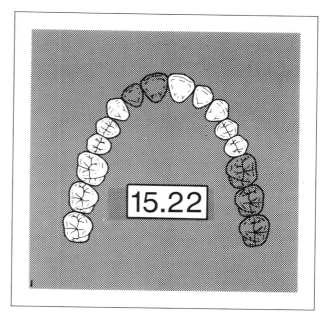

If the extension side varies from that shown, refer to cases 15.1 to 15.5 for the correct configuration.

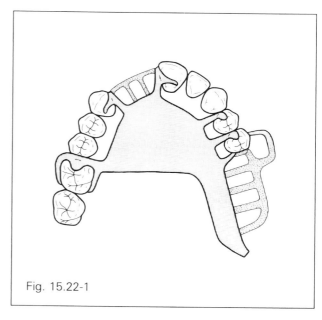

Fig. 15.22-1

The design for case 15.22 is essentially the same as that for case 15.1 with a two-tooth anterior modification space. Changes associated with the modification space are considered below. Refer to

case 15.1 for discussion of other aspects of the design.

Rests

The rest on the left first premolar is not absolutely essential since the rests on the central incisor and canine will act as indirect retainers.

Guide plates

Refer to case 15.21.

Major connector

Refer to case 15.18.

Minor connectors

Refer to case 15.1.

Retentive arms

Retentive arms on the central incisor and canine would be unesthetic and lie in front of the axis of rotation; they are rarely, if ever, indicated.

Denture base retentive elements/replacement teeth

Refer to case 15.21.

Case 15.23

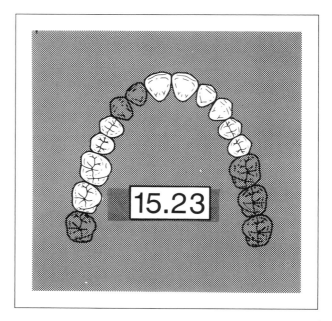

If the extension side varies from that shown, refer to cases 15.1 to 15.5 for the correct configuration.

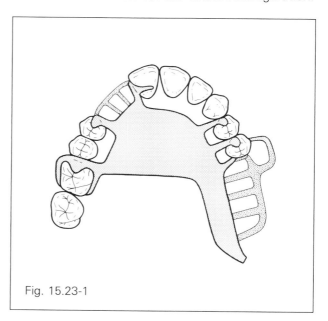

Fig. 15.23-1

The design for case 15.23 is essentially the same as that for case 15.1, with a two-tooth modification space. Changes associated with the modification space are considered below. Refer to case 15.1 for discussion of other aspects of the design.

Rests

The rest on the left first premolar is not absolutely necessary, because the rests on the central incisor and right first premolar will provide adequate indirect retention.

Guide plates

The guide plate on the first premolar and particularly that on the central incisor should be restricted to the linguoproximal surfaces so that they will not be visible from the labial aspect or interfere with positioning of the replacement teeth.

Major connector

Refer to case 15.18.

Minor connectors

Refer to case 15.1.

Retentive arms

Retentive arms on the central incisor and first premolar would be unesthetic and lie in front of the axis of rotation; they are seldom, if ever indicated.

Denture base retentive elements/replacement teeth

Refer to case 15.21.

Case 15.24

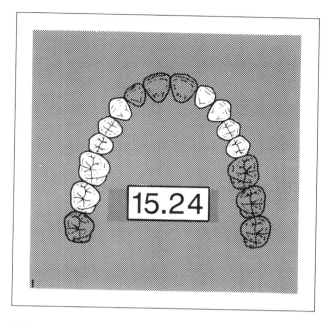

If the extension side varies from that shown, refer to cases 15.1 to 15.5 for the correct configuration.

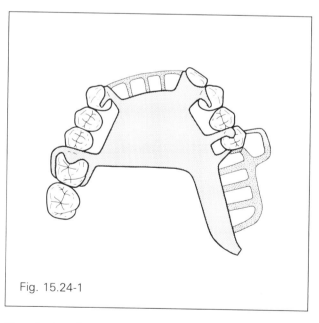

Fig. 15.24-1

The design for case 15.24 is essentially the same as that for case 15.1 with a three-tooth anterior modification space. Changes associated with the modification space are considered below. Refer to

case 15.1 for discussion of other aspects of the design.

Rests

If the left lateral incisor exhibits good bone support and a prominent cingulum, a rest seat and rest may be placed on it and the plating and rest on the adjacent canine omitted.

Guide plates

The anterior guide plates must be located on the linguoproximal surfaces so that they will not be visible from the labial aspect or interfere with positioning of the replacement teeth.

Major connector

Refer to case 15.18.

Minor connectors

Refer to case 15.1.

Retentive arms

Retentive arms on the central incisor and canine would be unesthetic and lie in front of the axis of rotation; they are rarely, if ever, indicated.

Denture base retentive elements/replacement teeth

With three teeth in the modification space, retentive network, denture teeth, and denture base would usually be used. However, if the residual ridge exhibits little resorption and the spacing is appropriate for the missing teeth, facings, tube teeth, or heat-cured or light-activated resin replacements may be selected.

Case 15.25

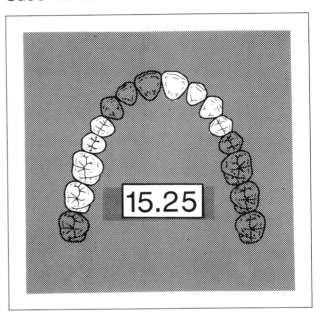

If the extension side varies from that shown, refer to cases 15.1 to 15.5 for the correct configuration.

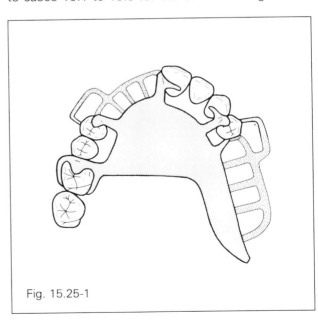

Fig. 15.25-1

The design for case 15.25 is essentially the same as that for case 15.2, with a three-tooth anterior modification space. Changes associated with the modification space are considered below. Refer to case 15.2 for other aspects of the design.

Rests

The rest on the left canine is not absolutely essential, because the rests on the central incisor and right first premolar will act as indirect retainers.

Guide plates

The guide plate on the premolar and particularly that on the central incisor should be located on the linguoproximal surfaces so that they will not be visible from the labial aspect or interfere with positioning of the replacement teeth.

Major connector

Refer to case 15.18.

Minor connectors

Refer to case 15.1.

Retentive arms

A retentive arm on the central incisor would be unesthetic and lie in front of the axis of rotation; it would rarely, if ever, be indicated.

With three teeth in the modification space, a retentive arm on the right first premolar might be necessary. A bar clasp would generally be preferred because the originating portion of a circumferential clasp would usually be located near the mesio-occlusal aspect of the tooth and could be esthetically objectionable. Since the bar clasp will lie in front of the axis of rotation, it should be long, tapered, and flexible.

Denture base retentive elements/replacement teeth

Refer to case 15.24.

Case 15.26

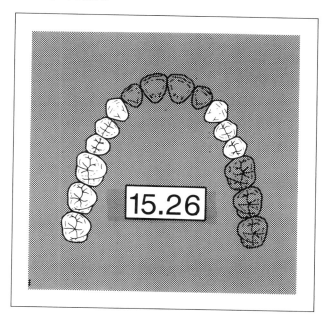

If the extension side varies from that shown, refer to cases 15.1 to 15.5 for the correct configuration.

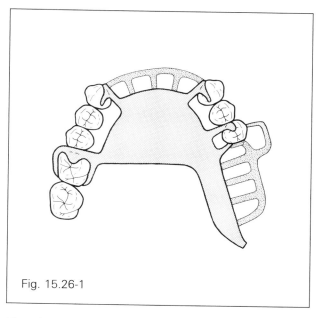

Fig. 15.26-1

The design for case 15.26 is essentially the same as that for case 15.1, with a four-tooth anterior modification space. Changes associated with the modification space are considered below. Refer to case 15.1 for other aspects of the design.

Rests

Rest location is almost always as shown in Fig. 15.26-1.

Guide plates

The guide plates on the canines should be located on the linguoproximal surfaces so that they will not be visible from the labial aspect or interfere with positioning of the replacement teeth.

Major connector

Refer to case 15.18.

Minor connectors

Refer to case 15.1.

Retentive arms

Because of esthetic considerations, clasps are not usually placed on the canines. If clasps are desired, I-bars are usually selected. They should be long, tapered, and flexible, because they lie in front of the axis of rotation. Wrought wire circumferential clasps have the desired flexibility but may be unesthetic because they often originate near the mesioincisal edges.

Denture base retentive elements/replacement teeth

With four teeth in the modification space, retentive network, denture base, and denture teeth are almost always used. However, if the residual ridge exhibits little resorption and if the width of the space is appropriate for the missing teeth, facings, tube teeth, or heat-cured or light-activated resin replacements may be selected.

Case 15.27

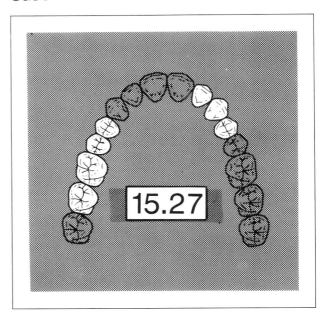

If the extension side varies from that shown, refer to cases 15.1 to 15.5 for the correct configuration.

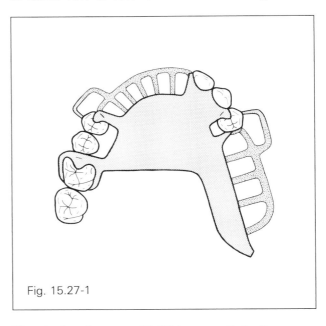

Fig. 15.27-1

The design for case 15.27 is essentially the same as that for case 15.2, with a four-tooth anterior modification space. Changes necessitated by the modification space are discussed below. Refer to case 15.2 for other aspects of the design.

Rests

The bone support and lingual anatomy of the lateral incisor are usually not sufficient to support such a large modification space. Therefore, it is often plated, and a definite cingulum rest seat is prepared on the canine.

Guide plates

Guide plates, particularly on the lateral incisor, should be located on the linguoproximal surfaces so that they will not be visible from the labial aspect or interfere with positioning of the replacement teeth.

Major connector

Refer to case 15.18.

Minor connectors

Refer to case 15.1.

Retentive arms

A retentive arm would seldom, if ever, be placed on the lateral incisor. Because of the size of the modification space, a bar clasp might be used on the first premolar. Because it lies in front of the axis of rotation, it should be long, tapered, and flexible. A wrought wire circumferential clasp could be used, except that it will often originate near the mesio-occlusal corner of the tooth and would be visible when the patient smiles.

Denture base retentive elements/replacement teeth

Refer to case 15.26.

Case 15.28

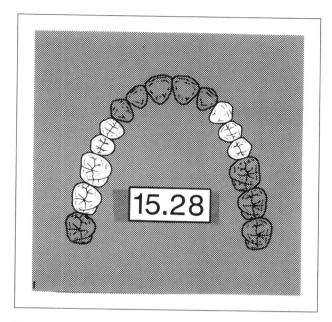

If the extension side varies from that shown, refer to cases 15.1 to 15.5 for the correct configuration.

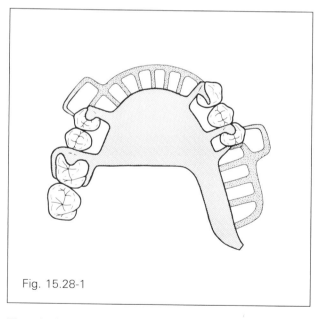

Fig. 15.28-1

The design for case 15.28 is essentially the same as that for case 15.27. The fact that the left lateral incisor is missing has little effect on the design principles utilized.

Case 15.29

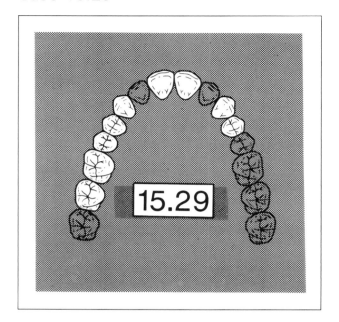

If the extension side varies from that shown, refer to cases 15.1 to 15.5 for the correct configuration.

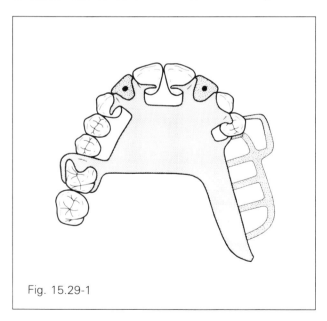

Fig. 15.29-1

The design for case 15.29 is essentially the same as that for case 15.19, except that the second lateral incisor is also missing. Refer to case 15.19 for design concepts and variations.

Case 15.30

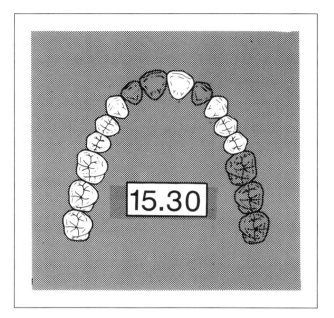

If the extension side varies from that shown, refer to cases 15.1 to 15.5 for the correct configuration.

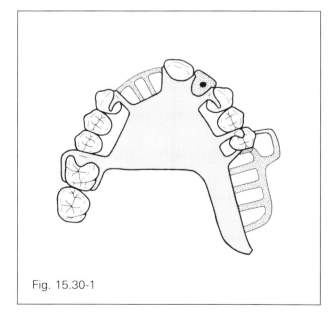

Fig. 15.30-1

The design for case 15.30 is essentially the same as that for case 15.1, with two anterior modification spaces. Changes necessitated by the modification spaces are considered below. Refer to case 15.1 for discussion of other aspects of the design.

The lone-standing central incisor often creates esthetic problems in both shade matching and spacing for the anterior replacement teeth. A good alternative would be to use the central incisor as a removable partial overdenture abutment. The root will provide an excellent vertical stop and there will be much more flexibility in replacement tooth selection and arrangement. The RPD design would then be the same as that for case 15.26.

Rests

The rests would almost always be as shown in Fig. 15.30-1.

Guide plates

The anterior guide plates should be located on the linguoproximal surfaces so that they will not be visible from the labial aspect or interfere with positioning of the replacement teeth.

Major connector

Refer to case 15.18.

Minor connectors

Refer to case 15.1.

Retentive arms

Retentive arms on the anterior teeth would be unesthetic and lie in front of the axis of rotation; they are rarely, if ever, indicated.

Denture base retentive elements/replacement teeth

A tube tooth, facing, or heat-cured or light-activated resin replacement would usually be used for the single-tooth space. The same options exist for the two-tooth space if the spacing is appropriate and if the residual ridge exhibits minimal resorp-

tion. Retentive network, denture teeth, and denture base are preferred for both anterior spaces if the spacing is unusual or if there has been extensive residual ridge loss.

Case 15.31

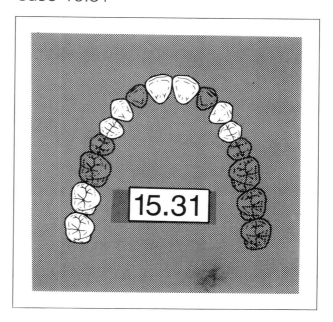

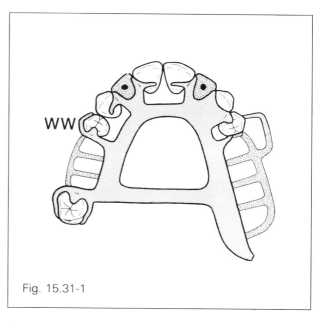

Fig. 15.31-1

Case 15.31 is one of a large number of possible

Class II arch forms with both anterior and posterior modification spaces. In order to arrive at the appropriate design, it will be necessary to integrate segments of two or more other designs. The extension area and anterior modification space(s) should usually be considered together (see cases 15.18 to 15.30), and the posterior modification space as a separate entity (see cases 15.6 to 15.16).

By consulting the "Case reference guide" and examining the partially edentulous arches, it is ev-

ident that the design for case 15.31 is a combination of those for cases 15.29 and 15.10. If all four incisors were missing, the design would be a combination of cases 15.26 and 15.10. Similarly, if all four incisors and the right first and second premolars and right first molar were missing, the design would be a combination of cases 15.26 and 15.13. In the last two examples, cases 15.1 to 15.5 would also need to be consulted for variations in the extension area.

Chapter 16

Maxillary Class III Designs

In our study of almost 2,000 maxillary partially edentulous arches for which removable partial dentures were fabricated, almost 40% were Class III. There were nearly 300 different arrangements of edentulous segments and the potential for variations was even greater. Discussion of every possible variation is not practical and, fortunately, not necessary. Because tooth-supported RPDs exhibit no functional motion, the designs are much less complicated and generally follow a fairly straightforward set of guidelines. Consequently, designs for partially edentulous arches not covered can be developed rather easily by extrapolation from or combining of the examples presented.

Case reference guide	
Both canines present	
Anterior edentulous segment(s) only	
Single anterior space: does not cross midline	16.1
Two anterior spaces	16.2 to 16.3
Posterior edentulous segment(s) only	
Without modification space	
Two teeth in segment	16.4 to 16.6
Three teeth in segment	16.7 to 16.8
Four teeth in segment	16.9
With modification space(s)	
Modification space on same side of arch	16.10 to 16.14
Modification space on opposite side of arch	
One tooth in space	16.15 to 16.18
More than one tooth in space	16.19
Both anterior and posterior edentulous segments	
Single anterior modification space	
One tooth in space	16.20 to 16.23
Two teeth in space	16.24 to 16.25
Three teeth in space	16.26
Four teeth in space	16.27 to 16.28
Two anterior modification spaces	16.29 to 16.30
One canine missing	16.31 to 16.36
Both canines missing	16.37 to 16.40

Case 16.1

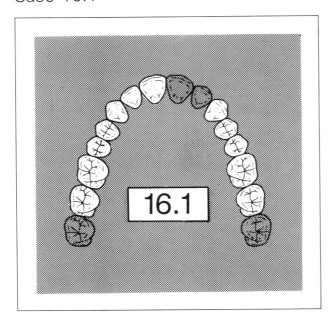

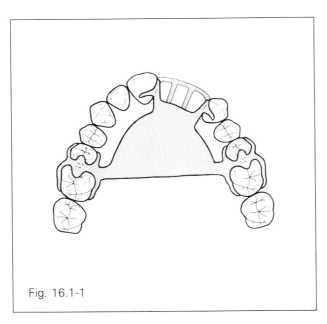

Fig. 16.1-1

Rests

The embrasure clasp assemblies may be moved one tooth forward or backward, depending on the location of undercuts and occlusal contacts. Cingulum rest seats and rests should always be included on the central incisor and canine.

Guide plates

Anterior guide plates must be located on the linguoproximal surfaces so they will not be visible from the labial aspect or interfere with positioning of the replacement teeth.

Major connector

An anterior-posterior palatal strap major connector is preferred if the palatal opening would be large enough to be of significant benefit (greater than 15 mm in an anterior-posterior dimension). This would most commonly occur when the embrasure clasps are placed on the first and second molars.

A U-shaped major connector may also be considered. Although there is some loss in rigidity, the edentulous segment is so small that the sacrifice is not of great importance.

Minor connectors

Design principles for minor connectors are the same as those discussed for case 14.1. No special considerations are necessary for Class III RPDs.

Retentive arms

Cast clasps are almost always used for Class III RPDs. With a small anterior edentulous space (as in case 16.1), anterior retentive arms are seldom used. However, a clasp can be placed on the canine if added retention is desired. A bar clasp would usually be selected if the approach arm will be hidden by the upper lip. If the approach arm will be visible crossing the gingiva, the clasp is normally omitted. A circumferential clasp on the canine is usually contraindicated because the originating portion of the arm is rigid, cannot be placed in an undercut, and will often lie very close to the mesioincisal edge. Rigid metal retention (dual path, rotational path) may also be considered for the anterior segment.

Circumferential (embrasure) clasps are almost always used to provide retention posteriorly, and the undercuts are invariably on the distobuccal surfaces. The clasp assembly may be moved forward or backward one tooth depending on the location of undercuts and occlusal contacts.

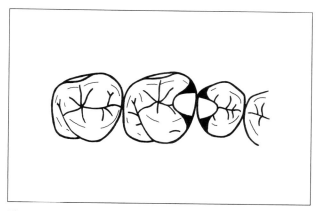

Fig. 16.1-2 Special care is required during mouth preparation for embrasure clasps. Access into and out of the rest seats *(shaded areas)* must be created by removal of tooth structure from the proximal inclines of the adjacent cusps. Fracture in these areas is extremely common when the space is not sufficient to ensure adequate strength of metal.

If the height of contour is very near the occlusal aspect of the buccal surface, minor recontouring may be required where retentive arms emerge from the embrasure. The originating portions of the arms are rigid and cannot be located in undercuts. Without recontouring, the arms would lie close to the occlusal surface, distort the normal form of the clasp, and possibly detract from esthetics.

Denture base retentive elements/replacement teeth

With a small anterior edentulous segment, several possiblities for replacement exist. Retentive network, denture teeth, and denture base would tend to be selected if the spacing is not appropriate for the missing teeth or if the residual ridge exhibits extensive resorption or incomplete healing. Facings, tube teeth, or heat-cured or light-activated resin replacements would be more appropriate if the residual ridge exhibits little resorption and large undercuts, if the spacing is correct, or if there is deep vertical overlap of the anterior teeth. In the last instance, metal backing should be used to reduce the potential for fracture.

Case 16.2

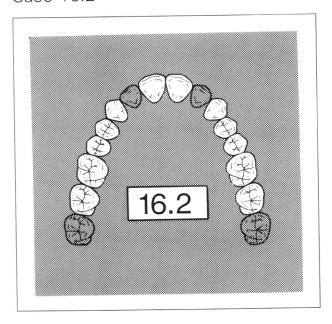

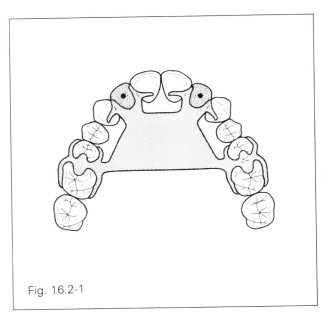

Fig. 16.2-1

Rests

The anterior rests are almost always placed as shown in Fig. 16.2-1. Although the central incisors may be plated, rest seats must be included beneath the plating.

The embrasure clasp assemblies may be moved one tooth forward or backward, depending on the location of undercuts and occlusal contacts.

Guide plates

Refer to case 16.1.

Major connector

Refer to case 16.1.

Minor connectors

Refer to case 16.1.

Retentive arms

Retentive arms would seldom, if ever, be used on the central incisors. Clasping options for the canines are the same as those for case 16.1. Also refer to case 16.1 for a discussion of the design of the embrasure clasps.

Denture base retentive elements/replacement teeth

Facings, tube teeth, or heat-cured or light-activated resin replacements would almost always be used for the two single-tooth anterior edentulous areas.

Case 16.3

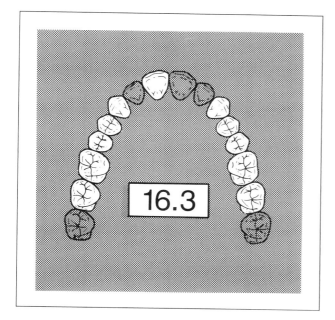

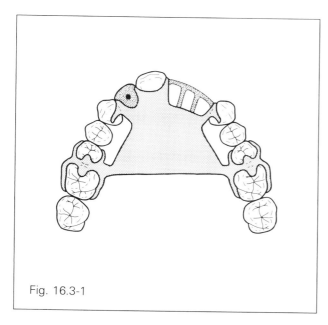

Fig. 16.3-1

Rests

The anterior rests are almost always placed as shown in Fig. 16.3-1. A rest seat should be prepared beneath the plating on the central incisor.

The embrasure clasp assemblies may be moved one tooth foward or backward depending on the location of undercuts and occlusal contacts. However, moving the assemblies forward may result in some loss of stability during incising.

Guide plates

Refer to case 16.1.

Major connector

Refer to case 16.1.

Minor connectors

Refer to case 16.1.

Retentive arms

A retentive arm would seldom, if ever, be placed on the central incisor. If clasps are needed on the canines, the options are the same as those described for case 16.1. Also refer to case 16.1 for a discussion of the design for the embrasure clasps.

Denture base retentive elements/replacement teeth

There are a number of possibilities for replacement of the missing anterior teeth. In Fig. 16.3-1 a combination of methods was used. In general, retentive network, denture teeth, and denture base would be selected if the spacing is unusual or if there has been extensive residual ridge resorption. Facings, tube teeth, or heat-cured or light-activated resin replacements would be more appropriate if the residual ridge exhibits little resorption and large undercuts, if the spacing is correct, or if there is a deep vertical overlap. In the last instance, metal backings should be used to reduce the potential for fracture.

Occasionally, the shape, position, or coloration of the lone-standing central incisor is such that an acceptable esthetic result is difficult to achieve. Rather than extract the central incisor, it would be preferable to perform root canal therapy and use the root as an "over partial denture" abutment. Such treatment will allow much greater freedom in tooth selection and arrangement, while at the same time providing an extremely good anterior vertical stop. Design options would then be the same as those for case 17.2.

Case 16.4

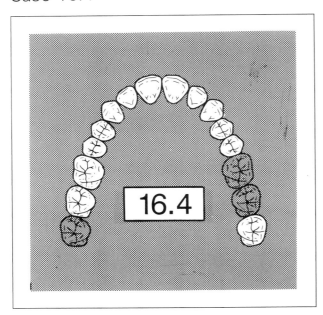

16.4

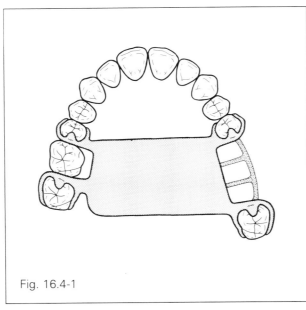

Fig. 16.4-1

Rests

The rest on the left second premolar may be moved to the mesial fossa or to the mesial or distal aspect of the first premolar if the occlusion precludes placement at the normal location.

On the right side, an embrasure clasp may be used on the second premolar and first molar or first molar and second molar. Some stability may be sacrificed because the rests will be closer together.

Guide plates

In Class III RPDs with posterior edentulous spaces, the path of insertion/dislodgement can be rather strictly defined. The degree of definition depends on the number, length, and parallelism of the guide surface–guide plate contacts. The general characteristics of the guide plates are the same as those described for case 14.1. However, since Class III RPDs do not exhibit functional motion, guide plates may be longer and may extend further lingually and above the survey line without creating adverse torquing forces on the abutments.

Major connector

With only two teeth in the edentulous segment, a palatal strap major connector would almost always be used. If the occlusion dictated that the rests be more widely separated, an anterior-posterior palatal strap could be considered. The opening between the straps should be 15 mm or more in an anterior-posterior dimension.

Minor connectors

Refer to case 16.1.

Retentive arms

Because there are no teeth missing on the right side, the considerations for the retentive arms are essentially the same as those described for the embrasure clasps of case 16.1.

On the left side, cast circumferential clasps are the retainers of choice if the undercuts are on the sides of the abutments away from the edentulous space. Bar clasps would be preferred if the undercuts are adjacent to the edentulous space.

Case 16.5

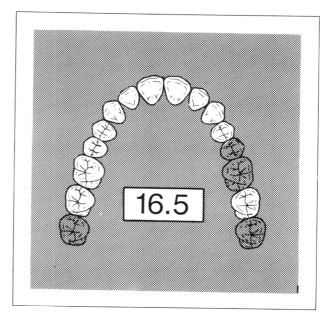

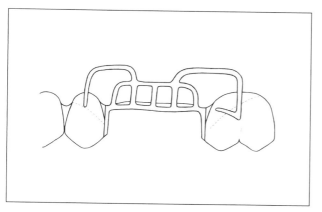

Fig. 16.4-2 If the undercut is located at the middle of the facial surface, an I-bar is the preferred retainer. If the undercut is adjacent to the edentulous space, a modified T-bar is more commonly selected.

Denture base retentive elements/replacement teeth

With two or more teeth in the edentulous space, retentive network, denture teeth, and denture base are most commonly used. A metal base with heat-cured or light-activated resin replacements may be indicated if vertical space is limited, if the metal base is not visible when the patient smiles, and if the residual ridge is well-healed.

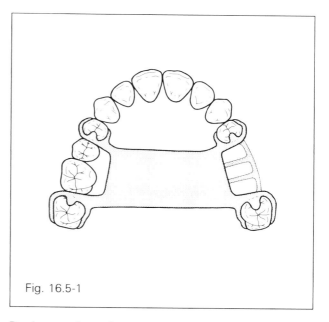

Fig. 16.5-1

Design options for case 16.5 are essentially the same as those for case 16.4. Because the anterior abutment on the left side is a first rather than a second premolar, there might be a greater tendency to use a bar clasp. Esthetics would improve as long as the approach arm is not visible crossing the gingiva. If appearance is an important factor,

279

the anterior circumferential clasp on the right side could also be moved to back to the second premolar.

The rest on the distal of the left first premolar may be moved to the mesial fossa or to the cingulum of the canine if occlusal interferences prevent normal placement.

Case 16.6

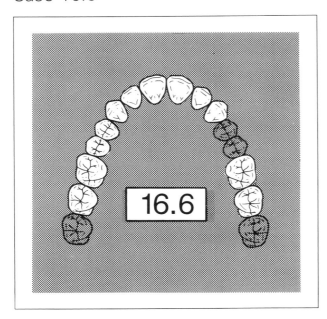

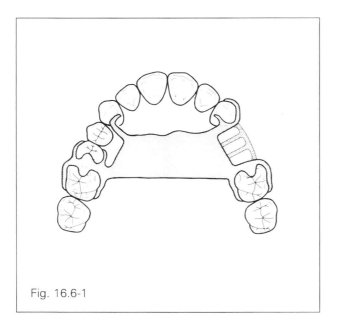

Fig. 16.6-1

Rests

The auxiliary rest on the right canine could be omitted if occlusal interferences exist. However, some compromise in stability and symmetry may occur.

Guide plates

Refer to case 16.4.

Major connector

Refer to case 16.4.

Minor connectors

Refer to case 16.1.

Retentive arms

A bar clasp on the left canine is preferred if the arm can be hidden behind the mesiodistal height of contour and/or if the approach portion of the arm is not visible crossing the gingiva.

A wrought wire circumferential clasp may be considered for the left canine if the increased flexibility will allow for utilization of an undercut greater than 0.01 in. Esthetics can then be improved by more gingival placement of the arm.

Refer to case 16.1 for a discussion of the embrasure clasp on the right side. The anterior component of the embrasure clasp may be moved to the first premolar if occlusion permits. The anterior rest would then be placed in the distal fossa and the clasp arm would engage a mesiofacial undercut.

Denture base retentive elements/replacement teeth

Refer to case 16.4.

Case 16.7

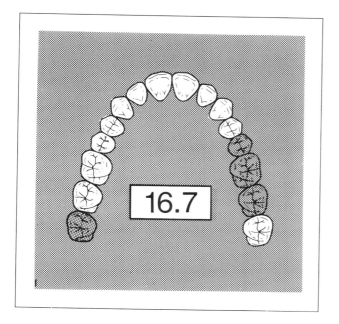

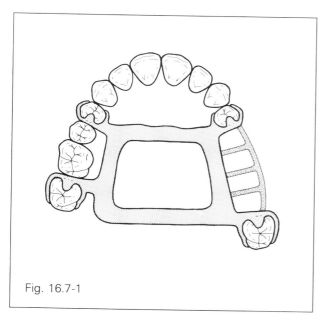

Fig. 16.7-1

Rests

The rests on the right side may be moved forward or backward depending on occlusal interferences and the location of undercuts for the clasp arms. However, stability tends to improve as the rests and clasps are more widely separated.

The rest on the left first premolar may be moved to the mesial fossa or to the cingulum of the canine if occlusion interferes with placement on the distal.

Guide plates

Refer to case 16.4.

Major connector

With three teeth in the edentulous space, an anterior-posterior palatal strap is the preferred major connector. However, if rest placement is such that the opening would be less than 15 mm in an anterior-posterior dimension, a single strap should be used.

Minor connectors

Refer to case 16.1.

Retentive arms

Refer to cases 16.5 and 16.1.

Denture base retentive elements/replacement teeth

Refer to case 16.4.

Case 16.8

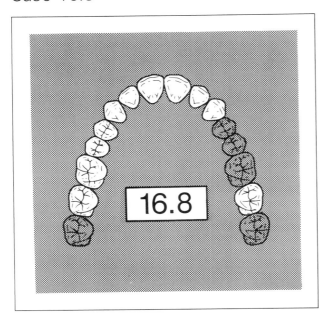

Fig. 16.8-1

Rests

Occlusion permitting, rests are usually placed as shown in Fig. 16.8-1. Although an embrasure clasp assembly may be used on the second premolar and first molar, it then becomes difficult to cross the palate at right angles with the major connector.

Guide plates

Refer to case 16.4.

Major connector

Refer to case 16.7.

Minor connectors

Refer to case 16.1.

Retentive arms

Refer to cases 16.5 and 16.1 for options for the right side and case 16.6 for options for the left side.

Denture base retentive elements/replacement teeth

Refer to case 16.4.

Case 16.9

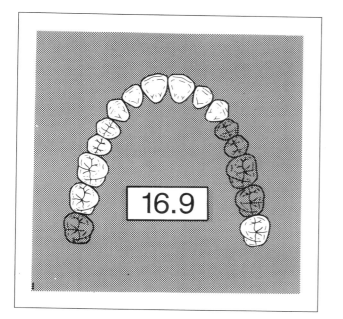

Case 16.10

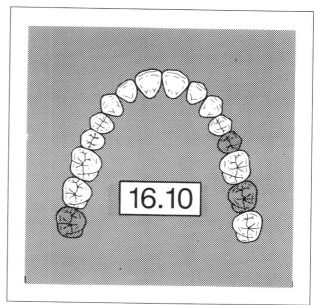

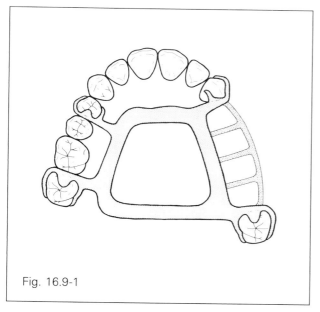

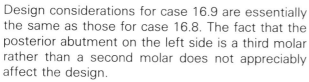

Fig. 16.9-1

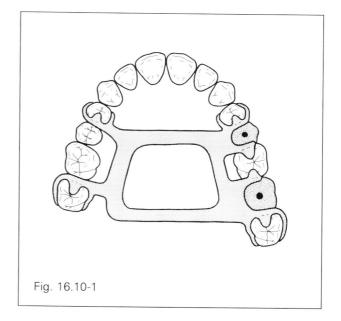

Fig. 16.10-1

Design considerations for case 16.9 are essentially the same as those for case 16.8. The fact that the posterior abutment on the left side is a third molar rather than a second molar does not appreciably affect the design.

Rests

One or both rests on the left first molar may be omitted if occlusal interferences exist. Refer to case 16.7 for options on the right side.

Guide plates

Refer to case 16.4.

Major connector

An anterior-posterior palatal strap is usually the preferred major connector. However, if the posterior border can be placed farther forward, a palatal strap may be selected.

Minor connectors

Refer to case 16.1.

Retentive arms

Clasping considerations for the right molar and premolar are the same as those discussed for cases 16.5 and 16.1. Refer to case 16.5 for clasping options for the left first premolar. If esthetics is a problem, the anterior clasp on the left side may be placed on the first molar rather than the first premolar.

Denture base retentive elements/replacement teeth

Tube teeth or heat-cured or light-activated resin replacements would usually be used for the two single-tooth posterior replacements. An all-metal tooth could be used to replace the second molar if vertical space is limited.

Case 16.11

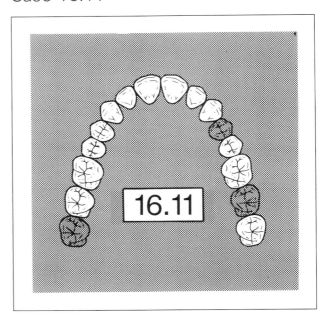

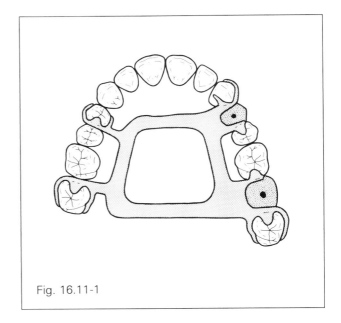

Fig. 16.11-1

Rests

The rests on the left second premolar and first molar could be omitted if occlusal interferences exist. Refer to case 16.7 for options on the right side.

Guide plates

Refer to case 16.4.

Major connector

An anterior-posterior palatal strap major connector would almost always be used.

Minor connectors

Refer to case 16.1.

Retentive arms

The clasp on the left canine could be moved back to the second premolar if esthetics is a major concern and if a distofacial undercut is available. Options for clasping the canine are the same as those for case 16.6.

Refer to cases 16.5 and 16.1 for a discussion of clasping on the right side.

Denture base retentive elements/replacement teeth

Refer to case 16.10.

Case 16.12

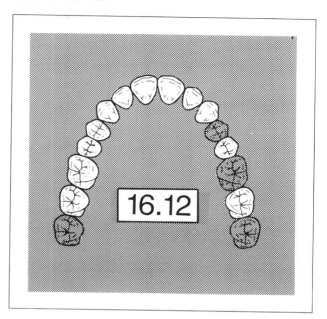

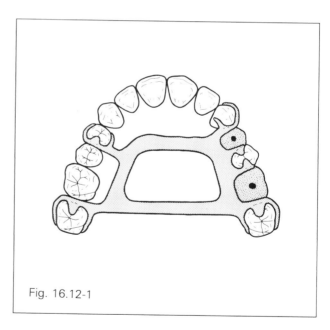

Fig. 16.12-1

Rests

One or both rests on the left second premolar could be omitted if occlusal interferences exist. Refer to case 16.7 for options on the right side.

Guide plates

Refer to case 16.4.

Major connector

Refer to case 16.7.

Minor connectors

Refer to case 16.1.

Retentive arms

Refer to case 16.6 for options for clasping the left canine. If esthetics is a major concern, a circumferential clasp, originating from the distal aspect and engaging a mesiobuccal undercut, may be used on the left second premolar and the clasp on the left canine omitted.

Refer to cases 16.5 and 16.1 for a discussion of clasps for the right side.

Denture base retentive elements/replacement teeth

Refer to case 16.10.

Case 16.13

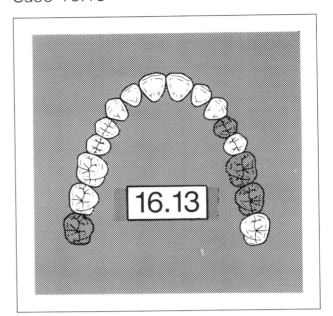

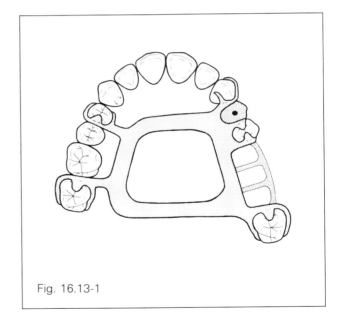

Fig. 16.13-1

Rests

One or both rests on the second premolar could be omitted if occlusal interferences exist. Refer to case 16.7 for options on the right side.

Guide plates

Refer to case 16.4.

Major connector

An anterior-posterior palatal strap would almost always be the preferred major connector.

Minor connectors

Refer to case 16.1.

Retentive arms

If esthetics is a major concern, a circumferential clasp, originating from the distal and engaging a mesiobuccal undercut, may be used on the left second premolar and the clasp on the canine omitted.

Refer to cases 16.5 and 16.1 for a discussion of clasping for the right side.

Denture base retentive elements/replacement teeth

Retentive network, denture teeth, and denture base would almost always be used for the posterior edentulous space. They may also be used for the anterior space, particularly when the space is wider than normal.

Case 16.14

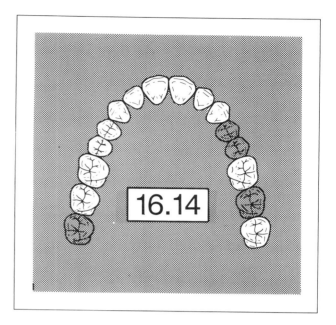

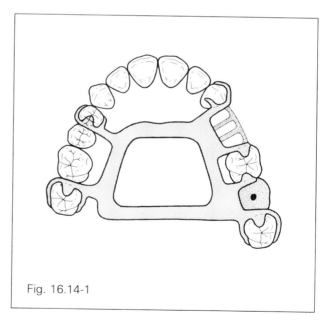

Fig. 16.14-1

Rests

One or both rests on the first molar could be omitted if occlusal interferences exist. Refer to case 16.7 for options on the right side.

Guide plates

Refer to case 16.4.

Major connector

An anterior-posterior palatal strap is almost always the major connector of choice.

Minor connectors

Refer to case 16.1.

Retentive arms

Clasping options for the canine are the same as those described for case 16.6. Options for the third molar are the same as those for case 16.4. If the third molar does not possess a usable undercut, a circumferential clasp may be placed on the first molar. It would usually originate from the mesial and engage a distofacial undercut.

Refer to cases 16.5 and 16.1 for a discussion of clasping for the right side.

Denture base retentive elements/replacement teeth

A tube tooth, heat-cured or light-activated resin replacement would usually be used for the single-tooth posterior space. However, retentive network, a denture tooth, and denture base may also be used and is particularly indicated if the space is wider than normal. An all-metal replacement is indicated if vertical space is limited.

Tube teeth or resin replacements may also be used to replace the premolars if the residual ridge is well-healed and exhibits minimal resorption.

Case 16.15

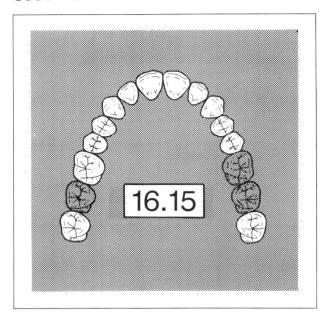

If the left side varies from that shown, refer to cases 16.4 to 16.14 for the correct configuration.

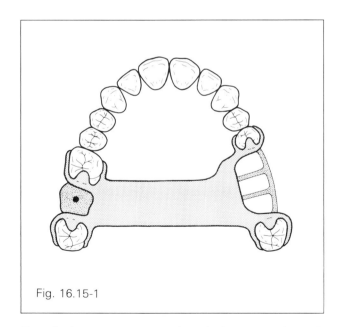

Fig. 16.15-1

For design concepts and variations on the left side, refer to cases 16.4 to 16.14. Options related to the right-side modification space are discussed below.

Rests

The rest on the distal of the right first molar could be moved forward to the mesial fossa or to the distal fossa of the second premolar if occlusal interferences preclude normal placement.

Guide plates

Refer to case 16.4.

Major connector

A palatal strap would almost always be used.

Retentive arms

Modified T-bars are the retainers of choice on the right first and third molar if the only usable undercuts are adjacent to the edentulous space.

Denture base retentive elements/replacement teeth

With a single tooth in the modification space, a tube tooth or heat-cured or light-activated resin replacement would usually be used. If the width of the space is narrowed by drifting, or if vertical space is limited, an all-metal replacement should be considered.

Case 16.16

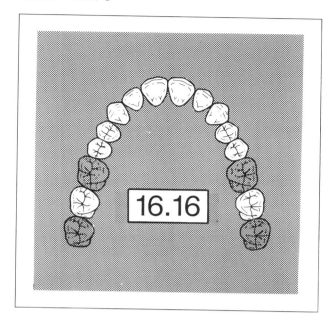

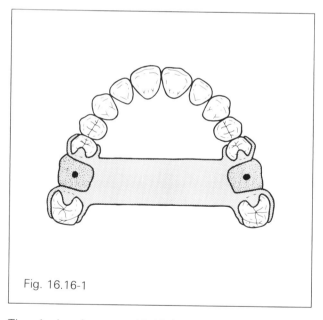

Fig. 16.16-1

The design for case 16.16 is a combination of the right side of case 16.15 and its mirror image. Refer to case 16.15 for design concepts and variations.

Case 16.17

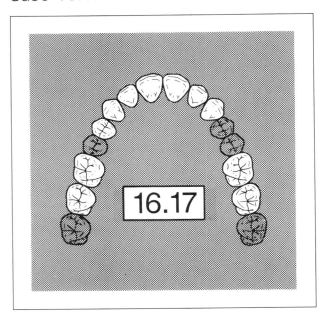

If the left side varies from that shown, refer to cases 16.4 to 16.14 for the correct configuration.

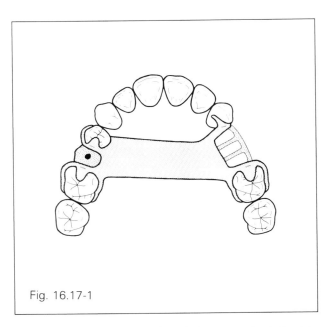

Fig. 16.17-1

For design concepts and variations on the left side refer to cases 16.4 to 16.14. Options related to the right-side modification space are discussed below.

Rests

The rest on the right first premolar can be moved to the mesial fossa or to the cingulum of the canine if occlusal interferences contraindicate placement on the distal. The mesial rest on the first molar may also be moved to the distal if necessary.

Guide plates

Refer to case 16.4.

Major connector

A palatal strap would almost always be used. The right first premolar is plated to facilitate crossing the palate at right angles to the midline. However, a lingual bracing arm is an acceptable alternative.

Minor connectors

Refer to case 16.1.

Retentive arms

A modified T-bar would be the retainer of choice for the first molar or first premolar if the undercut is adjacent to the edentulous space.

A bar clasp would also be the retainer of choice for the first premolar if it would be less visible than a circumferential clasp.

With relatively small edentulous spaces, a retainer on the left canine could usually be omitted, particularly if the four guide surface–guide plate contacts are parallel and restrict the path of insertion/dislodgement.

Denture base retentive elements/replacement teeth

With a single tooth in the modification space, a tube tooth or heat-cured or light-activated resin replacement would usually be used. Retentive network, a denture tooth, and denture base could be considered if the residual ridge is still in the process of recontouring or if the space is considerably wider than normal.

Case 16.18

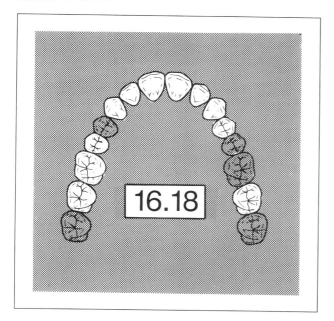

If the left side varies from that shown, refer to cases 16.4 to 16.14 for the correct configuration.

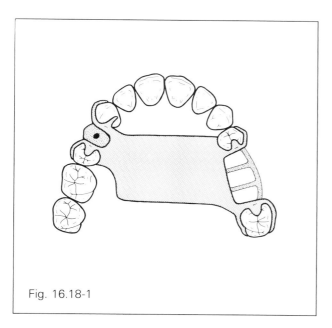

Fig. 16.18-1

For design concepts and variations on the left side refer to cases 16.4 to 16.14. Options for the right-side modification space are essentially the same as those for case 16.17.

The retentive arm on the right canine may be omitted, particularly if the four guide surface–guide plate contacts restrict the path of insertion/dislodgement. If a clasp on the canine is necessary, the options are the same as those discussed for the left canine of case 16.6.

Case 16.19

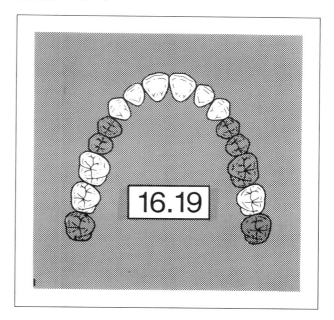

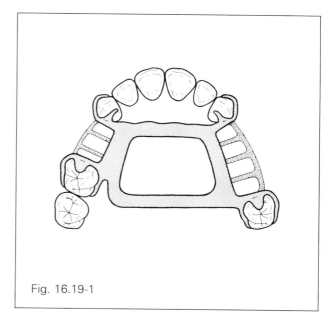

Fig. 16.19-1

Case 16.19 is one example of a large number of possible Class III arch forms with bilateral posterior tooth-bounded edentulous areas.

The designs for bilateral tooth-supported RPDs can be created by combining portions of the designs for cases 16.4 to 16.14 (or their mirror images). It will be necessary to consult the "Case reference guide" at the beginning of the chapter in order to locate the design for a specific segment. In the example of case 16.19, the edentulous space on the left side is missing three teeth and would correspond to the left side of case 16.7 or 16.8. The right side of the arch is missing two teeth and would correspond to the mirror image of the left side of case 16.4, 16.5, or 16.6. Examination of the individual arches reveals that the design for case 16.19 is a composite of those for case 16.8 and the mirror image of case 16.6. Designs for similar cases can be developed by the same process. Although some extrapolation will be necessary, the principles are similar throughout and the process should not be too difficult.

Case 16.20

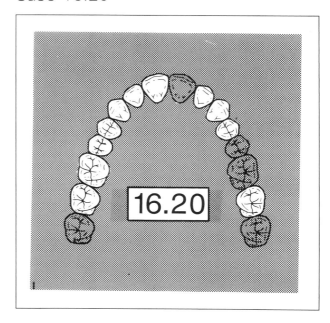

If the left posterior edentulous segment varies from that shown, refer to cases 16.4 to 16.14 for the correct configuration.

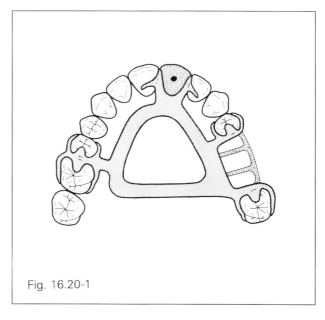

Fig. 16.20-1

The design for case 16.20 is the same as that for case 16.5 with a single-tooth anterior modification space. Changes associated with the anterior modification space are considered below. Refer to case 16.5 for a discussion of other aspects of the design.

Rests

If the lateral incisor exhibits poor bone support or severely sloped lingual anatomy, it should be plated and a cingulum rest placed on the canine. A rest seat and rest should always be placed on the central incisor.

Guide plates

Anterior guide plates must be located on the linguoproximal surfaces so that they will not be visible from the labial aspect or interfere with positioning of the replacement teeth.

Major connector

Although an anterior-posterior palatal strap would usually be selected, the opening should be eliminated if its anterior-posterior dimension is less than 15 mm. Also refer to case 16.1.

Retentive arms

Retentive arms on the central or lateral incisor would be unesthetic; they are rarely, if ever, indicated.

Denture base retentive elements/replacement teeth

With only one tooth in the anterior edentulous space, a facing, tube tooth, or heat-cured or light-activated resin replacement would almost always be used. Retentive network, a denture tooth, and denture base should be considered if the residual ridge exhibits incomplete healing or extensive resorption or if the space is wider than normal for the missing tooth.

Case 16.21

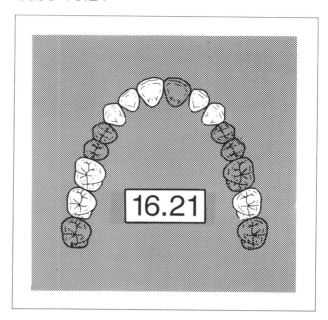

If the posterior segments vary from those shown, refer to cases 16.4 to 16.14 for the correct configuration.

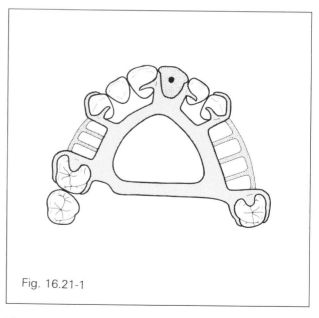

Fig. 16.21-1

The design for case 16.21 is a composite of those for case 16.8 (left posterior), the mirror image of case 16.5 (right posterior), and case 16.20 (anterior). Refer to cases 16.8, 16.5, and 16.20 for design concepts and variations.

Case 16.22

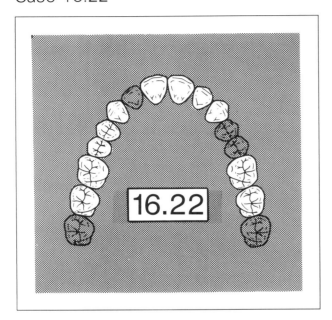

If the left posterior edentulous segment varies from that shown, refer to cases 16.4 to 16.14 for the correct configuration.

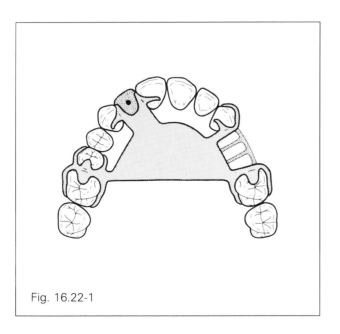

Fig. 16.22-1

The design for case 16.22 is the same as that for case 16.6 with a single-tooth anterior modification space. Changes associated with the anterior modification space are considered below. Refer to case 16.6 for a discussion of other aspects of the design.

Rests

Rest seats and rests should always be placed on the central incisor and canine adjacent to the anterior edentulous space.

Guide plates

Refer to case 16.20.

Retentive arms

Retentive arms on the central incisor and canine are seldom needed or indicated. If a retentive arm is desired for the canine, refer to case 16.1 for design options.

Denture base retentive elements/replacement teeth

Refer to case 16.20.

Case 16.23

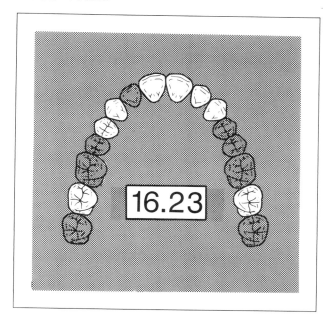

rior). Refer to cases 16.8, 16.5, and 16.22 for design concepts and variations.

Case 16.24

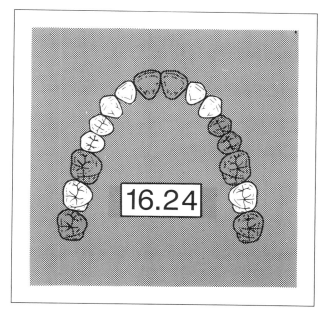

If the posterior segments vary from those shown, refer to cases 16.4 to 16.14 for the correct configuration.

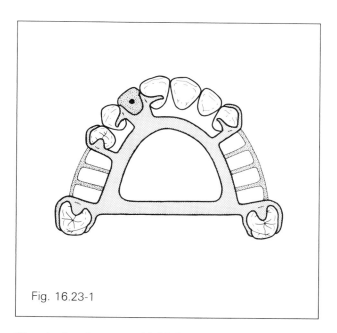

Fig. 16.23-1

The design for case 16.23 is a composite of those for case 16.8 (left posterior), the mirror image of case 16.5 (right posterior), and case 16.22 (ante-

If the posterior segments vary from those shown, refer to cases 16.4 to 16.14 for the correct configuration.

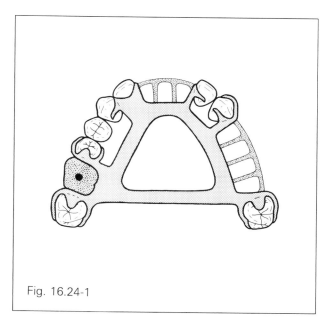

Fig. 16.24-1

The design for case 16.24 is a composite of those for case 16.8 (left posterior) and case 16.16 (right posterior) combined with a two-tooth anterior modification space. Changes associated with the modification space are considered below. Refer to cases 16.8 and 16.16 for a discussion of other aspects of the design.

Rests

If the right lateral incisor exhibits acceptable bone support and lingual anatomy, a rest seat and rest may be placed on it and the rest on the right canine omitted.

If the left lateral incisor is periodontally weak or possesses a steep lingual slope, both it and the canine should be plated. A rest seat must be prepared beneath the plating, at least on the canine.

Guide plates

Refer to case 16.20.

Major connector

Refer to case 16.20.

Retentive arms

Retentive arms on the lateral incisors would be unesthetic; they are rarely, if ever, indicated. If proximal undercuts on the lateral incisors can be utilized for rigid metal retention (dual path, rotational path), the retentive arm on the left canine can be omitted.

Denture base retentive elements/replacement teeth

With a small anterior edentulous segment, several possibilities for replacement exist. Retentive network, denture teeth, and denture base would tend to be selected if the spacing is not appropriate for the missing teeth or if the residual ridge exhibits extensive resorption or incomplete healing. Facings, tube teeth, or heat-cured or light-activated resin replacements would be more appropriate if the residual ridge exhibits little resorption and large undercuts, if the spacing is correct, or if there is deep vertical overlap of the anterior teeth. In the last instance, metal backings should be used to reduce the potential for fracture.

Case 16.25

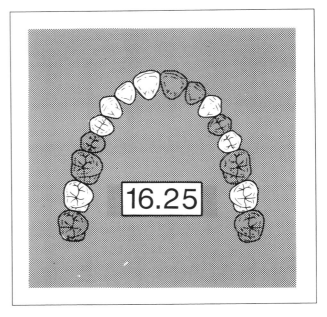

If the posterior segments vary from those shown, refer to cases 16.4 to 16.14 for the correct configuration.

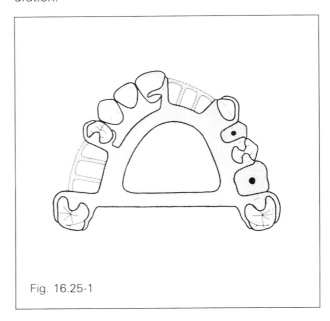

Fig. 16.25-1

The design for case 16.25 is a composite of those for cases 16.12 (left posterior), 16.5 (right posterior), and 16.1 (anterior). Refer to these cases for design concepts and variations.

Case 16.26

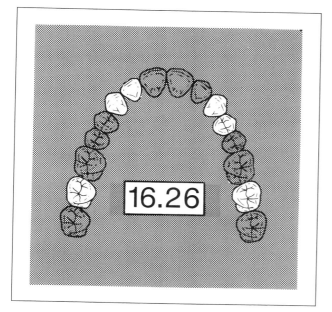

If the posterior segments vary from those shown, refer to cases 16.4 to 16.14 for the correct configuration.

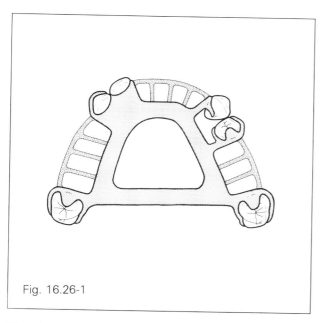

Fig. 16.26-1

The design for case 16.26 is a composite of those for case 16.5 (left posterior) and the mirror image of case 16.8 (right posterior), combined with a three-tooth anterior modification space. Changes associated with the modification space are considered below. Refer to cases 16.5 and 16.8 for a discussion of other aspects of the design.

Rests

If the right lateral incisor exhibits exceptionally good bone support and acceptable lingual contour, cingulum rests may be placed on it and the adjacent canine. The plating would then be omitted.

Guide plates

Refer to case 16.20.

Major connector

Refer to case 16.20.

Retentive arms

A retentive arm would seldom, if ever, be located on the lateral incisor. If necessary, a clasp may be placed on the right canine. Refer to case 16.1 for design options.

If proximal undercuts on the lateral incisor and canine permit the use of rigid metal retention (dual path, rotational path), the clasps on the anterior teeth and possibly the left first premolar can be omitted.

Denture base retentive elements/replacement teeth

With three missing teeth in the anterior modification space, retentive network, denture teeth, and denture base would usually be selected. However, facings, tube teeth, or heat-cured or light-activated resin replacements could be used if the residual ridge exhibits little resorption and complete healing and if the spacing is correct for the missing teeth.

Case 16.27

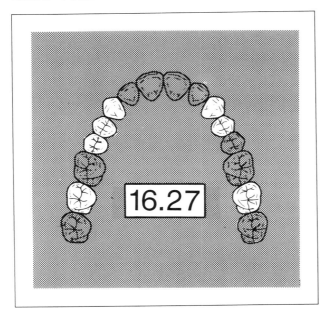

If the posterior segments vary from those shown refer to cases 16.4 to 16.14 for the correct configuration.

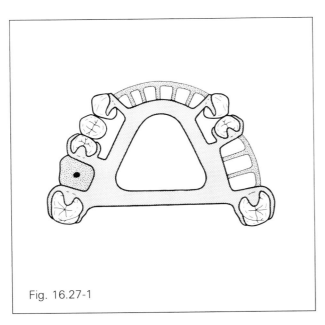

Fig. 16.27-1

The design for case 16.27 is a composite of those for case 16.5 (left posterior) and case 16.16 (right posterior), combined with a four-tooth anterior

modification space. Changes associated with the modification space are considered below. Refer to cases 16.5 and 16.16 for other aspects of the design.

Rests

Rests are almost always placed as shown in Fig. 16.27-1. Rest seats must be prepared beneath the plating on the canines.

Guide plates

Refer to case 16.20.

Major connector

Refer to case 16.20.

Retentive arms

Clasp arms can be omitted from the premolars if mesial proximal undercuts can be utilized for rigid metal retention (dual path, rotational path).

Denture base retentive elements/replacement teeth

With four missing teeth in the anterior modification space, retentive network, denture teeth, and denture base would almost always be used. However, facings, tube teeth, or heat-cured or light-activated resin replacements may be considered if the residual ridge exhibits little resorption and complete healing and if the spacing is correct for the missing teeth.

Case 16.28

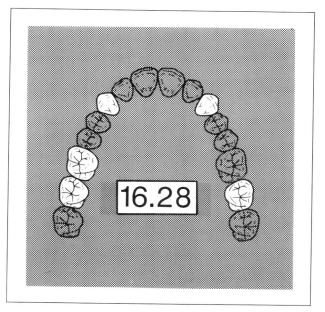

If the posterior segments vary from those shown, refer to cases 16.4 to 16.14 for the correct configuration.

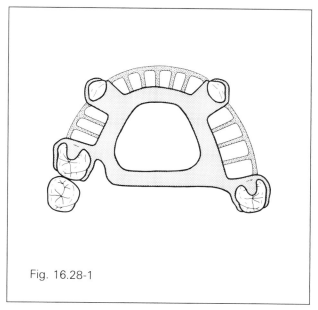

Fig. 16.28-1

The design for case 16.28 is a composite of those for case 16.8 (left posterior), the mirror image of case 16.6 (right posterior), and case 16.28 (anterior). Refer to these cases for design concepts and variations.

Case 16.29

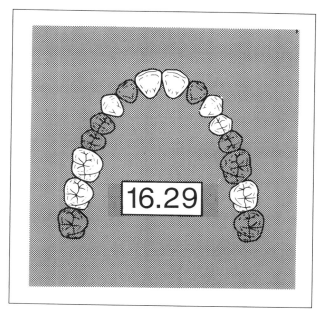

If the posterior segments vary from those shown, refer to cases 16.4 to 16.14 for the correct configuration.

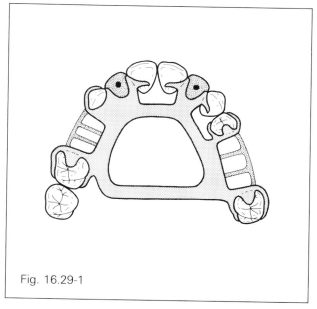

Fig. 16.29-1

The design for case 16.29 is a composite of those for case 16.5 (left posterior), the mirror image of case 16.6 (right posterior), and case 16.2 (anterior).

rior). Refer to these cases for design concepts and variations.

Case 16.30

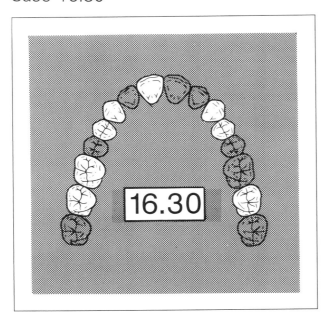

If the posterior segments vary from those shown, refer to cases 16.4 to 16.14 for the correct configuration.

The design for case 16.30 is a composite of those for case 16.5 (left posterior), case 16.17 (right posterior), and case 16.3 (anterior). Refer to these cases for design concepts and variations.

Case 16.31

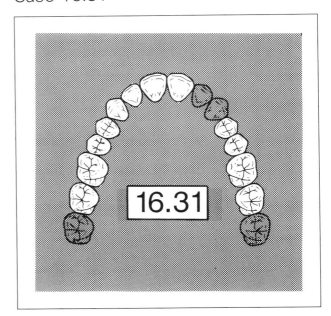

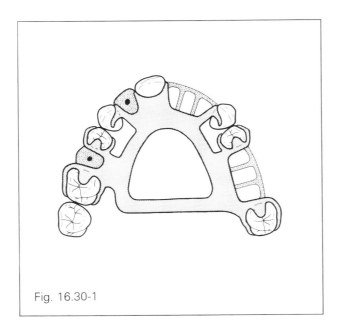

Fig. 16.30-1

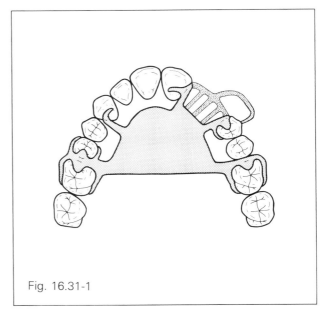

Fig. 16.31-1

Ceroplast Ltd.

Specialists in Technical Dentistry
11 Bromyard Terrace, Worcester WR2 5BW.
Tel: 01905 425151 Fax: 01905 425858

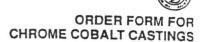

**ORDER FORM FOR
CHROME COBALT CASTINGS**

Name	Patient's Name

Remarks

Date Sent	Date Required
Teeth to be Replaced	
Clasps Required	
Rests Required	

**Type of Connector
Please Tick**

Upper

- Full Coverage ☐
- Horse Shoe ☐
- Single Bar ☐
- Double Bar ☐
- Skel/Plate ☐
- Ring with Covered Gingival Margins ☐
- Rochet Bridge ☐

Lower

- Plate ☐
- Lingual Bar ☐
- Double Bar/ Continuous Clasps ☐
- Labial Bar ☐
- Sub Lingual Bar ☐
- Rochet Bridge ☐

Enclosures (Please Tick)

Upper Model ☐	Set-Up ☐
Lower Model ☐	Additional ☐
Bite Block ☐	

Office Use Only

Conditions of models on arrival

Please Tick Here ☐ if you do not agree to grind teeth that oppose Occlusal Rests

Rests

The embrasure clasp assemblies may be moved one tooth forward or backward, depending on the location of undercuts and occlusal contacts. The rest on the right canine is not absolutely necessary and would almost certainly be omitted if the right embrasure clasp is moved forward.

Guide plates

The guide plate on the central incisor must be located on the linguoproximal surface so that it will not be visible from the labial aspect or interfere with positioning of the replacement teeth.

Major connector

An anterior-posterior palatal strap major connector would be preferred if the opening were large enough to be of significant benefit (greater than 15 mm in an anterior-posterior dimension). This would most commonly occur when the embrasure clasps are placed on the first molars and second molars.

A U-shaped major connector may also be considered if there is an inoperable palatal torus or if the patient cannot tolerate normal palatal coverage by the major connector. Although there is some loss in rigidity, the edentulous segment is so small that the sacrifice is not significant.

Minor connectors

Refer to case 16.1.

Retentive arms

If an anterior component is added to the embrasure clasp on the left side, the retentive arm on the first premolar can be omitted. If the embrasure clasp assemblies are moved forward, the anterior retentive arm on the left side would engage a mesiofacial undercut on the first premolar. A clasp would seldom, if ever, be included on the central incisor.

In the design shown in Fig. 16.31-1, a bar clasp was selected for the left first premolar primarily for esthetic reasons. However, if the approach arm is visible crossing the gingiva, one of the options noted above should be selected. A circumferential clasp, emanating from the mesial aspect and engaging a distofacial undercut, would usually be esthetically unacceptable because the originating portion would be very near the mesio-occlusal aspect of the facial surface.

Refer to case 16.1 for other design considerations relating to the embrasure clasps.

Denture base retentive elements/replacement teeth

Refer to case 16.1.

Case 16.32

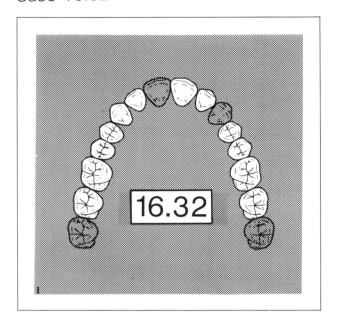

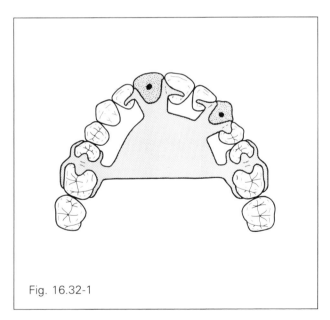

Fig. 16.32-1

Rests

The embrasure clasp assemblies may be moved one tooth forward or backward, depending on the location of undercuts and occlusal contacts. If the lateral incisors exhibit extensive bone loss or poor lingual anatomy for rest preparations, they should be plated. A cingulum rest would then be placed on the right canine. The left central incisor would also be plated. A rest seat must be prepared beneath the plating on at least the central incisor.

Guide plates

The anterior guide plates must be located on the linguoproximal surfaces so that they will not be visible from the labial aspect or interfere with positioning of the replacement teeth.

Major connector

Refer to case 16.31.

Minor connectors

Refer to case 16.1.

Retentive arms

Retentive arms would seldom, if ever, be placed on the central or lateral incisors. Options for posterior retention are essentially the same as those described for case 16.31.

Denture base retentive elements/replacement teeth

Facings, tube teeth, or heat-cured or light-activated resin replacements would almost always be used for the two single-tooth anterior edentulous areas. Retentive network, denture teeth, and denture base could be considered if the residual ridge exhibits incomplete healing or extensive resorption or if the space is wider than normal.

Case 16.33

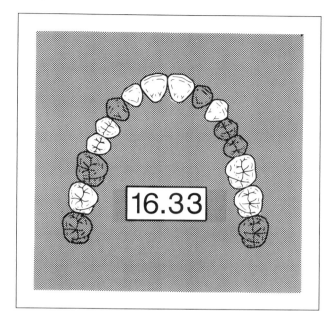

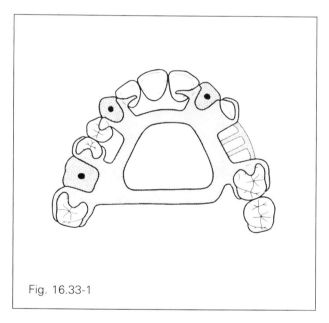

Fig. 16.33-1

Rests

The rest on the right second premolar may be omitted if occlusal interferences exist. If the lateral incisor exhibits extensive bone loss or lingual anatomy inconsistent with rest seat preparation, it may be plated, and a rest placed on the adjacent central incisor.

Guide plates

Refer to case 16.32.

Major connector

An anterior-posterior palatal strap is the major connector of choice. A U-shaped major connector may be considered if there is an inoperable palatal torus or if the patient cannot tolerate the posterior palatal strap.

Minor connectors

Refer to case 16.1.

Retentive arms

Retentive arms would seldom, if ever, be placed on the right lateral incisor or left central incisor. Options for clasping the left canine are the same as those for case 16.6. A retentive arm would usually be omitted from the right first premolar unless no usable undercut existed on the second premolar. If a retentive arm is needed for the first premolar, a bar clasp is usually selected. A circumferential clasp would originate near the mesio-occlusal aspect of the facial surface and could compromise esthetics.

Denture base retentive elements/replacement teeth

With both single and multiple edentulous segments, a variety of possibilities for replacement exist. Retentive network, denture teeth, and denture base would tend to be selected if the spacing is not appropriate for the missing teeth or if the residual ridge exhibits extensive resorption or incomplete healing. Facings, tube teeth, or heat-cured or light-activated resin replacements would be more appropriate if the residual ridge exhibits little resorption and large undercuts, if the spacing is correct, or if there is a deep vertical overlap of the anterior teeth. In the last instance, metal backings should be used to reduce the potential for fracture.

Case 16.34

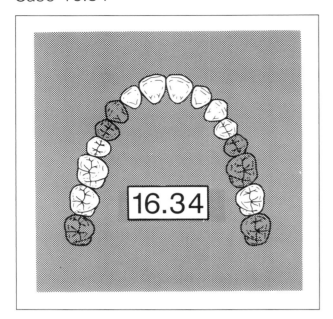

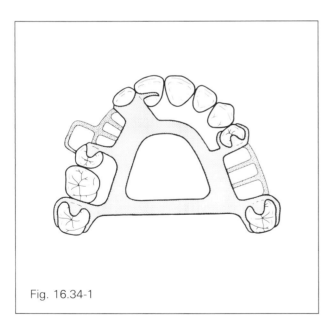

Fig. 16.34-1

Rests

If the right lateral incisor exhibits exceptionally good bone support and a prominent cingulum, a

rest may be placed on it and the plating and rest on the central incisor omitted.

An embrasure clasp assembly may be placed on the second premolar and first molar. The mesial rest on the second premolar could then be omitted.

Guide plates

The distal guide plate on the lateral incisor must be located on the linguoproximal surface so that it will not be visible from the labial or interfere with positioning of the replacement teeth.

Major connector

Refer to case 16.33.

Minor connectors

Refer to case 16.1.

Retentive arms

A retentive arm would seldom, if ever, be placed on the right lateral incisor.

A circumferential clasp, originating from the mesial aspect and engaging a distofacial undercut, may be used on the right second premolar. However, the origin of the arm may be near the occlusal surface and may compromise esthetics. Another option would be to place an embrasure clasp assembly on the second premolar and first molar. The anterior retentive arm would then originate on the distal surface of the second premolar and engage a mesiofacial undercut.

Denture base retentive elements/replacement teeth

Retentive network, denture teeth, and denture base would ordinarily be used for both edentulous areas. Facings, tube teeth, or heat-cured or light-activated resin replacements may be considered for the anterior area if the residual ridge is large and completely healed. They would also tend to be indicated if the residual ridge is undercut or if vertical space is limited.

Case 16.35

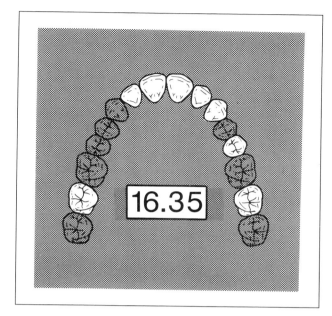

If the left side varies from that shown, refer to cases 16.4 to 16.14 for the correct configuration.

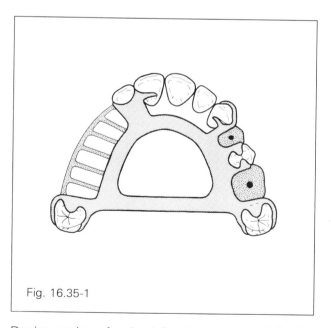

Fig. 16.35-1

Design options for the left side are essentially the same as those for case 16.12. Variations for the right side are discussed below.

Rests

With the large edentulous segment on the right side, the lateral incisor would seldom be used as a single anterior abutment. If possible, a rest seat should be prepared beneath the plating on the lateral incisor.

Guide plates

Refer to case 16.34.

Major connector

Refer to case 16.33.

Minor connectors

Refer to case 16.1.

Retentive arms

Because of esthetic considerations, a clasp arm is not usually placed on the lateral incisor. Undoubtedly, some sacrifice in overall retention results. If esthetics is unimportant or if the patient exhibits a very low lipline during smiling or speaking, a clasp could be included. A bar clasp would usually be selected because of its decreased visibility.

Options for the retentive arm on the right molar are the same as those discussed for case 16.4.

Denture base retentive elements/replacement teeth

Retentive network, denture teeth, and denture base would always be used on the right side and should also be used on the left side if there has been extensive residual ridge resorption or if the single-tooth spaces are wider than normal.

Case 16.36

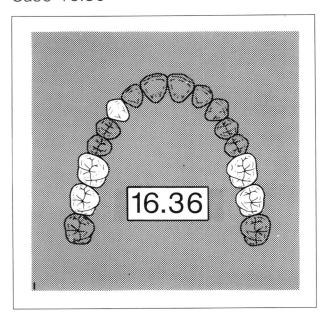

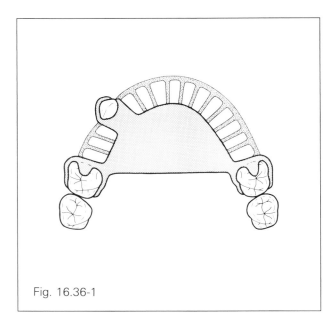

Fig. 16.36-1

Rests

Posterior rests would be located in the distal fossae of the first molars and mesial fossae of the second molars if embrasure clasps were utilized. A rest seat must be placed on the canine beneath the plating.

Guide plates

The mesial guide plate on the canine must be located on the linguoproximal surface so that it will not be visible from the labial aspect or interfere with positioning of the replacement teeth.

Major connector

An anterior-posterior palatal strap could be selected, particularly if embrasure clasp assemblies were used on the first and second molars.

Minor connectors

Refer to case 16.1.

Retentive arms

Refer to case 16.6 for clasping options for the canine. Refer to case 16.4 for clasping options for the molars.

Denture base retentive elements/replacement teeth

Because of the size of the edentulous segments, retentive network, denture teeth, and denture base would always be used.

Case 16.37

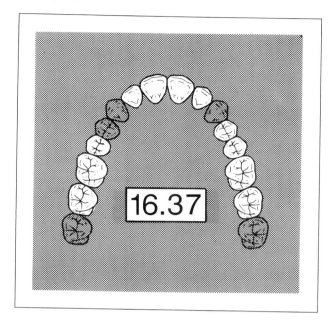

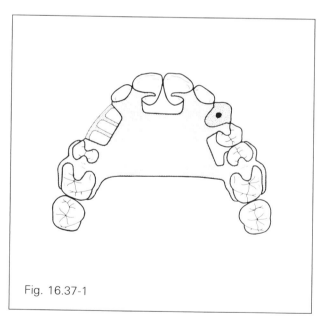

Fig. 16.37-1

Rests

The mesial rests on the right second premolar and left first premolar could be omitted if occlusal interferences exist. Rests may be placed on the lateral incisors if they exhibit good bone support and acceptable lingual contours.

Guide plates

The distal guide plate on the lateral incisor must be located on the linguoproximal surface so that it will not be visible from the labial aspect or interfere with positioning of the replacement teeth.

Major connector

An anterior-posterior palatal strap could be selected if the opening were large enough to be of significant benefit (greater than 15 mm in an anterior-posterior dimension). A U-shaped major connector should only be used to circumvent an inoperable palatal torus or if the patient cannot tolerate the posterior extensions of the other major connectors.

Minor connectors

Refer to case 16.1.

Retentive arms

A retentive arm would seldom, if ever, be placed on the lateral incisor. If additional retention is necessary, a bar clasp may be placed on the left first premolar. A circumferential clasp would usually be avoided because the mesial originating portion of the arm would lie close to the occlusal surface and could compromise esthetics.

Denture base retentive elements/replacement teeth

Refer to case 16.33.

Case 16.38

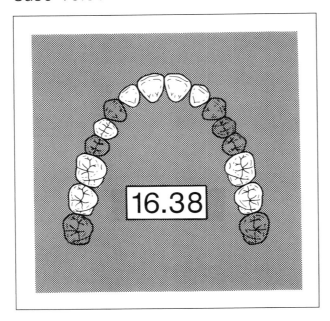

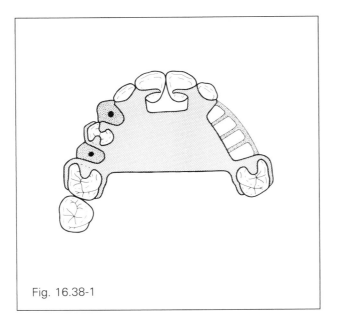

Fig. 16.38-1

Rests

One of the rests on the right first premolar could be omitted if occlusal interferences exist. If the lateral incisors exhibit exceptionally good bone support and acceptable lingual contours, rests may be placed on them and the rests on the central incisors omitted.

Guide plates

Refer to case 16.37.

Major connector

Refer to case 16.37.

Minor connectors

Refer to case 16.1.

Retentive arms

Retentive arms would seldom be placed on the lateral incisors. However, if the patient's upper lip will conceal the clasps during smiling and speech, they may be incorporated into the design. Bar clasps would usually be selected because they would tend to be less visible than circumferential clasps.

Clasping options for the posterior teeth are essentially the same as those described for case 16.4.

Denture base retentive elements/replacement teeth

Refer to case 16.33.

Case 16.39

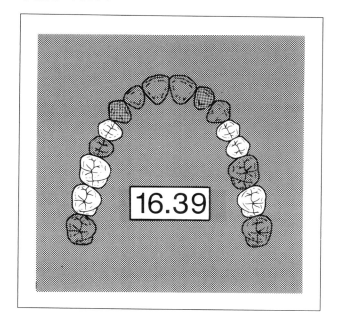

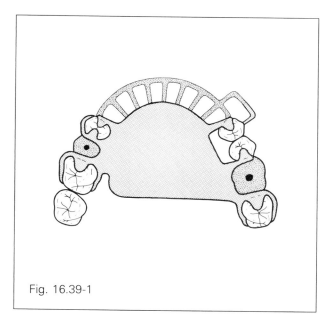

Fig. 16.39-1

Rests

The location of rests for case 16.39 depends largely on whether or not the RPD is considered an anterior extension. If the residual ridge provides substantial support, the RPD could be considered tooth supported and the design shown in Fig. 16.39-1 would be appropriate. However, if the quality of the residual ridge is poor, the retentive arm on the left first premolar would have the potential for creating torquing stresses. The best solution would seem to be omitting the mesial rest. The retentive arm would then lie in front of the axis of rotation and would release when the anterior extension moves toward the residual ridge. As an alternative, the mesial rest could be moved to the distal fossa. The mechanics of the clasp assembly would be acceptable but the proximity of the minor connectors might compromise oral hygiene. The design on the right first premolar is acceptable even if the RPD is considered an anterior extension. The retentive tip lies so close to the axis of rotation that little torque will be developed. However, if a bar clasp is used to engage a midfacial or distofacial undercut, the mesial rest should be deleted.

Guide plates

If the RPD is considered an anterior extension, the guide plates on the mesial surfaces of the premolars should not extend above the height of contour or they will preempt the planned rests.

Major connector

Refer to case 16.37.

Minor connectors

Refer to case 16.1.

Retentive arms

For a discussion of retentive arms for the premolars, refer to "Rests," above. Clasping considerations for the molars are the same as those for the molars of case 16.4. Although the clasps on the molars are behind the axis of rotation, the teeth are relatively strong and the forces applied are in a vertical direction.

Denture base retentive elements/replacement teeth

Because residual ridge support is important for the anterior segment, retentive network, denture teeth, and denture base would always be used in this area. They could also be used for the single-tooth posterior edentulous segments if the residual ridge exhibits incomplete healing, extensive resorption, or if the width of the spaces is greater than normal.

Case 16.40

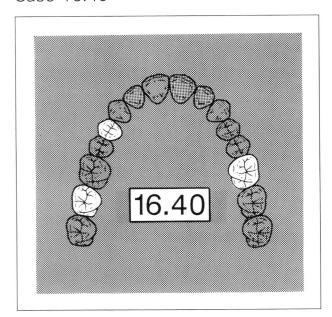

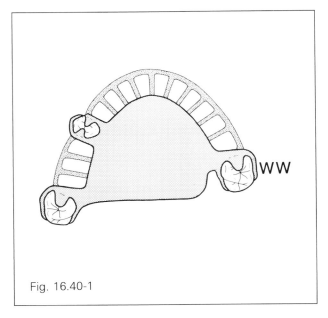

Fig. 16.40-1

Quite frequently, the three remaining teeth would be extracted and a maxillary conventional complete denture or overdenture fabricated. A design is being presented for the sake of completeness and for those cases when a partial denture might be fabricated. An RPD might be indicated if (1) the residual ridge exhibits considerable resorption, (2) bone support for the teeth is good, (3) oral hygiene is acceptable, (4) the patient has a debilitating disease (e.g., diabetes), (5) the patient exhibits poor neuromuscular control, or (6) the patient has a fear of losing the remaining teeth or a strong desire to keep them.

Rests

Since the RPD for case 16.40 should definitely be regarded as an anterior-extension prosthesis, the location of rests on the premolars is intimately associated with the type of clasp arms selected. Refer to the discussion in "Retentive arms," below.

Guide plates

If a bar clasp is used on the right first premolar, the mesial rest will be omitted and the mesial guide plate must not extend above the height of contour.

Major connector

Palatal coverage should be used to improve the degree of palatal support. If an I-bar is used on the right first premolar, plating should be avoided if at all possible.

Minor connectors

Refer to case 16.1.

Retentive arms

The clasp assembly on the right first premolar will apply minimal torquing forces because the retentive tip of the cast circumferential arm lies almost directly under the axis of rotation (which passes through the mesial rest). If a bar clasp is used to engage a midfacial or distofacial undercut, the mesial rest should be omitted. The tip of the clasp will then move distally and gingivally and will release when the anterior extension moves toward the residual ridge.

The buccal retentive arm on the left first molar should be flexible (wrought wire) because it lies behind but very close to the axis of rotation and has the potential for torquing the abutment. Although the clasp on the right second molar also lies behind the axis of rotation, the stresses applied to it will be in a vertical direction, greatly reducing the potential for damage.

Denture base retentive elements/replacement teeth

Retentive network, denture teeth, and denture base would always be used.

Maxillary Class IV Designs

According to Applegate's rules for applying the Kennedy Classification, Class IV removable partial dentures cannot have modification spaces. A posterior modification space would take precedence in nomenclature, resulting in a Class III RPD. Thus, the frequency of Class IV RPDs is quite low. In our study of almost 2,000 maxillary arches for which RPDs were fabricated, less than 5% were truly Class IV. Considering frequency of occurrence, the 16 cases discussed in chapter 17 cover over 95% of these partially edentulous arches (or their mirror images). The partially edentulous arch discussed in case 17.2 comprised over one half of the total.

Case reference guide	
Symmetrical	
Two teeth in space	17.1
Four teeth in space	17.2
Six teeth in space	17.3
Eight teeth in space	17.4
Ten teeth in space	17.5
Asymmetrical	
Three teeth in space	17.6
Four teeth in space	17.7
Five teeth in space	17.8 to 17.9
Six teeth in space	17.10 to 17.11
Seven teeth in space	17.12 to 17.13
Eight teeth in space	17.14
Nine teeth in space	17.15 to 17.16

Case 17.1

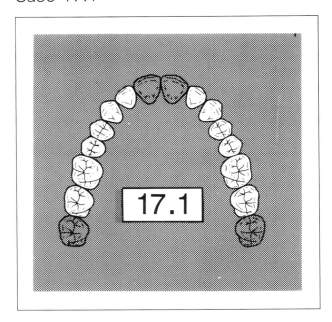

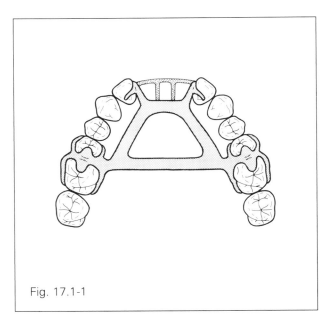

Fig. 17.1-1

Rests

Rests may be placed on the lateral incisors if the bone support is adequate and the lingual anatomy is appropriate for positive rest seat preparations. If either of these factors is unacceptable, the lateral incisors should be plated and cingulum rest seats and rests placed on the canines.

The embrasure clasp assemblies may be moved one tooth forward or backward, depending on the location of undercuts and occlusal contacts (see "Retentive arms," below).

Guide plates

Guide plates on the anterior teeth must be located on the linguoproximal surfaces so they will not be visible from the labial aspect or interfere with positioning of the replacement teeth.

Major connector

An anterior-posterior palatal strap is the major connector of choice if the A-P dimension of the opening is 15 mm or more. If the embrasure clasp assemblies are moved forward one tooth, the opening will be very small and is usually omitted. The lateral and posterior border of the major connector will remain as shown in Fig. 17.1-1.

A U-shaped major connector may also be considered. Although there is some loss in rigidity, the edentulous segment is so small that this sacrifice is not of great significance.

Refer to case 14.1 for further discussion of major connectors.

Minor connectors

Considerations for minor connectors are the same as those discussed for case 14.1. No special considerations are necessary for Class IV RPDs.

Retentive arms

Cast clasps are usually used for Class IV RPDs, especially when the edentulous segment is not so large that the prosthesis is considered an anterior extension.

If the edentulous space is small (as in case 17.1) anterior retentive arms are usually omitted. When there are proximal undercuts bordering the edentulous space, rigid metal retention (dual path, rotational path) may be used.

Circumferential (embrasure) clasps are almost always used to provide retention posteriorly, and the undercuts are invariably on the buccal surfaces. The clasp assembly may be moved forward or backward one tooth, depending on the location of undercuts and occlusal contacts.

Refer to case 16.1 for additional information.

Denture base retentive elements/replacement teeth

With a small edentulous segment, several possibilities for replacement exist. Retentive network, denture teeth, and denture base would tend to be selected if the spacing is not appropriate for the missing teeth or if the residual ridge exibits extensive resorption or incomplete healing. Facings, tube teeth, or heat-cured or light-activated resin replacements would be more appropriate if the residual ridge exhibits little resorption and large undercuts, if the spacing is correct, or if there is deep vertical overlap of the anterior teeth. In the last instance, a metal lingual backing should be used to reduce the potential for fracture.

Case 17.2

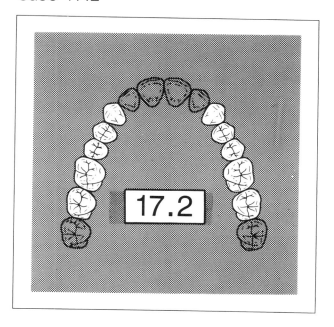

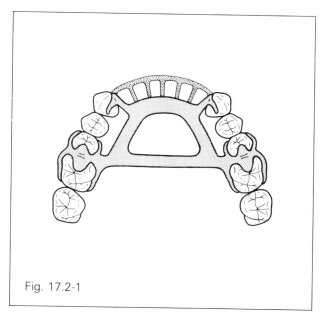

Fig. 17.2-1

Rests

Variations in the location of the embrasure clasp assemblies are essentially the same as those for case 17.1, except that moving the assembly forward is seldom acceptable because of a decrease in the resistance to biting forces on the anterior segment.

If the lingual anatomy of the canines is too steep for adequate rest seat preparations, the canines may be plated and mesial rests placed on the first premolars.

Guide plates

Refer to case 17.1.

Major connector

An anterior-posterior palatal strap is the major connector of choice. The opening would be eliminated only in the rare instance when the embrasure clasp assemblies are moved forward. Because of the size of the edentulous segment, a U-shaped major connector should only be considered if a torus extends within 6 to 8 mm of the vibrating line or if the patient cannot tolerate the posterior palatal strap. The U-shaped connector generally lacks rigidity, or if made broad enough to possess rigidity, will cover excessive tissue in an area prone to the development of inflammatory papillary hyperplasia.

Minor connectors

Refer to case 17.1.

Retentive arms

Rigid metal retention (dual path, rotational path) should be considered if mesioproximal undercuts are present on the canines.

I-bars may be used on the canines if they will be hidden by the patient's lip. Circumferential clasps are seldom indicated because the origin of the arms would usually be near the incisal edge and would therefore be esthetically unacceptable.

Retention posteriorly is essentially the same as that discussed for case 17.1, except that the embrasure clasp assembly would seldom be moved forward.

Denture base retentive elements/replacement teeth

The options are the same as described for case 17.1. However, with four teeth in the modification space, there is a greater tendency to use retentive network, denture teeth and denture base.

Case 17.3

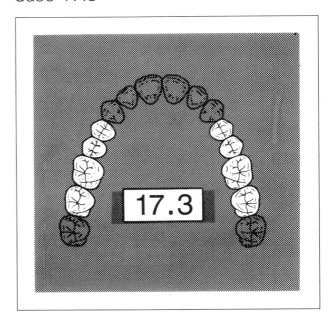

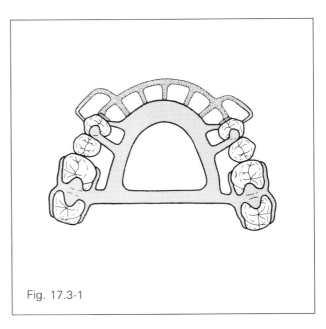

Fig. 17.3-1

With both canines missing, the prosthesis should be considered an anterior extension RPD. The principles for clasp assemblies are the same as those discussed for distal extension RPDs except the extension area is reversed.

The anterior abutments are most subject to torquing forces. Thus, in these areas, clasp design should be such that the retentive arms will either release or flex during functional movements of the extension base. Although the posterior embrasure clasps will lie opposite the axis of rotation from the extension area, the molars are relatively strong teeth and the forces applied to them will be nearly vertical. Fortunately, they seldom show the effects of adverse functional forces.

Rests

Rests for the embrasure clasps should be placed on the first and second molars if possible. They may be located on the second premolar and first molar but stability on incising may decrease considerably.

The rests on the first premolars should ideally be placed in the distal fossae (opposite from the extension area). Then, the bar clasps will release when functional forces are applied (see "Retentive arms," below).

Guide plates

The mesial guide plates on the first premolars should have the same design as the distal guide plates on the premolars for distal extension cases (refer to case 14.1). Physiologic relief at the framework try-in is essential so that the guide plates will not preempt the planned rests during functional movements of the anterior extension.

Major connector

An anterior-posterior palatal strap is the major connector of choice. The opening may be eliminated if additional palatal support is required. A U-shaped major connector should only be selected if an inoperable palatal torus extends to within 6 to 8 mm of the vibrating line, so that the posterior strap cannot be placed posterior to the torus.

The second premolars and first premolars may be plated if necessary. However, plating of the first premolars should be avoided if possible. When they are plated, the metal must end exactly at the survey line. If the plating extends above the survey line, it will preempt the planned distal rests, and torquing forces will be applied to the abutments.

Minor connectors

Refer to case 17.1.

Retentive arms

With the large edentulous area, clasps would almost always be placed on the first premolars. Bar clasps are preferred because they will release during functional movements of the anterior segment (if distal rests are used), and because they are less apt to be visible when the patient smiles. I-bars would be used if the undercuts are located on the midfacial or distofacial surfaces and modified T-bars if the undercuts are on the mesiofacial surfaces.

Circumferential clasps often originate near the occlusal aspect of the mesiofacial surface and would therefore be esthetically objectionable. If circumferential clasps are selected, they should be flexible (wrought wire) and the rest should be moved to the mesial fossa. Conversely, if the rest must be placed in the mesial fossa due to occlusal interferences with a distal location, a wrought wire circumferential clasp should be selected.

Denture base retentive elements/replacement teeth

Retentive network, denture teeth and denture base would almost always be used because residual ridge support is needed for the anterior extension area.

317

Case 17.4

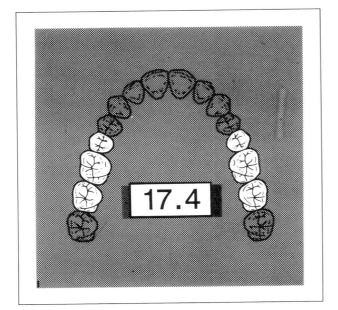

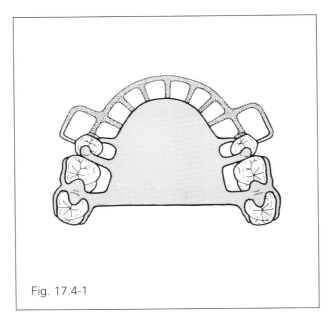

Fig. 17.4-1

Case 17.5

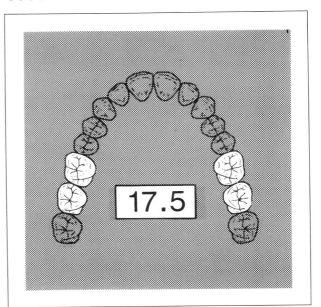

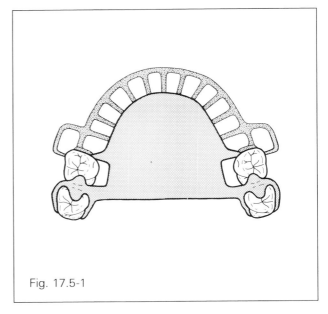

Fig. 17.5-1

The design principles for case 17.4 are essentially the same as those for case 17.3. Lingual bracing arms on the first molars are not necessary because the combination of mesial and distal minor connectors provides adequate bracing and prevents lingual migration of the teeth.

The design principles for case 17.5 are essentially the same as those for case 17.3. However, with the very large anterior extension area, there is considerable potential for the development of torquing forces on all the molars, particularly if the quality of the residual ridge is poor. In addition, it could be argued that because of the few teeth remaining and the extent of the edentulous area, a complete denture would be more retentive and stable than a partial denture. The choice between a complete and partial denture would depend on *(1)* the size and quality of the residual ridge, *(2)* the condition and position of the abutments, *(3)* the opposing occlusion, and *(4)* patient preference.

For design concepts and variations, refer to case 17.1 for the right side and case 17.2 for the left side.

Case 17.6

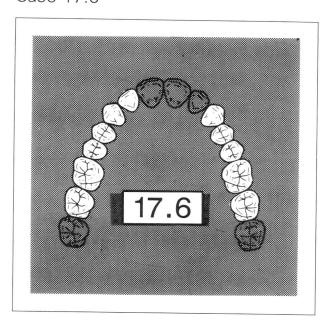

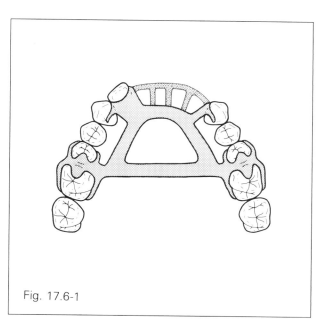

Fig. 17.6-1

Case 17.7

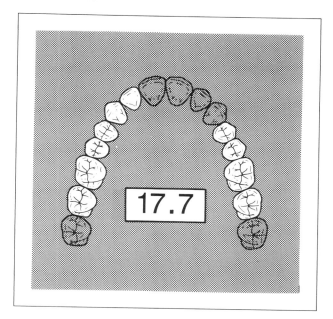

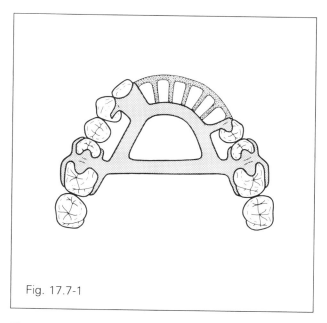

Fig. 17.7-1

The design for case 17.7 is essentially a combination of those for cases 17.1 and 17.3.

Because of the size of the edentulous segment, the right lateral incisor has been plated and a rest placed on the canine. If possible, a rest seat should also be prepared on the lateral incisor.

The design for the left side will vary, depending on whether the RPD is considered an anterior extension and whether retention on the first premolar is necessary. If the residual ridge possesses good mass and contour, and retention on the first premolar is unnecessary, the design will be as shown in Fig. 17.7-1. However, if retention on the first premolar is desired and the anterior residual ridge is poor in quantity and quality, the RPD should be considered an anterior extension; retention on the first premolar would be the same as that described for case 17.3.

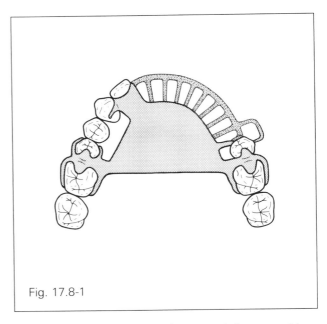

Fig. 17.8-1

Case 17.8

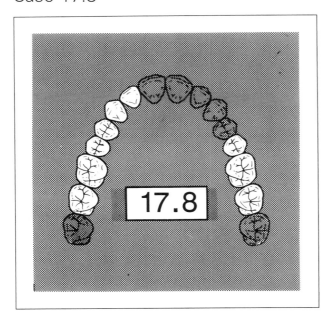

The design for case 17.8 is essentially a combination of those for cases 17.1 and 17.4.

Because of the size of the edentulous space, the right lateral incisor has been plated and a rest placed on the canine. If possible, a small rest seat should also be prepared on the lateral incisor.

With the canine and premolar both missing on the left side, the prosthesis should be considered an anterior extension. The retentive arm on the left side should either release or flex during functional movement of the extension base. Refer to case 17.4 for design options.

Case 17.9

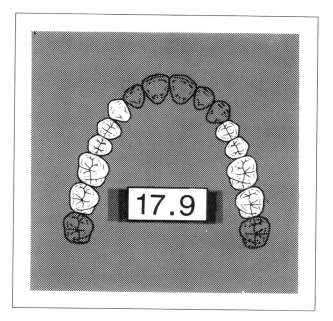

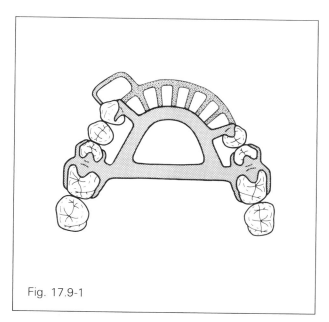

Fig. 17.9-1

The design for case 17.9 is essentially a combination of those cases 17.2 and 17.3.

The clasp arm on the right canine may be omitted if rigid metal retention (dual path, rotational path) can be used, or if esthetics is more important than retention.

A clasp arm on the left first premolar has been omitted because the circumferential clasp on the second premolar should provide adequate retention without sacrificing esthetics. If the embrasure clasps are moved backward to the first and second molars, a retentive arm would usually be placed on the first premolar; the options for the clasp assembly are the same as those described in case 17.3.

Case 17.10

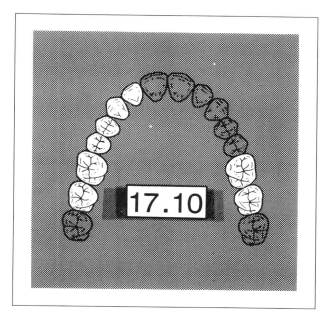

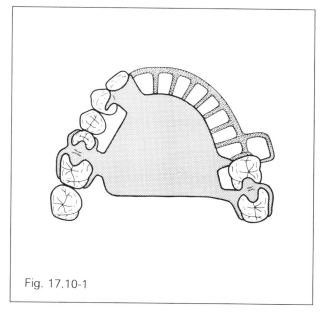

Fig. 17.10-1

The design for case 17.10 is essentially a combination of those for cases 17.1 and 17.5.

Because of the size of the edentulous space, the right lateral incisor has been plated and a rest placed on the canine. If possible, a small rest seat should also be prepared on the lateral incisor.

The prosthesis should be considered an anterior extension and the clasp on the first molar should either release or flex during tissueward movement of the anterior area.

Case 17.11

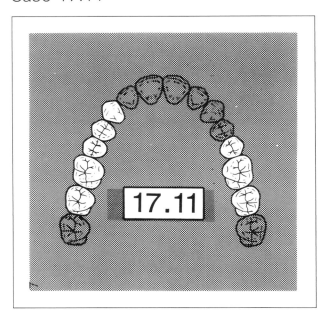

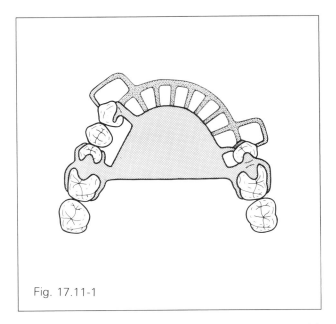

Fig. 17.11-1

The design for case 17.11 is essentially a combination of those for cases 17.2 and 17.4.

The clasp arm on the right canine may be omitted if rigid metal retention (dual path, rotational path) can be used, or if esthetics is more important than retention.

Stability of the anterior segment during function might improve if the embrasure clasp assemblies were moved to the first and second molars. This option should be considered if the undercuts are appropriately located and if the occlusion does not interfere with this location.

Case 17.12

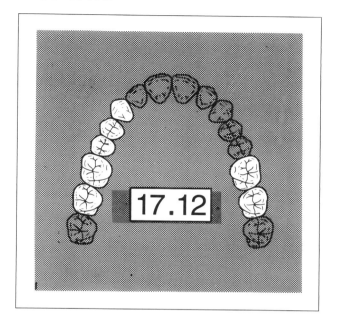

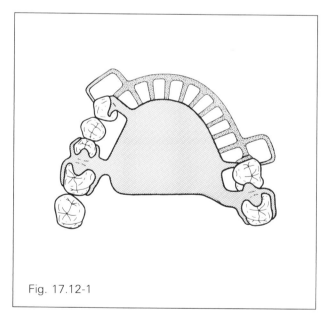

Fig. 17.12-1

The design for case 17.12 is essentially a combination of those for cases 17.2 and 17.5; refer to these cases for design concepts and variations.

Case 17.13

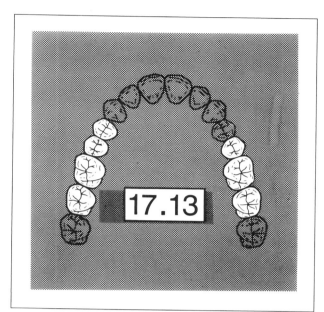

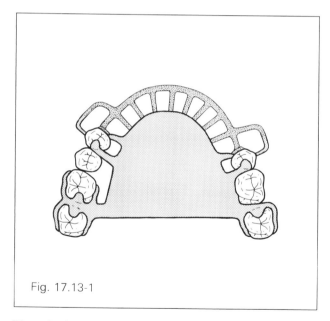

Fig. 17.13-1

The design for case 17.13 is a combination of those for cases 17.3 and 17.4; refer to these cases for design concepts and variations.

Case 17.14

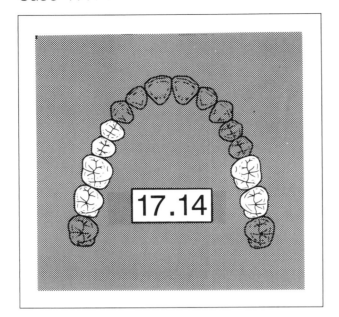

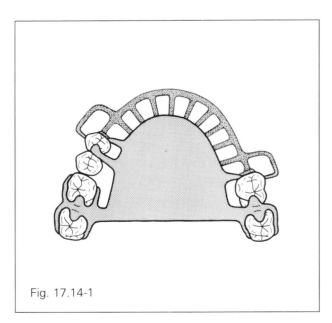

Fig. 17.14-1

Case 17.15

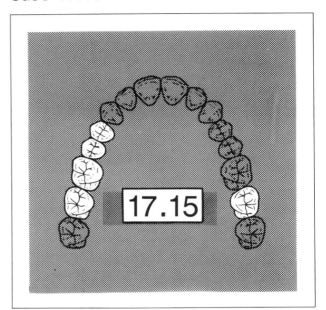

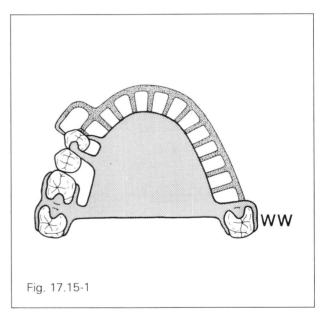

Fig. 17.15-1

The design for case 17.14 is a combination of those for cases 17.3 and 17.5; refer to these cases for design concepts and variations.

The design for the right side is essentially the same as that for case 17.3.

With only one molar remaining on the left side, it is very difficult to design a clasp assembly that will release during functional movement of the anterior extension. Because the circumferential arm shown in Fig. 17.15-1 will not release, it must be flexible (wrought wire).

Case 17.16

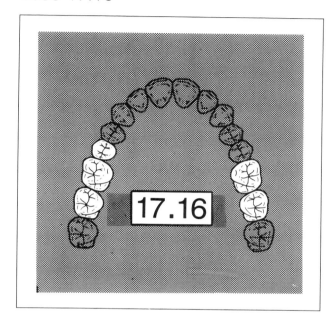

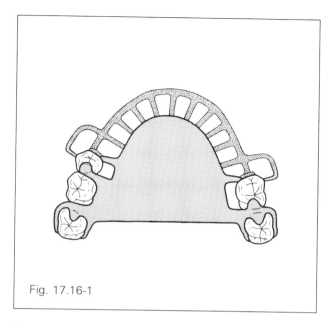

Fig. 17.16-1

The design for case 17.16 is a combination of those for cases 17.4 and 17.5; refer to these cases for design concepts and variations.

Selected Reading Resources

The following list of selected readings is included for students or practitioners who wish to further their knowledge in removable partial denture design.

Abel, L. F., and Manly, R. S. Masticatory function of partial denture patients among Navy personnel. J. Prosthet. Dent. 3:382–392, 1953.

Akers, P. E. A new and simplified method of partial denture prosthesis. J. Am. Dent. Assoc. 12:711–715, 1925.

Anderson, J. N., and Bates, J. F. The cobalt-chromium partial denture—a clinical survey. Br. Dent. J. 107:57–62, 1959.

Anderson, J. N., and Lammie, G. A. A clinical survey of partial dentures. Br. Dent. J. 92:59–67, 1952.

Anthony, L. P. American Textbook of Prosthetic Dentistry. 7th ed. Philadelphia: Lea & Febiger, 1942.

Antos, E. W. An update on clasp design for removable partial dentures. Quint. Dent. Technol. 9:115–117, 1985.

Applegate, O. C. Use of the paralleling surveyor in modern partial denture construction. J. Am. Dent. Assoc, 27:1397–1407, 1940.

Applegate, O. C. The removable partial denture in the general practice of tomorrow. J. Prosthet. Dent. 8:609–622, 1958.

Applegate, O. C. An evaluation of the support for the removable partial denture. J. Prosthet. Dent. 10:112–123, 1960.

Applegate, O. C. The rationale of partial denture choice. J. Prosthet. Dent. 10:891–907, 1960

Applegate, O. C. Essentials of Removable Partial Denture Prosthesis. 3rd ed. Philadelphia: W. B. Saunders Co., 1965.

Applegate, O. C., and Nissle, R. D. Keeping the partial denture in harmony with biologic limitations. J. Am. Dent. Assoc. 43:409–419, 1951.

Askinas, S. W. Facings in removable partial dentures. J. Prosthet. Dent. 633–636, 1975.

Atkinson, H. F. Partial denture problems: designing about a path of withdrawal. Aust. Dent. J. 37:187–190, 1953.

Atkinson, H. F. Partial denture problems: surveyors and surveying. Aust. Dent. J. 59:28–31, 1955.

Atkinson, R. A., and Elliott, R. W., Jr. Removable partial dentures designed for laboratory fabrication by recent dental school graduates. A survey. J. Prosthet. Dent. 22:429–435, 1969.

Augsberger, R. H. Evaluating removable partial dentures by mathematical equations. J. Prosthet. Dent. 22:528–543, 1969.

Avant, W. E. Indirect retention in partial denture design. J. Prosthet. Dent. 16:1103–1110, 1966.

Avant, W. E. Fulcrum and retention lines in planning removable partial dentures. J. Prosthet. Dent. 25:162–166, 1971.

Avant, W. E. A universal classification for removable partial denture situations. J. Prosthet. Dent. 16:533–539, 1966.

Axinn, S. Preparation of retentive areas for clasps in enamel. J. Prosthet. Dent. 34:405–407, 1975.

Bates, J. F. Cast clasps for partial dentures. Int. Dent. J. 13:610–614, 1963.

Bates, J. F. The mechanical properties of the cobalt-chromium alloys and their relation to partial denture design. Br. Dent. J. 119:389–396, 1965.

Bates, J. F. Studies related to the fracture of partial dentures. Br. Dent. J. 120:79–83, 1966.

Bates, J. F. Studies on the retention of cobalt-chromium partial dentures. Br. Dent. J. 125:97–102, 1968.

Bates, J. F. Removable Partial Denture Construction. 2nd ed. Littleton, Mass.:John Wright & Sons Ltd., 1978.

Bates, J. F., Neill, D. J., and Preiskel, H. W. Restoration of the Partially Dentate Mouth: Proceedings of the International Prosthodontic Symposium. Berlin: Quintessence Publ. Co., 1984.

Beckett, L. S. The influence of saddle classification on the design of partial removable restorations. J. Prosthet. Dent. 3:506–516, 1953.

Beder, O. E. An evaluation of conventional circumferential clasps. J. Prosthet. Dent. 3:88–95, 1953.

Benson, D., and Spolsky, V. W. A clinical evaluation of removable partial dentures with I-bar retainers. Part I. J. Prosthet. Dent. 41:246–254, 1979.

Berg, T., Jr. I-bar: myth and countermyth. Dent. Clin. North Am. 23:65–75, 1979.

Berg, T., Jr., and Caputo, A. A. Anterior rests for maxillary removable partial dentures. J. Prosthet. Dent. 39:139–142, 1978.

Bergman, B., Hugoson, A., and Olsson, C. Periodontal and prosthetic conditions in patients treated with removable partial dentures and artificial crowns. Acta Odontol. Scand. 29:621–638, 1971.

Bergman, B., Hugoson, A., and Olsson, C. Caries and periodontal status in patients fitted with removable partial dentures. J. Clin. Periodontol. 4:134–146, 1977.

Bickley, R. W. Combined splint-stress breaker removable partial denture. J. Prosthet. Dent. 21:509–512, 1969.

Bissada, N. F., Ibrahim, S. I., and Barsoum, W. M. Gingival response to various types of removable partial dentures. J. Periodontol. 45:651–659, 1974.

Blatterfein, L. A study of partial denture clasping. J. Am. Dent. Assoc. 43:169–185, 1951.

Blatterfein, L. A new approach to partial denture design for unilaterally remaining lower teeth. J. Prosthet. Dent. 28:145–163, 1972.

Blatterfein, L., Pearce, R. L., and Jackson, J. T. Minimum acceptable procedures for satisfactory removable partial denture service. J. Prosthet. Dent. 27:84–87, 1972.

Boero, E., and Forbes, W. Considerations in design of removable prosthetic devices with no posterior abutments. J. Prosthet. Dent. 28:253–263, 1972.

Boitel, R. H. The parallelometer, a precision instrument for the prosthetic laboratory. J. Prosthet. Dent. 12:732–736, 1962.

Bolouri, A. Removable partial denture design for a few remaining natural teeth. J. Prosthet. Dent. 39:346–348, 1978.

Bonwill, W. G. A. New methods of clasping artificial dentures to human teeth without injury, versus immobile bridges. Dent. Items Interest, 21:656–670, 1899.

Boucher, L. J., and Renner, R. P. Treatment of Partially Edentulous Patients. St. Louis: The C. V. Mosby Co., 1982.

Bowman, J. F. Removable partial prosthodontics comparison surveys. J. Dent. Educ. 34:93–97, 1970.

Brill, N., et al. Ecologic changes in the oral cavity caused by removable partial dentures. J. Prosthet. Dent. 38:138–148, 1977.

Brown, E. T., III. The dentist, the laboratory technician, and the prescription law. J. Prosthet. Dent. 15:1132–1138, 1965.

Brudvik, J. S., and Morris, H. F. Stress-relaxation testing. III. Influence of wire alloys, gauges, and lengths on clasp behavior. J. Prosthet. Dent. 46:374–379, 1981.

Brudvik, J. S., and Wormley, J. H. Construction techniques for wrought wire retentive clasp arms as related to clasp flexibility. J. Prosthet. Dent. 30:769–774, 1973.

Buckner, H., and Lavelle, W. E. Metal backings for denture teeth. J. Prosthet. Dent. 32:579–581, 1974.

Campbell, L. D. Subjective reactions to major connector designs for removable partial dentures. J. Prosthet. Dent. 37:507–516, 1977.

Carlsson, G. E., Hedegard, B., and Koivumaa, K. K. Studies in partial dental prosthesis. II. An investigation of mandibular partial dentures with double extension saddles. Acta Odontol. Scand. 19:215–237, 1961.

Carlsson, G. E., Hedegard, B., and Koivumaa, K. K. Studies in partial dental prosthesis. III. A longitudinal study of mandibular partial dentures with double extension saddles. Acta Odontol. Scand. 20:95–119, 1962.

Carlsson, G. E., Hedegard, B., and Koivumaa K. K. Studies in partial dental prosthesis. IV. Final results of a 4 year longitudinal investigation of dentogingivally supported partial dentures. Acta Odontol. Scand. 23:443–472, 1965.

Carlsson, G. E., Hedegard, B., and Koivumaa, K. K. The current place of removable partial dentures in restorative dentistry. Dent. Clin. North Am. 14:553–568, 1970.

Carlsson, G. E., Hedegard, B., and Koivumaa, K. K. Late results of treatment with partial dentures. An investigation by questionnaire and clinical examination 13 years after treatment J. Oral Rehabil. 3:267–272, 1976.

Casey, D. M., and Lauciello, F. R. A method for marking the functional depth of the floor of the mouth. J. Prosthet. Dent. 43:108–111, 1980.

Cecconi, B. T. Lingual bar design. J. Prosthet. Dent. 29:635–639, 1973.

Cecconi, B. T. Effect of rest design on transmission of forces to abutment teeth. J. Prosthet. Dent. 32:141–151, 1974

Cecconi, B. T., Asgar, K., and Dootz, E. The effect of partial denture clasp design on abutment tooth movement. J. Prosthet. Dent. 25:44–56, 1971.

Cecconi, B. T., Asgar, K., and Dootz, E. Removable partial denture abutment tooth movement as affected by inclination of residual ridges and type of loading. J. Prosthet. Dent. 25:375–381, 1971.

Cecconi, B. T., Asgar, K., and Dootz, E. Fit of the removable partial denture base and its effect on abutment tooth movement. J. Prosthet. Dent. 25:515–519, 1971.

Cecconi, B. T., Asgar, K., and Dootz, E. Clasp assembly modifications and their effect on abutment tooth movement. J. Prosthet. Dent. 27:160–167, 1972.

Chandler, J. A., and Brudvik, J. S. Clinical evaluation of patients eight to nine years after placement of removable partial dentures. J. Prosthet. Dent. 51:736–743, 1984.

Chestner, S. B. A methodical approach to the analysis of study casts. J. Prosthet. Dent. 4:622–624, 1954.

Chick, A. O. The correct location of clasps and rests on dentures without stress-breakers. Br. Dent. J. 95:303–309, 1953.

Christidou, L., Osborne, J., and Chamberlain, J. The effects of partial denture design on the mobility of abutment teeth. Br. Dent. J. 135:9–18, 1973.

Clayton, J., and Jaslow, C. A measurement of clasp forces on abutment teeth. J. Prosthet. Dent. 25:21–43, 1971.

Collett, H. A. A biologic approach to clasp partial dentures. Dent. Digest 61:309–313, 1955.

Costa, E. A simplified system for identifying partially edentulous arches. J. Prosthet. Dent. 32:639–645, 1974.

Coy, R. E., and Arnold, P. D. Survey and design of diagnostic casts for removable partial dentures. J. Prosthet. Dent. 32:103–106, 1974.

Craddock, F. W., and Bottomley, G. A. Second thoughts on clasp surveying. Br. Dent. J. 96:134–137, 1954.

Craig, R. G., and Farah, J. W. Stresses from loading distal extension removable partial dentures. J. Prosthet. Dent. 39:274–277, 1978.

Demer, W. J. An analysis of mesial rest–I-bar clasp designs. J. Prosthet. Dent. 36:243–253, 1976.

Derry, A., and Bertram, U. A clinical survey of removable partial dentures after two years usage. Acta Odontol. Scand. 28:581–598, 1970.

DeVan, M. M. Embrasure saddle clasp—its principle and design. J. Am. Dent. Assoc. 22:1352–1362, 1935.

DeVan, M. M. The nature of the partial denture foundation: suggestions in preservation. J. Prosthet. Dent. 2:210–218, 1952.

DeVan, M. M. Preserving natural teeth through the use of clasps. J. Prosthet. Dent. 5:208–214, 1955.

Dunn, B. W. Treatment planning for removable partial dentures. J. Prosthet. Dent. 11:247–255, 1961.

Dunny, J. A., and King, G. E. Minor connector designs for anterior acrylic resin bases: a preliminary study. J. Prosthet. Dent. 34:496–502, 1975.

Dykema, R. W., Cunningham, D. M., and Johnston, J. F. Modern Practice in Removable Partial Prosthodontics. Philadelphia: W. B. Saunders Co., 1969.

Eich, F. A. The role of removable partial dentures in the destruction of the natural dentition. Dent. Clin. North Am. 6:717–731, 1962.

Eliason, C. M. RPA clasp design for distal extension removable partial dentures. J. Prosthet. Dent. 49:25–27, 1983.

Elliott, F. C. A method that simplifies the design of partial dentures. J. Am. Dent. Assoc. 27:1263–1268, 1940.

Farah, J. W., MacGregor, A. R., and Miller, T. P. G. Stress analysis of disjunct removable partial dentures. J. Prosthet. Dent. 42:271–275, 1979.

Farrell, J., and Selby, G. Wrought wire retainers—a method of increasing their flexibility. Br. Dent. J. 131:327, 1971.

Fenner, W., Gerber, A., and Muhlemann, H. R. Tooth mobility changes during treatment with partial denture prostheses. J. Prosthet. Dent. 6:520–525, 1956.

Firtell, D. N. Effect of clasp design upon retention of removable partial dentures. J. Prosthet. Dent. 20:43–52, 1968.

Firtell, D. N., and Jacobson, T. E. Removable partial dentures with rotational paths of insertion: problem analysis. J. Prosthet. Dent. 50:8–15, 1983.

Firtell, D. N., Grisius, R. J., and Muncheryan, A. M. Reaction of the anterior abutment of a Kennedy Class II removable partial denture to various clasp arm designs: an in vitro study. J. Prosthet. Dent. 53:77–82, 1985.

Firtell, D. N., Herzberg, T. W., and Walsh, J. F. Root retention and removable partial denture design. J. Prosthet. Dent. 42:131–134, 1979.

Fish, E. W. A new principle in partial denture design. Br. Dent. J. 92:135–144, 1952.

Fish, E. W. Periodontal diseases: occlusal trauma and partial dentures. Br. Dent. J. 95:199–206, 1953.

Fisher, R. L. Factors that influence the base stability of mandibular distal-extension removable partial dentures: a longitudinal study. J. Prosthet. Dent. 50:167–171, 1983.

Fisher, R. L., and Jaslow, C. The efficiency of an indirect retainer. J. Prosthet. Dent. 34:24–30, 1975.

Frank, R. P., and Nicholls, J. I. An investigation of the effectiveness of indirect retainers. J. Prosthet. Dent. 38:494–506, 1977.

Frank R. P., and Nicholls, J. I. A study of the flexibility of wrought wire clasps, J. Prosthet. Dent. 45:259–267, 1981.

Frank, R. P., Brudvik, J. S., and Nicholls, J. I. A comparison of the flexibility of wrought wire and cast circumferential clasps. J. Prosthet. Dent. 49:471–476, 1983.

Frantz, W. R. Variability in dentists' designs of a removable maxillary partial denture. J. Prosthet. Dent. 29:172–182, 1973.

Frantz, W. R. Variations in a removable maxillary partial denture design by dentists. J. Prosthet. Dent. 34:625–633, 1975.

Frechette, A. R. Partial denture planning with special reference to stress distribution. J. Prosthet. Dent. 1:710–724, 1951.

Frechette, A. R. The influence of partial denture design on distribution of force to abutment teeth. J. Prosthet. Dent. 6:195–212, 1956.

Friedman, J. The ABC classification of partial denture segments. J. Prosthet. Dent. 3:517–524, 1953.

Friedman, J. Abutment sites and spaces in partial denture case analysis. J. Prosthet. Dent. 4:803–812, 1954.

Garver, D. G. A new clasping system for unilateral distal extension removable partial dentures. J. Prosthet. Dent. 39:268–273, 1978.

Gaston, G. W. Rest area preparations for removable partial dentures. J. Prosthet. Dent. 10:124–134, 1960.

Geissler, P. R., and Watt, D. M. Disjunct dentures for patients with teeth of poor prognosis. Dent. Pract. Record 15:421–423, 1965.

Girardot, R. L. History and development of partial denture design. J. Am. Dent. Assoc. 28:1399–1408, 1941.

Girardot, R. L. The physiologic aspects of partial denture restorations. J. Prosthet. Dent. 3:689–698, 1953.

Glann, G. W., and Appleby, R. C. Mouth preparations for removable partial dentures. J. Prosthet. Dent. 10:698–706, 1960.

Glossary of Prosthodontic Terms. 4th ed. St. Louis: The C. V. Mosby Co., 1977.

Gomes, B. C., Renner, R. P., and Bauer, P. N. Periodontal considerations in removable partial dentures. J. Am. Dent. Assoc. 101:496–498, 1980.

Goodkind, R. J. The effects of removable partial dentures on abutment tooth mobility: a clinical study. J. Prosthet. Dent. 30:139–146, 1973.

Grasso, J. E. A new removable partial denture clasp assembly. J. Prosthet. Dent. 43:618–621, 1980.

Granger, E. R. Mechanical principles applied to partial denture

construction. J. Am. Dent. Assoc. 28:1943–1951, 1941.

Handlers, M., Lenchner, N. H., and Weissman, B. A retaining device for partial dentures. J. Prosthet. Dent. 7:483–488, 1957.

Hanson, J. G., Axinn, S., and Kopp, E. N. Surveying. J. Am. Dent. Assoc. 91:826–828, 1975.

Hardy, I. R. Partial lower denture design. Dent. Digest 44:56–61, 1938.

Hardy, I. R. Partial dentures that function—partial dentures that fail. J. Am. Dent. Assoc. 25:562–566, 1938.

Henderson, D. Major connectors—united it stands. Dent. Clin. North Am. 17:661–678, 1973.

Henderson, D. Major connectors for mandibular removable partial dentures: design and function. J. Prosthet. Dent. 30:532–548, 1973.

Henderson, D., and Seward, T. Design and force distribution with removable partial dentures: a progress report. J. Prosthet. Dent. 17:350–364, 1967.

Henderson, D., and Steffel, V. L. McCracken's Removable Partial Prosthodontics. 6th ed. St. Louis: The C. V. Mosby Co., 1981.

Henderson, D., McGivney, G. P., and Castleberry, D. J. McCracken's Removable Partial Prosthodontics. 7th ed. St. Louis: The C. V. Mosby Co., 1985.

Highton, R., and Caputo, A. A. Force transmission by labial and lingual I-bar partial dentures. J. Dent. Res. (IADR abstr.) 59:940, 1980.

Highton, R., Caputo, A. A., and Rhodes, S. Force transmission and retentive capabilities utilizing labial and palatal I-bar partial dentures. J. Dent. Res. (IADR abstr.) 60:613, 1981.

Hindels, G. W. Stress analysis in distal extension partial dentures. J. Prosthet. Dent. 7:197–205, 1957.

Holmes, J. B. Preparation of abutment teeth for removable partial dentures. J. Prosthet. Dent. 20:396–406, 1968.

Holt, J. E. Guiding planes: when and where. J. Prosthet. Dent. 46:4–6, 1981.

Jacobson, T. E., and Krol, A. J. Rotational path removable partial denture design. J. Prosthet. Dent. 48:370–376, 1982.

Jermyn, A. C. Center-poise balanced partial denture construction for rehabilitation of mobile teeth. Dent. Digest 67:420–426, 1961.

Jochen, D. G. Achieving planned parallel guiding planes for removable partial dentures. J. Prosthet. Dent. 27:654–661, 1972.

Johnson, D. L., and Stratton, R. J. Fundamentals of Removable Prosthodontics. Chicago: Quintessence Publ. Co., 1980.

Johnson, D. L., Stratton, R. J., and Duncanson, M. G. J. The effect of single plane curvature on half-round cast clasps. J. Dent. Res. 62:833–836, 1983.

Johnston, J. F. Preparation of mouth for fixed and removable partial dentures. J. Prosthet. Dent. 11:456–462, 1961.

Jones, R. R. The lower partial denture. J. Prosthet. Dent. 2:219–229, 1952.

Jordan, L. G. Partial dentures. J. Am. Dent. Assoc. 29:169–183, 1942.

Jordan, L. G. Designing removable partial dentures with external attachments (clasps). J. Prosthet. Dent. 2:716–722, 1952.

Kabcenell, J. L. Effective clasping of removable partial dentures. J. Prosthet. Dent. 12:104–110, 1962.

Kaires, A. K. Effect of partial denture design on bilateral force distribution. J. Prosthet. Dent. 6:373–385, 1956.

Kaires, A. K. Effect of partial denture design on unilateral force distribution. J. Prosthet. Dent. 6:526–533, 1956.

Kaires, A. K. Partial denture design and its relations to force distribution and masticatory performance. J. Prosthet. Dent. 6:672–683, 1956.

Kaires, A. K. A study of partial denture design and masticatory pressures in a mandibular bilateral extension case. J. Prosthet. Dent. 8:340–350, 1958.

Katulski, E. M., and Appleyard, W. N. Biological concepts of the use of the mechanical cast surveyor. J. Prosthet. Dent. 9:629–634, 1959.

Kelly, E. K. The physiologic approach to partial denture design. J. Prosthet. Dent. 3:699–710, 1953.

Kennedy, E. Partial Denture Construction. 2nd ed. Brooklyn: Dental Items of Interest, 1944.

King, G. E. Dual path design for removable partial dentures. J. Prosthet. Dent. 39:392–395, 1978.

King, G. E., Barco, M. T., and Alson, R. J. Inconspicuous retention for removable partial dentures. J. Prosthet. Dent. 39:505–507, 1978.

Knapp, J. G., Shotwell, J. L., and Kotowicz, W. E. Technique for recording dental cast–surveyor relations. J. Prosthet. Dent. 41:352–354, 1979.

Knowles, L. E. The biomechanics of removable partial dentures and its relationship to fixed prostheses. J. Prosthet. Dent. 8:426–430, 1958.

Kotowitz, W. E., et al. The combination clasp and the distal extension removable partial denture. Dent. Clin. North Am. 17:651–660, 1973.

Kratochvil, F. J. Influence of occlusal rest position and clasp design on movement of abutment teeth. J. Prosthet. Dent. 13:114–124, 1963.

Kratochvil, F. J. Maintaining supporting structures with a removal partial prosthesis. J. Prosthet. Dent. 25:167–174, 1971.

Kratochvil, F. J., and Caputo, A. A. Photoelastic analysis of pressure on teeth and bone supporting removable partial dentures. J. Prosthet. Dent. 32:52–61, 1974.

Kratochvil, F. J., and Vig, R. G. Principles of Removable Partial Dentures. Los Angeles: UCLA School of Dentistry, 1979.

Kratochvil, F. J., Davidson, P. N., and Guijt, J. Five year survey of treatment with removable partial dentures. J. Prosthet. Dent. 48:237–244, 1982.

Kratochvil, F. J., Thompson, W. D., and Caputo, A. A. Photoelastic evaluation of removable partial dentures. In W. Lefkowitz (ed.) Proceedings of the Second International Prosthodontic Conference. St. Louis: The C. V. Mosby Co., 1979.

Krikos, A. A. Artificial undercuts for teeth which have unfavorable shapes for clasping. J. Prosthet. Dent. 22:301–306, 1969.

Krikos, A. A. Preparing guide planes for removable partial dentures. J. Prosthet. Dent. 34:152–155, 1975.

Krol, A. J. RPI clasp retainer and its modifications. Dent. Clin. North Am. 17:631–649, 1973.

Krol, A. J. Clasp design for extension-base removable partial dentures. J. Prosthet. Dent. 29:408–415, 1973.

Krol, A. J. Removable Partial Denture Design Outline Syllabus. 3rd ed. San Francisco: University of the Pacific School of Dentistry, 1981.

Kydd, W. L., Dutton, D. A., and Smith, D. W. Lateral forces exerted on abutment teeth by partial dentures. J. Am. Dent. Assoc. 68:859–863, 1964.

Lammie, G. A., and Osborne, J. The bilateral free-end saddle lower denture. J. Prosthet. Dent. 4:640–652, 1954.

Langer, A. Combinations of diverse retainers in removable partial dentures. J. Prosthet. Dent. 40:378–384, 1978.

LaVere, A. M. A simplified procedure for survey and design of diagnostic casts. J. Prosthet. Dent. 37:680–683, 1977.

LaVere, A. M., and Krol, A. J. Selection of a major connector for the extension-base removable partial denture. J. Prosthet. Dent. 30:102–105, 1973.

Lefkowitz, W. (ed.) Proceedings of the Second International Prosthodontic Congress. St. Louis: The C.V. Mosby Co., 1979.

Mahler, D. B., and Terkla, L. G. Analysis of stress in dental structures. Dent. Clin. North Am. 2:789–798, 1958.

Mann, A. W. The lower distal extension partial denture using the Hart-Dunn attachment. J. Prosthet. Dent. 8:282–288, 1958.

Matsumoto, M., and Gotto, T. Lateral force distribution in partial denture design. J. Dent. Res. 49:359–364, 1970.

Maxfield, J. B., Nicholls, J. I., and Smith, D.E. The measurement of forces transmitted to abutment teeth of removable partial dentures. J. Prosthet. Dent. 40:134–142, 1979.

McCall, J. O. The periodontist looks at the clasp partial denture. J. Am. Dent. Assoc. 43:439–443, 1951.

McCartney, J. W. Lingual plating for reciprocation. J. Prosthet. Dent. 42:624–625, 1979.

McCartney, J. W. Motion vector analysis of an abutment for a distal extension removable partial denture: a pilot study. J. Prosthet. Dent. 43:15–21, 1980.

McCracken, W. L. A comparison of tooth-borne and tooth-tissue-borne removable partial dentures. J. Prosthet. Dent. 3:375–381, 1953.

McCracken, W. L. Mouth preparations for partial dentures. J. Prosthet. Dent. 6:39–52, 1956.

McCracken, W. L. Contemporary partial denture designs. J. Prosthet. Dent. 8:71–84, 1958.

McCracken, W. L. Survey of partial denture designs by commercial laboratories. J. Prosthet. Dent. 12:1089–1110, 1962.

McDowell, G. C. Force transmission by indirect retainers during unilateral loading. J. Prosthet. Dent. 39:616–621, 1978.

McDowell, G. C., and Fisher, R. L. Force transmission by indirect retainers when a unilateral dislodging force is applied. J. Prosthet. Dent. 47:360–365, 1982.

Miller, E. L. Systems for classifying partially edentulous arches. J. Prosthet. Dent. 24:25–40, 1970.

Miller, E. L. The cingulum rest. J. Prosthet. Dent. 28:369–372, 1972.

Miller, E. L., and Grasso, J. E. Removable Partial Prosthodontics. 2nd ed. Baltimore: Williams & Wilkins Co., 1981.

Mills, M. L. Mouth preparation for the removable partial denture. J. Am. Dent. Assoc. 60:154–159, 1960.

Monteith, B. D. Management of loading forces on mandibular distal extension prostheses. Part I. Evaluation of concepts for design. J. Prosthet. Dent. 52:673–681, 1984.

Monteith, B. D. Management of loading forces on mandibular distal extension prostheses. Part II. Classification for matching modalities to clinical situations. J. Prosthet. Dent. 52:832–836, 1984.

Morris, H. F., et al. Stress distribution within circumferential clasp arms. J. Oral Rehabil. 3:387–394, 1976.

Morris, H. F., Asgar, K., and Tillotson, E. Stress-relaxation testing. Part I. A new approach to the testing of removable partial denture alloys, wrought wires, and clasp behavior. J. Prosthet. Dent. 46:133–144, 1981.

Morris, H. F., et al. Stress-relaxation testing. Part II. Comparison of bending profiles, microstructures, microhardnesses, and surface characteristics of several wrought wires. J. Prosthet. Dent. 46:256–262, 1981.

Morris, H. F., Asgar, K., and Brudvik, J. S. Stress-relaxation testing. Part IV: Clasp pattern dimensions and their influence on clasp behavior. J. Prosthet. Dent. 50:319–326, 1983.

Nairn, R. I. The problem of free-end denture bases. J. Prosthet. Dent. 16:522–532, 1966.

Nally, J. Methods of handling abutment teeth in Class I partial dentures. J. Prosthet. Dent. 30:561–566, 1973.

Neill, D. J., and Walter, J. D. The problem of the lower free-end removable partial denture. J. Prosthet. Dent. 8:623–634, 1958.

Neurohr, F. G. Health conservation of the periodontal tissues by a method of functional partial denture design. J. Am. Dent. Assoc. 31:59–70, 1944.

Oddo, V. J., Jr. The movable-arm clasp for complete passivity in partial denture construction. J. Am. Dent. Assoc. 74:1008–1015, 1967.

Osborne, J., and Lammie, G. A. Partial Dentures. 4th ed. Oxford: Blackwell Scientific Publications, 1974.

Perry, C. A philosophy of partial denture design. J. Prosthet. Dent. 6:775–784, 1956.

Perry, C. F., and Applegate, S. G. The occlusal rest: an important part of a partial denture. J. Mich. Dent. Soc. 29:24–25, 1947.

Potter, R. B., Appleby, R. C., and Adams, C. D. Removable partial denture design: a review and a challenge. J. Prosthet. Dent. 17:63–68, 1967.

Pound, E. Cross-arch splinting vs. premature extractions. J. Prosthet. Dent. 16:1058–1068, 1966.

Pruden, W. H. The role of study casts in diagnosis and treatment planning. J. Prosthet. Dent. 10:707–710, 1960.

Quinn, I. Status of the dental laboratory work authorization. J. Am. Dent. Assoc. 79:1189–1190, 1969.

Rad, M. N., and Yarmand, M. A. Design of a direct retainer for removable partial dentures. J. Prosthet. Dent. 31:457–459, 1974.

Reitz, P. V., Sanders, J. L., and Caputo, A. A. A photoelastic study of a split palatal major connector. J. Prosthet. Dent. 51:19–23, 1984.

Roach, F. E. Principles and essentials of bar clasp partial dentures. J. Am. Dent. Assoc. 17:124–138, 1930.

Roach, F. E. Mouth survey and design of partial dentures. J. Am. Dent. Assoc. 21:1166–1176, 1934.

Robinson, C. R. Clasp design and rest placement for the distal extension removable partial denture. Dent. Clin. North Am. 14:583–594, 1970.

Rudd, K. D. The prevention of tissue injury from removable partial dentures. Dent. Clin. North Am. 16:805–813, 1972.

Rudd, K. D., and O'Leary, T. J. Stabilizing periodontally weakened teeth by using guide plane removable partial dentures: a preliminary report. J. Prosthet. Dent. 16:721–727, 1966.

Rudd, J.D., Morrow, R. M., and Eissman, H. F. Dental Laboratory Procedures. Vol. 3. Removable Partial Dentures. St. Louis: The C. V. Mosby Co., 1981.

Rybeck, S. A., Jr. Simplicity in a distal extension partial denture. J. Prosthet. Dent. 3:783–806, 1953.

Sauser, C. W. Pretreatment evaluation of partially edentulous patients. J. Prosthet. Dent. 11:886–893, 1961.

Schmidt, A. H. Planning and designing removable partial dentures. J. Prosthet. Dent. 3:783–806, 1953.

Schopper, A. F. Value of stressbreakers for unilateral partial dentures with free end saddles. J. Am. Dent. Assoc. 38:183–187, 1949.

Schopper, A. F. Partial dentures and its relation to periodontics. J. Am. Dent. Assoc. 45:415–421, 1952.

Schorr, L., and Clayton, L. H. Reshaping abutment teeth for reception of partial denture clasps. J. Prosthet. Dent. 4:625–633, 1954.

Schulte, J. K., and Smith, D. E. Clinical evaluation of swinglock removable partial dentures. J. Prosthet. Dent. 44:595–603, 1980.

Schuyler, C. H. Stress distribution as the prime requisite to the success of a partial denture. J. Am. Dent. Assoc. 20:2148–2154, 1933.

Schuyler, C. H. The partial denture as a means of stabilizing abutment teeth. J. Am. Dent. Assoc. 28:1121–1125, 1941.

Schuyler, C. H. An analysis of the use and relative value of the precision attachment and the clasp in partial denture planning. J. Prosthet. Dent. 3:711–714, 1953.

Schwalm, C. A., Smith, D. E., and Erickson, J. D. A clinical study of patients 1 to 2 years after placement of removable partial dentures. J. Prosthet. Dent. 38:380–391, 1977.

Seemann, S. K. A study of the relationship between periodontal disease and the wearing of partial dentures. Austr. Dent. J. 8:206–208, 1963.

Seiden, A. Occlusal rests and rest seats. J. Prosthet. Dent. 8:431–440, 1958.

Simmons, J. J. Swing-lock stabilization and retention. Texas Dent. J. 81:10–12, 1963.

Singer, F., and Schön, F. Partial Dentures. Berlin: Quintessence Publ. Co., 1973.

Shohet, H. Relative magnitude of stress on abutment teeth with different retainers. J. Prosthet. Dent. 21:267–282, 1969.

Skinner, D. N. A classification of removable partial dentures based upon the principles of anatomy and physiology. J. Prosthet. Dent. 9:240–246, 1959.

Smith, B. J. Esthetic factors in removable partial prosthodontics. Dent. Clin. North Am. 23:53–63, 1979.

Smith, G. P. Cast clasps: their uses, advantages, and disadvantages. Am. J. Orthodont. Oral Surg. 33:479–483, 1947.

Smith, G. P. The responsibility of the dentist toward dental laboratory procedures in fixed and removable partial denture prosthesis. J. Prosthet. Dent. 13:295–301, 1963.

Smyd, E. S. The role of torque, torsion, and binding in prosthodontic failures. J. Prosthet. Dent. 11:95–101, 1961.

Solle, W. An improved dental surveyor. J. Am. Dent. Assoc. 60:727–731, 1960.

Spielberger, M. C., et al. Effect of retentive arm clasp design on gingival health: a feasibility study. J. Prosthet. Dent. 52:397–401, 1984.

Steffel, V. L. Simplified clasp partial dentures designed for maximum function. J. Am. Dent. Assoc. 32:1093–1100, 1945.

Steffel, V. L. Fundamental principles involved in partial denture design. J. Am. Dent. Assoc. 42:534–544, 1951.

Steffel, V. L. Planning removable partial dentures. J. Prosthet. Dent. 12:524–535, 1962.

Steffel, V. L. Clasp partial dentures. J. Am. Dent. Assoc. 66:803–811, 1963.

Steffel, V. L. Current concepts in removable partial denture service. J. Prosthet. Dent. 20:387–395, 1968.

Stern, W. J. Guiding planes in clasp reciprocation and retention. J. Prosthet. Dent. 34:408–414, 1975.

Stewart, K. L., and Rudd, K. D. Stabilizing periodontally weakened teeth with removable partial dentures. J. Prosthet. Dent. 19:475–482, 1968.

Stewart, K. L., Rudd, K. D., and Kuebker, W. A. Clinical Removable Partial Prosthodontics. St. Louis: The C. V. Mosby Co., 1983.

Stone, E. R. The tripping action of clasps. Dent. Cosmos 124:960–967, 1932.

Stone, E. R. Tripping action of bar clasps. J. Am. Dent. Assoc. 23:596–617, 1936.

Stratton, R. J., and Wiebelt, F. W. Surveying in removable partial denture design. Quint. Dent. Technol. 8:237–242, 1984.

Stratton, R. J., and Wiebelt, F. W. Major connectors for removable partial dentures. I. Quint. Dent. Technol. 9:297–301, 1985.

Stratton, R. J., and Wiebelt, F. W. Major connectors for removable partial dentures. II. Quint. Dent. Technol. 9:359–

331

363, 1985.

Sykora, O., and Calikkocaoglu, S. Maxillary removable partial denture designs by commercial dental laboratories. J. Prosthet. Dent. 23:633–640, 1970.

Taylor, D. T., Pflughoeft, F. A., and McGivney, G. P. Effect of two clasping assemblies on arch integrity as modified by base adaptation. J. Prosthet. Dent. 47:120–125, 1982.

Tebrock, O. C., et al. The effect of various clasping systems on the mobility of abutment teeth for distal extension removable partial dentures. J. Prosthet. Dent. 41:511–516, 1979.

Tench, R. W. Fundamentals of partial denture design. J. Am. Dent. Assoc. 23:1087–1092, 1936.

Terkla, L. G., and Laney, W. R. Partial Dentures. 3rd ed. St. Louis: The C. V. Mosby Co., 1963.

Thompson, W. D., Kratochvil, F. J., and Caputo, A. A. Evaluation of photoelastic stress patterns produced by various designs of bilateral distal extension removable partial dentures. J. Prosthet. Dent. 38:261–273, 1977.

Tomlin, H. R., and Osborne, J. Cobalt-chromium partial dentures—a clinical survey. Br. Dent. J. 110:307–310, 1961.

Trainor, J. E., Elliott, R. W., and Bartlett, S. O. Removable partial dentures designed by dentists before and after graduate level instruction: a comparative study. J. Prosthet. Dent. 27:509–514, 1972.

Trapozzano, V.R., and Winter, G. R. Periodontal aspects of partial denture design. J. Prosthet. Dent. 2:101–107, 1952.

Tsao, D. H. Designing occlusal rests using mathematical principles. J. Prosthet. Dent. 23:154–163, 1970.

von Gonten, A. S., and Nelson, D. R. Laboratory pitfalls that contribute to embrasure clasp failure. J. Prosthet. Dent. 53:136–138, 1985.

von Gonten, A. S., and Palik, J. F. Tooth preparation guide for embrasure clasp designs. J. Prosthet. Dent. 53:281–282, 1985.

Wagner, A. G., and Forgue, E. G. A study of four methods of recording the path of insertion of removable partial dentures.

J. Prosthet. Dent. 35:267–272, 1976.

Wagner, A. G., and Traweek, F. C. Comparison of major connectors for removable partial dentures. J. Prosthet. Dent. 47:242–245, 1982.

Walsh, J. The professions's responsibility. Int. Dent. J. 17:75–82, 1967.

Warr, J. A. An analysis of clasp design in partial dentures. Physics Med. Biol. 3:212–232, 1959.

Warren, A. B., and Caputo, A. A. Load transfer to alveolar bone as influenced by abutment designs for tooth-supported dentures. J. Prosthet. Dent. 33:137–148, 1975.

Weinberg, L. A. Lateral force in relation to the denture base and clasp design. J. Prosthet. Dent. 6:785–800, 1956.

White, J. T. Visualization of stress and strain related to removable partial denture abutments. J. Prosthet. Dent. 40:143–151, 1978.

Wiebelt, F. W., and Stratton, R. J. Bracing and reciprocation in removable partial denture design. Quint. Dent. Technol. 9:15–17, 1985.

Wong, R., Nicholls, J. I., and Smith, D. E. Evaluation of prefabricated lingual rest seats for removable partial dentures. J. Prosthet. Dent. 48:521–526, 1982.

Yilmaz, G. Optical surveying of casts for removable partial dentures. J. Prosthet. Dent. 34:292–296, 1975.

Zach, G. A. Advantages of mesial rests for removable partial dentures. J. Prosthet. Dent. 33:32–35, 1975.

Zarb, G. A., and MacKay, H. F. Cosmetics and removable partial dentures: the Class IV partially edentulous patient. J. Prosthet. Dent. 46:360–368, 1981.

Zarb, G. A., et al. Prosthodontic Treatment for Partially Edentulous Patients. St. Louis: The C. V. Mosby Co., 1978.

Zoeller, G. N. Block form stability in removable partial dentures. J. Prosthet. Dent. 22:633–637, 1969.

Zoeller, G. N., and Kelly, W. J., Jr. Block form stability in removable prosthodontics. J. Prosthet. Dent. 26:141–145, 1971.

Index